Mohs Surgery

Guest Editors

ALLISON T. VIDIMOS, RPh, MD
CHRISTINE POBLETE-LOPEZ, MD
CHRISTOPHER C. GASBARRE, DO

DERMATOLOGIC CLINICS

www.derm.theclinics.com

Consulting Editor
BRUCE H. THIERS, MD

April 2011 • Volume 29 • Number 2

SAUNDERS an imprint of ELSEVIER, Inc.

W.B. SAUNDERS COMPANY
A Division of Elsevier Inc.

1600 John F. Kennedy Boulevard • Suite 1800 • Philadelphia, PA 19103-2899

http://www.theclinics.com

DERMATOLOGIC CLINICS Volume 29, Number 2
April 2011 ISSN 0733-8635, ISBN-13: 978-1-4557-0437-8

Editor: Stephanie Donley

Dermatologic Clinics (ISSN 0733-8635) is published quarterly by Elsevier Inc., 360 Park Avenue South, New York, NY 10010-1710. Months of publication are January, April, July, and October. Business and editorial offices: 1600 John F. Kennedy Blvd., Suite 1800, Philadelphia, PA 19103-2899. Customer service office: 11830 Westline Drive, St. Louis, MO 63146. Periodicals postage paid at New York, NY, and additional mailing offices. Subscription prices are USD 317.00 per year for US individuals, USD 474.00 per year for US institutions, USD 371.00 per year for Canadian individuals, USD 568.00 per year for Canadian institutions, USD 434.00 per year for international individuals, USD 568.00 per year for international institutions, USD 148.00 per year for US students/residents, and USD 214.00 per year for Canadian and international students/residents. International air speed delivery is included in all *Clinics* subscription prices. All prices are subject to change without notice. **POSTMASTER:** Send address changes to *Dermatologic Clinics*, Elsevier Health Sciences Division, Subscription Customer Service, 3251 Riverport Lane, Maryland Heights, MO 63043. **Customer Service: 1-800-654-2452 (U.S. and Canada); 314-447-8871 (outside U.S. and Canada). Fax: 314-447-8029. E-mail: journalscustomerservice-usa@elsevier.com (for print support); journalsonlinesupport-usa@elsevier.com (for online support).**

Reprints. For copies of 100 or more, of articles in this publication, please contact the Commercial Reprints Department, Elsevier Inc., 360 Park Avenue South, New York, New York 10010-1710. Tel.: (212) 633-3813; Fax: (212) 462-1935; Email: repritns@elsevier.com.

The *Dermatologic Clinics* is covered in *MEDLINE/PubMed (Index Medicus)*, *Current Contents/Clinical Medicine*, *Excerpta Medica*, *Chemical Abstracts*, and *ISI/BIOMED*.

Printed and bound by CPI Group (UK) Ltd, Croydon, CR0 4YY

Transferred to Digital Print 2011

Contributors

CONSULTING EDITOR

BRUCE H. THIERS, MD
Professor and Chairman, Department
of Dermatology and Dermatologic Surgery,
Medical University of South Carolina,
Charleston, South Carolina

GUEST EDITORS

ALLISON T. VIDIMOS, RPh, MD
Staff, Section of Dermatologic Surgery and
Cutaneous Oncology, and Chairman,
Department of Dermatology; Vice Chair,
Dermatology and Plastic Surgery Institute,
Cleveland Clinic, Cleveland, Ohio

CHRISTINE POBLETE-LOPEZ, MD
Staff, Section of Dermatologic Surgery and
Cutaneous Oncology, Department of
Dermatology; Program Director, Dermatology
Residency, Cleveland Clinic, Cleveland, Ohio

CHRISTOPHER C. GASBARRE, DO
Associate Professor, Dermatologic Surgery
and Cutaneous Oncology, Cleveland Clinic
Foundation, Cleveland, Ohio

AUTHORS

CHRISTIE T. AMMIRATI, MD
Associate Professor of Dermatology,
Penn State Hershey Department of
Dermatology, Penn State Milton S.
Hershey Medical Center, Hershey,
Pennsylvania

PHILIP L. BAILIN, MD, MBA, FACP
Head, Section of Dermatologic Surgery
and Cutaneous Oncology, Department
of Dermatology, Dermatology and Plastic
Surgery Institute, Cleveland Clinic,
Cleveland, Ohio

BARBARA BECK, HT/HTL(ASCP)
Director, Mohs Technical Consulting, Inc,
Highlands, North Carolina;
President, American Society
of Mohs Histotechnology

DANIEL BELKIN
Research Fellow, Department of
Dermatology, Weill Cornell Medical College,
New York, New York

PAUL X. BENEDETTO, MD
Resident, Department of Dermatology,
Cleveland Clinic Foundation,
Cleveland, Ohio

JEREMY S. BORDEAUX, MD, MPH
Assistant Professor, Director of Mohs
and Dermatologic Surgery; Director of
Melanoma Program, Department of
Dermatology, Case Western Reserve
University School of Medicine,
University Hospitals Case Medical
Center, Orange Village, Ohio

NAVID BOUZARI, MD
Clinical Fellow in Mohs Surgery and Clinical
Oncology, Department of Dermatology,
Lahey Clinic, Burlington; Harvard Medical
School, Boston, Massachusetts

JOHN A. CARUCCI, MD, PhD
Chief, Mohs Micrographic and Dermatologic
Surgery; Associate Professor of Dermatology,
New York University Langone Medical Center,
New York, New York

ROBERT H. COOK-NORRIS, MD
Fellow in Dermatologic Surgery, Department
of Dermatology, Mayo School of Graduate
Medical Education, College of Medicine,
Mayo Clinic, Rochester, Minnesota

STEPHANIE A. DIAMANTIS, MD
Fellow, Procedural Dermatology, Department
of Dermatology, Geisinger Health System,
Danville, Pennsylvania

MICHAEL A. FRITZ, MD
Department of Otolaryngology–Head and
Neck Surgery, Head and Neck Institute,
Cleveland Clinic, Cleveland, Ohio

EDWARD M. GALICZYNSKI, DO
Resident, Department of Dermatology,
Cleveland Clinic Foundation,
Cleveland, Ohio

JORGE GARCIA-ZUAZAGA, MD, MS, FAAD
Department of Dermatology, Case Western
Reserve University; Director, Mohs
Micrographic Surgery and Cutaneous
Oncology, University Hospitals Westlake
Medical Center, Cleveland, Ohio

CHRISTOPHER C. GASBARRE, DO
Associate Professor, Dermatologic Surgery
and Cutaneous Oncology, Cleveland Clinic
Foundation, Cleveland, Ohio

JUDAH N. GREENBERG, MD
Department of Medicine, Emory University
School of Medicine, Atlanta, Georgia

KYLE L. HORNER, MD, MS
Fellow, Dermatologic Surgery and Cutaneous
Oncology, Cleveland Clinic Foundation,
Cleveland, Ohio

MICHAEL HUBAND, DDS
Staff, Maxillofacial Prosthetics, Section of
Dentistry, Head and Neck Institute,
Cleveland Clinic, Cleveland, Ohio

ROHUN HULYALKAR
School of Humanities and Sciences, Stanford
University, Stanford, California

HILLARY JOHNSON-JAHANGIR, MD, PhD
Volunteer Instructor, Department of
Dermatology, Columbia University Medical
Center, New York, New York

RICHELLE M. KNUDSON, MD
Resident in Dermatology, Department
of Dermatology, Mayo School of Graduate
Medical Education, College of Medicine,
Mayo Clinic, Rochester, Minnesota

SOON-YOU KWON, MD
Resident in Dermatology, Department
of Dermatology, University of Maryland,
Baltimore, Maryland

W. ELLIOT LOVE, DO
Department of Dermatology, MetroHealth
Medical Center; Assistant Professor, Case
Western Reserve University School of
Medicine, Pepper Pike, Ohio

JENNIFER LUCAS, MD
Department of Dermatology, Dermatology
and Plastic Surgery Institute, Cleveland Clinic,
Cleveland Ohio

VICTOR J. MARKS, MD
Associate, Department of Dermatology,
Geisinger Health System, Danville,
Pennsylvania

JON G. MEINE, MD
Department of Dermatology, Cleveland Clinic
Foundation, Cleveland, Ohio

CHRISTOPHER J. MILLER, MD
Director of Dermatologic Surgery;
Assistant Professor of Dermatology,
Perelman Center for Advanced Medicine,
University of Pennsylvania, Philadelphia,
Pennsylvania

STANLEY J. MILLER, MD
Associate Professor of Dermatology and
Otolaryngology–Head and Neck Surgery,
Part-Time, Johns Hopkins Hospital,
Baltimore, Maryland

TERRI NUNNCIATO
Mohs Surgery Histotechnician, Department of Dermatology, University of Pennsylvania, Philadelphia, Pennsylvania

SUZANNE OLBRICHT, MD
Chair, Department of Dermatology, Lahey Clinic, Burlington; Associate Professor of Dermatology, Harvard Medical School, Boston, Massachusetts

CHRISTINE POBLETE-LOPEZ, MD
Staff, Section of Dermatologic Surgery and Cutaneous Oncology, Department of Dermatology; Program Director, Dermatology Residency, Cleveland Clinic, Cleveland, Ohio

TINA RAKKHIT, MD
Department of Dermatology, Case Western Reserve University, Cleveland, Ohio

DÉSIRÉE RATNER, MD
Professor of Clinical Dermatology, Director of Dermatologic Surgery, Department of Dermatology, Columbia University Medical Center, New York, New York

PETER C. REVENAUGH, MD
Department of Otolaryngology–Head and Neck Surgery, Head and Neck Institute, Cleveland Clinic, Cleveland, Ohio

RANDALL K. ROENIGK, MD
Robert H. Kieckhefer Professor of Dermatology; Consultant, Department of Dermatology, College of Medicine, Mayo Clinic, Rochester, Minnesota

ADAM R. SCHMITT, BA
Department of Dermatology, Case Western Reserve University School of Medicine, Cleveland, Ohio

RAHUL SETH, MD
Department of Otolaryngology–Head and Neck Surgery, Head and Neck Institute, Cleveland Clinic, Cleveland, Ohio

JOSEPH F. SOBANKO, MD
Assistant Professor of Dermatology, University of Pennsylvania, Philadelphia, Pennsylvania

TODD W. STULTZ, DDS, MD
Staff, Section of Neuroradiology, Imaging Institute, Cleveland Clinic Foundation, Cleveland, Ohio

SHARON L. THORNTON, MD
Director, Columbus Skin Surgery Center, Inc, Dublin; Clinical Assistant Professor, Division of Dermatology, Department of Internal Medicine, The Ohio State University, Columbus, Ohio

LEONID B. TROST, MD, FAAD
Associate Staff, Department of Dermatology, Dermatology and Plastic Surgery Institute, Cleveland Clinic, Cleveland, Ohio

CHRISTOPHER R. URBAN, MD
Resident, Department of Medicine, Pennsylvania Hospital, Philadelphia, Pennsylvania

ALLISON T. VIDIMOS, RPh, MD
Staff, Section of Dermatologic Surgery and Cutaneous Oncology, and Chairman, Department of Dermatology; Vice Chair, Dermatology and Plastic Surgery Institute, Cleveland Clinic, Cleveland, Ohio

LANCE D. WOOD, MD
Penn State Hershey Department of Dermatology, Penn State Milton S. Hershey Medical Center, Hershey, Pennsylvania

JEREMY S. YOUSE, MD
Fellow in Dermatologic Surgery, Department of Dermatology, Mayo School of Graduate Medical Education, College of Medicine, Mayo Clinic, Rochester, Minnesota

ALEXANDRA Y. ZHANG, MD
Department of Dermatology, Cleveland Clinic Foundation, Cleveland, Ohio

XIAODONG ZHU
Mohs Surgery Histotechnician, Department of Dermatology, University of Pennsylvania, Philadelphia, Pennsylvania

FIONA O. ZWALD, MD, MRCPI
Assistant Professor, Mohs Micrographic Surgery, Transplant Dermatology, Department of Dermatology; Division of Transplantation, Department of Surgery, Emory University School of Medicine, Atlanta, Georgia

Contents

Leonid B. Trost and Philip L. Bailin

> Mohs micrographic surgery (MMS) has become the gold standard for treating many forms of primary and recurrent contiguous skin cancers and offers the highest cure rates and maximum tissue conservation compared with other modalities. Developed by Dr Frederic E. Mohs in the 1930s, it was initially called chemosurgery and used zinc chloride paste in a process called fixed tissue technique. Although this technique had high cure rates, it could take days to complete, and it gradually gave way to fresh tissue technique, renamed MMS. Now, MMS is practiced widely as part of a multidisciplinary approach for treating skin cancer.

Paul X. Benedetto and Christine Poblete-Lopez

> This article provides a protocol for the systematic approach to the technique of Mohs micrographic surgery. Each step, from tumor excision and tissue mapping, to specimen processing and histologic interpretation, through wound closure and postoperative management, is covered. The advantages of Mohs surgery over other treatment modalities are observed histologic margin control, superior cure rates, and maximal tissue-sparing potential. The increased preservation of normal tissue leads to smaller surgical defects, optimal reconstructive results, and diminished risk of poor surgical outcomes. Overall, the risks of the procedure are few, the benefits numerous, and the outcomes worth the time and effort spent in learning the technique.

Lance D. Wood and Christie T. Ammirati

> This article reviews Mohs micrographic surgery for basal cell carcinoma. Its evolution to the present day technique, indications, and limitations are discussed, along with future expectations for the procedure.

Daniel Belkin and John A. Carucci

> Cutaneous squamous cell carcinoma (SCC) is the second most common human cancer and can behave aggressively. Mohs micrographic surgery offers the highest cure rates for high-risk SCCs and is particularly useful for SCCs on challenging anatomic sites.

Soon-You Kwon and Stanley J. Miller

> Mohs micrographic surgery is a valuable option for the treatment of melanoma in situ, especially lesions of the lentigo maligna subtype that are clinically ill defined. Complete peripheral margin assessment of a tumor's borders by means of frozen

or permanent sections can help reduce the surgical defect size and maximize cure rate as compared with standard excision with preset 5-mm margins. This article reviews the different variations of Mohs micrographic surgery that are currently used for melanoma in situ.

Microcystic adnexal carcinoma is a rare neoplasm with a propensity for slow growth and extensive local invasion. Pathology is characterized by multiple islands of basaloid epithelial cells, ductal structures, and keratinizing cysts, located intradermally but often extending deep as thin strands of tumor cells intercalating between collagen bundles. Perineural and intramuscular invasion are common. Treatment with Mohs surgery allows for fewer procedures with increased likelihood of long-term cure and tissue conservation.

Dermatofibrosarcoma protuberans (DFSP) is a rare soft-tissue tumor that most commonly presents on the trunk and extremities of adults. It is characterized by low metastatic potential and a favorable prognosis, but extensive subclinical growth can contribute to a high risk of local recurrence. Surgical excision is the first-line treatment, using Mohs micrographic surgery or wide local excision with careful evaluation of the peripheral and deep surgical margins. Adjuvant therapy may be beneficial in patients with unresectable, recurrent, or metastatic DFSP. Historically, adjuvant radiation therapy has been used to reduce the risk of local recurrence when residual disease is present after surgery. The advent of targeted molecular therapies, such as the selective tyrosine kinase inhibitor, imatinib mesylate, has provided new effective and safe options for adjuvant treatment of DFSP.

Atypical fibroxanthoma, malignant fibrous histiocytoma, sebaceous carcinoma, and extramammary Paget disease are rare cutaneous tumors. Their recognition and diagnosis are critical in decreasing long-term morbidity and mortality. Surgical excision is the treatment of choice for these tumors, and Mohs micrographic surgery has been shown to be as favorable or better than wide local excision in providing long-term clearance rates.

Reconstruction of Mohs surgical defects is a challenging venture. A thorough understanding of skin physiology and anatomy (cosmetic subunits, relaxed skin tension lines, underlying neurovascular structures at risk, potential functional compromise, character of adjacent skin, and so forth), careful wound analysis, and meticulous operative techniques is key to a successful reconstruction. This article discusses in detail the use of local skin flaps and graft reconstruction.

Solid-organ transplant recipients are at increased risk for the development of skin cancers. A promising strategy for managing these complex patients involves a multidisciplinary approach that incorporates clinicians from various specialties, which provides the optimal milieu for patient education, treatment, and follow-up. The multidisciplinary clinic also facilitates communication between dermatologists and transplant physicians regarding such crucial concerns as revision of immuno-suppression. This article reviews the problem of skin cancer in solid-organ trans-plant recipients, outlines preventive measures, discusses therapeutic modalities, and reinforces the advantage of a multidisciplinary approach in the management of this population.

An overview of currently available imaging modalities is presented. Indications for imaging in cutaneous nonmelanoma skin cancers, selection of the most appropriate and cost-effective study, limitations, and risks are discussed. Finally, representative cases are discussed with emphasis on choice of imaging study for preoperative staging and treatment planning.

The success of the Mohs procedure depends on the reliability of each step in the technique. Pitfalls in histologic preparation of the tissue specimens may occur dur-ing debulking, excising, orienting, creating the map, sectioning, inking, tissue flatten-ing and freezing, cutting, slide fixation, staining, and mapping the tumor. Challenges are also present in interpreting the slides. Diagnostic pitfalls include floaters, inflam-matory conditions resembling tumor, and perineural invasion. The technique re-quires time, teaching, and a sufficient quantity of cases from which to learn, as well as attention to the pitfalls that occur while processing tissue specimens and in-terpreting and mapping the histology.

The excellent cure rates associated with Mohs micrographic surgery depend on accurate interpretation of complete and high-quality microscopic frozen sections. Reliable interpretation of microscopic slides is only possible if the surgeon can dis-tinguish tumor cells from surrounding normal tissue. By highlighting tumor cells with a chromogen that is visible on light microscopy, immunostaining allows the Mohs surgeon to distinguish tumor from normal cells in these challenging scenar-ios. This article focuses on practical aspects involving the most commonly used immunostains in dermatologic surgery, including MART-1 for melanocytic neo-plasms, cytokeratin stains for keratinocytic neoplasms, and CD34 stains for der-matofibrosarcoma protuberans.

Dermatologic Clinics

THE CLINICS ARE NOW AVAILABLE ONLINE!

Access your subscription at:
www.theclinics.com

Preface

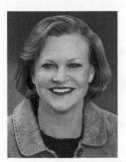 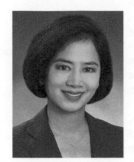 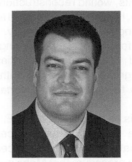

Allison T. Vidimos, RPh, MD   Christine Poblete-Lopez, MD   Christopher C. Gasbarre, DO

Guest Editors

Dr Frederic E. Mohs was a visionary who changed the way skin cancer is treated when he pioneered micrographic surgery in the 1930s. The surgical procedure for skin cancer that bears his name has proven optimal cure rates and tissue sparing for many types of skin cancer that grow in continuity. The American College of Mohs Surgery has over 800 fellowship-trained members who continue to educate the public on the importance of skin cancer prevention and treatment, train future Mohs surgeons, and improve skin cancer therapy.

We have assembled experts in the field of skin cancer to provide an update on the Mohs surgery technique, indications, histologic pitfalls, use of immunohistochemical stains, preoperative and postoperative radiologic imaging, Multidisciplinary management of aggressive skin

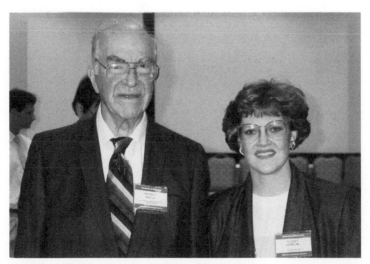

Fig. 1. Dr Frederic E. Mohs and Dr Allison T. Vidimos, Mohs Surgery conference, University of Wisconsin at Madison; July, 1994.

Dermatol Clin 29 (2011) xiii–xiv
doi:10.1016/j.det.2011.02.009

tumors, management of skin cancer in organ transplant recipients, wound reconstruction, prosthetic rehabilitation, histology lab setup and accreditation, and coding for Mohs surgery. Other treatment options for skin cancer, including radiation therapy and nonsurgical modalities, are reviewed. We are grateful to all of our authors for their contributions to this issue of *Dermatologic Clinics*.

We dedicate this text to Dr Frederic E. Mohs, whose innovative ideas, perseverance, and compassion for patients with skin cancer gave birth to the surgical procedure that Mohs surgeons around the world use today to deliver optimal care to our patients.

Allison T. Vidimos, RPh, MD
Christine Poblete-Lopez, MD
Christopher C. Gasbarre, DO

Section of Dermatologic Surgery and
Cutaneous Oncology
Department of Dermatology
Cleveland Clinic
9500 Euclid Avenue
Cleveland, OH 44195, USA

E-mail addresses:
vidimoa@ccf.org (A.T. Vidimos)
lopezc@ccf.org (C. Poblete-Lopez)
gasbarc@ccf.org (C.C. Gasbarre)

History of Mohs Surgery

Leonid B. Trost, MD[a], Philip L. Bailin, MD, MBA[b],*

KEYWORDS

- Mohs • Surgery • Basal cell carcinoma
- Squamous cell carcinoma • Melanoma

BEGINNINGS

Dr Frederic E. Mohs first conceived of the concepts underlying Mohs micrographic surgery (MMS) in the 1930's while he was a Brittingham Research Assistant to Professor Michael F. Guyer, Chairman of the Department of Zoology at the University of Wisconsin. They were studying the potential curative effects of injecting various substances into different neoplasms. During one experiment, a 20% solution of zinc chloride was injected and inadvertently caused tissue necrosis. Microscopic analysis showed that the tissue retained its microscopic structure as if it had been excised and processed for routine pathologic examination. Dr Mohs realized that this in situ fixation effect could be coupled with surgical excision to remove neoplasms in a microscopically controlled serial manner. In addition, he conceived of the idea of using horizontal frozen sections to evaluate 100% of the specimen margins (deep and peripheral) rather than traditional vertical sections or random step sections, which examine only 0.01% of the total surface area of an excised tumor.[1,2]

FIXED TISSUE TECHNIQUE

Mohs tested numerous in situ fixatives before choosing zinc chloride. Arsenic trioxide, phenol, and mercuric chloride were associated with systemic toxicity. Antimony trichloride was found to distort tissue structures. Sodium hydroxide and potassium hydroxide liquefied tissue and resulted in loss of tissue structures. Zinc chloride was chosen because (1) it preserved necessary microscopic features for analysis, (2) had good penetration into the tissues with precise control of fixation depth when the thickness of paste applied and the time interval between application and excision were varied, (3) lacked interference with subsequent second-intention healing, (4) lacked systemic toxicity, (5) was safe to handle, and (6) lacked odor.[3] In addition, the fixation process stopped spontaneously after about 18 hours. This property resulted in the separation of fixed tissue from the underlying healthy tissue with its vasculature intact, allowing for rapid healing and epithelialization.[4] Mohs and Guyer[5] also demonstrated in murine models that exposure to zinc chloride was not associated with an increased risk of metastasis.

Next, Mohs with the aid of an 85-year-old owner of a local pharmacy developed a vehicle (paste) to topically deliver and release the zinc chloride. After some modifications, Mohs chose a mixture of zinc chloride, stibnite (a granular antimony ore), and *Sanguinaria canadensis* (bloodroot) powder. In an effort to limit untrained physicians from inappropriately using this material, Mohs patented the paste, sold the rights to the Wisconsin Alumni Research Foundation for $1 in 1944, and arranged for the Department of Pharmacy at the University of Wisconsin to supply it to physicians who were certified to use it properly.[6]

Finally, Mohs made several other improvements that increased the effectiveness and efficiency of

Financial disclosures: The authors have nothing to disclose.
[a] Department of Dermatology, Dermatology and Plastic Surgery Institute, Cleveland Clinic, 9500 Euclid Avenue, A-61, Cleveland, OH 44195, USA
[b] Section of Dermatologic Surgery and Cutaneous Oncology, Department of Dermatology, Dermatology and Plastic Surgery Institute, Cleveland Clinic, 9500 Euclid Avenue, A-61, Cleveland, OH 44195, USA
* Corresponding author.
E-mail address: BAILINP@CCF.ORG

Dermatol Clin 29 (2011) 135–139
doi:10.1016/j.det.2011.01.010

the procedure, such as orienting the excised tissue layer so as to produce complete horizontal sections,[7] putting multiple sections on a single slide, and color coding the tissue edges for proper orientation.[6]

Initially, Mohs wanted to name the technique microsurgery, but this term was already used to describe the dissection of small structures using a microscope. He then chose the name chemosurgery because the skin cancers that were being treated were first chemically fixed in situ before being excised.[6]

Mohs treated his first human patient on June 23, 1936[8] in the dermatology clinic at the Wisconsin General Hospital.[4] In 1941, he published his first clinical article in the *Archives of Surgery* in which he reported the treatment of 440 consecutive patients over a period of 4 years.[9] Because Mohs[10–13] was describing a surgical technique, the first series of articles were published in surgical journals. Despite this choice of surgical journals, few surgeons contacted Mohs about his technique. Because the most accessible and common tumors that he had treated were on the skin, he turned his attention to the dermatologic community. After his lecture at the 1946 meeting of the American Academy of Dermatology, publication of an article in *Archives of Dermatology*,[14] and his lecture to the Dermatology Section of the California Medical Association in 1948,[15] Mohs came to believe that dermatologists would accept the technique more readily than any other specialty. In fact, literally hundreds of dermatologists came to visit Mohs in Madison and learn his technique.[6]

In addition to introducing chemosurgery to the medical community, he also popularized using second-intention wound healing extensively. Until then, tradition stated that first-intention surgical repairs were always superior to second-intention wound healing. Mohs found that in many instances, especially on concave surfaces, second-intention healing had comparable and sometimes even superior cosmetic outcomes when compared with first-intention surgical repairs.[2]

FRESH TISSUE TECHNIQUE

Although the fixed tissue technique had higher cure rates than conventional excision, there were limitations to the technique. Each layer took 1 day to complete because of the time required for the paste to fix the tissue before excision, and patients with large tumors requiring excision of multiple layers had to return daily, sometimes for many days. The paste was painful and caused local inflammation and often fever and lymphadenopathy. Although Mohs usually used second-intention healing, when some patients needed surgical reconstruction there would be delays because of postoperative sloughing of the final fixed tissue layer which could take 5 to 7 days to complete.[16,17] Trying to solve these problems led to the development of the fresh tissue technique.

Mohs actually used the fresh tissue technique in some of his original cases when performing the fixed tissue technique. For example, if cartilage on the ear or nasal ala were being approached, the final layer was excised without prior fixation to avoid damage to the underlying cartilage.[6]

In 1951, one of Mohs' trainees, Dr R. R. Allington, showed him his technique for first debulking a cancer and then achieving hemostasis with dichloroacetic acid. Mohs was so impressed with the idea that he started using it himself. In 1953, he began to make movies of this technique. While filming the removal of a pigmented basal cell carcinoma from a lower eyelid, removal of small extensions of the carcinoma was delaying the filming. To speed up the process, Mohs removed the next 2 layers using local anesthesia without any fixation in what is now known as the fresh tissue technique. After that, he started using the technique for most eyelid cancers and some cancers in other locations.[6] He first wrote about the technique in the book *Skin Surgery* in 1956.[18] He also presented this technique and a series of 70 patients at the 1969 meeting of the American College of Chemosurgery and published the results in *Bulletin of the American College of Chemosurgery*.[19]

The publication by Tromovitch and Stegman[20] of a series of 102 patients in 1974 in *Archives of Dermatology* is generally recognized by many authorities as being the turning point at which the fresh tissue technique became widely accepted.[2,21] The investigators initially named the technique microscopically controlled excision to differentiate it from the fixed tissue technique, which then was called Mohs' chemosurgery, and they presented the first series of patients treated with the fresh tissue technique at the American College of Chemosurgery meeting in 1970.[22] The fresh tissue technique had clear advantages over the fixed tissue technique. The fresh tissue technique eliminated the need for the zinc chloride paste, which could cause the patient considerable discomfort; a tumor requiring excision of multiple layers could usually be removed in a single day; reconstruction could be performed the same day without waiting for the eschar caused by the zinc chloride paste to separate from the underlying viable tissue; unnecessary and uncontrolled fixation beyond the final required surgical margin was avoided. This final aspect was important because it could, in some cases, prevent uncontrolled perforation of underlying structures such as the nose.[20] Mohs[23] later published a much larger series of 3466 patients undergoing fresh tissue technique in which he reported a 99.8% cure rate for nonmelanoma skin cancers.

Although the fresh tissue technique had become the predominant way of performing MMS, Mohs continued to use the fixed tissue technique for melanoma, large extensive neoplasms involving bone, osteomyelitis, penile carcinoma, and gangrene. He thought that because the incisions for layers was made only through fixed tissue containing nonviable melanocytes, the risk of disseminating the malignant melanocytes and possibly causing metastasis was lower than for the fresh tissue technique. For extensive neoplasms involving bone and osteomyelitis, he thought that the bone could more easily be removed with the fixed tissue technique. For penile carcinoma, hemostasis was less problematic with the fixed tissue technique. For removing gangrene and other necrotic processes, Mohs found that the fixed tissue technique caused fixation a few millimeters beyond the area of necrosis and produced healthy granulation tissue, which could lead to faster healing.[6]

EXPANSION OF USE

Roughly a quarter of a century after he first published his technique in 1967, Mohs founded the American College of Chemosurgery whose first meeting was held in Chicago before the national meeting of the American Academy of Dermatology. In 1986, the College was renamed American College of Mohs Micrographic Surgery and Cutaneous Oncology. In addition, formal fellowship training programs were instituted by the College in the early 1980's to replace the existing informal preceptorships. Mohs always hoped that other specialists, including otolaryngologists, oculoplastic surgeons, and plastic surgeons, would become involved. However, primarily, dermatologists have performed the procedure, perhaps because they are more comfortable with dermatopathology and interpreting their own histologic specimens than other specialties.[6]

MMS is now also practiced extensively in Europe, including Germany, Spain, the United Kingdom, Belgium, Italy, and Sweden. There is a European Society for Micrographic Surgery.[24] In addition, the technique is practiced in Argentina,[25] Australia,[26] Brazil,[27] Canada,[28] Israel, and Portugal.[29]

In addition to the original application to basal cell and squamous cell skin cancers, MMS has been used successfully for an ever-growing number of neoplasms, including atypical fibroxanthoma,[30] dermatofibrosarcoma protuberans,[31] microcystic adnexal carcinoma,[32] sebaceous carcinoma,[33] Merkel cell carcinoma,[34] extramammary Paget disease,[35] and leiomyosarcoma among others.[36] MMS may not be as effective in noncontiguous tumors or tumors that cannot be identified well on routine frozen sections. However, such tumors can be even more difficult to identify with standard surgical and histologic techniques, and this limitation can be overcome by performing the slow Mohs that involves sending each excised layer for routine formalin-fixed tissue processing. However, this technique can slow down the procedure dramatically and may make the entire procedure take days to complete if multiple layers need to be excised.[2]

Mohs surgery has also been found to be cost-effective, resulting in an average cost similar to that of standard office-based excision with permanent section margin control and a cost lower than that of office-based excision with frozen section margin control or excision with frozen section margin control in an ambulatory surgical facility.[37]

SUMMARY

MMS has become the gold standard for treating many forms of primary and recurrent contiguous skin cancers and offers the highest cure rates coupled with tissue conservation compared with other modalities. Originally developed by Dr Frederic E. Mohs at the University of Wisconsin in the 1930s, it was initially called chemosurgery and used zinc chloride paste preoperative in situ fixation in a process called the fixed tissue technique. Although it offered a high cure rate, it could take days to complete. This technique gradually gave way to the fresh tissue technique, and the procedure was renamed MMS. Initially promoted to surgeons, MMS was not widely accepted. However, dermatologists readily accepted the technique and helped promulgate its use, and now, MMS is practiced all over the world as part of a multidisciplinary approach to treating skin cancer.

DR FREDERIC E. MOHS

Frederic E. Mohs, MD (March 1, 1910–July 1, 2002) spent his entire professional career at the University of Wisconsin. He treated literally thousands of patients with cancer and enthusiastically taught his techniques to hundreds of physicians who came to visit him from all over the world.[8,38]

He was an imposing figure in both stature and personality. Like many scientific pioneers, he had a vision and the courage and strength to bring it to fruition. Early in his career, he encountered not only skepticism regarding his concepts and techniques but also actual censure by organized medicine. Still he persevered, and when faced with almost universal rejection by his surgical colleagues, he had the flexibility to seek another audience in the specialty of dermatology.

Dr Mohs believed that everyone who treated skin cancer should learn and use MMS. He was skeptical about any regulations or prohibitions on practice, which likely stemmed from his early negative experiences with the medical hierarchy of his day. When his own creation, the American College of Chemosurgery, in the early 1980's established formal fellowship guidelines requiring 1 to 2 years of training, he was very vocal in his opposition. He truly believed that the guidelines would limit the spread of the technique and effectively marginalize it. Only several years later did he admit that the formal fellowships had put MMS on a solid and academic base, which was essential for its acceptance by organized medicine and regulatory bodies. Today, there are nearly 70 approved fellowship programs and the American College of Mohs Surgery (the direct descendant of the American College of Chemosurgery) has more than 500 members. Moreover, the spread of MMS and its resultant focus on reconstruction and cosmesis has led to the development of dermatologic surgery as an important pillar of the specialty as it is practiced today.

Perhaps the 2 most symbolic moments for the author (P.L.B.) in a quarter century relationship with Dr Mohs as his fellow and then his colleague came at national meetings. The first was in New Orleans at a world symposium on skin cancer and facial reconstructive surgery. Dr Mohs was the designated the guest of honor, scheduled to receive an award and the key to the city from the mayor. Unfortunately, he was assaulted and robbed just outside the hotel and had to be taken to a physician's office where he had a severe head wound sutured. Another lesser man might have requested a delay in the proceedings, but Dr Mohs went directly from the office to the hotel auditorium and bloodied but unbowed, with full head wrap in place and blood stains on his suit, he received the key to the city of New Orleans.

Much later in his life, he was a victim of progressing myasthenia gravis. Although too weakened to be able to present a full paper at the annual Mohs meeting he still took the podium

and delivered as much of the paper as he physically was able, then let his current fellow finish the presentation. His dedication to advancing the field and to his colleagues was unwavering.

These 2 moments symbolize the courage, passion, intensity, and dedication that allowed Fred Mohs to father a specialty that literally revolutionized the treatment of skin cancer around the world.

REFERENCES

1. Mohs F. Chemosurgery in cancer, gangrene, and infections. Springfield (IL): Charles C. Thomas; 1956.
2. Otley C, Roenigk R. Mohs surgery. In: Bolognia J, Jorizzo J, Rapini R, editors. Dermatology. 2nd edition. St Louis (MO): Mosby; 2008. p. 2269–79.
3. Mohs F. History of Mohs micrographic surgery. In: Roenigk R, Roenigk H, editors. Dermatologic surgery, principles and practice. New York: Marcel Dekker, Inc; 1989. p. 783–9.
4. Mohs F. Mohs micrographic surgery, a historical perspective. Dermatol Clin 1989;7(4):609–11.
5. Mohs F, Guyer M. Pre-excisional fixation of tissues in the treatment of cancer in rats. Cancer Res 1941;1: 49–51.
6. Mohs F. Origin and progress of Mohs micrographic surgery. In: Snow S, Mikhail G, editors. Mohs micrographic surgery. 2nd edition. Madison (WI): University of Wisconsin Press; 2004. p. 3–13.
7. Mohs F. The preparation of frozen sections for use in the chemosurgical technique for the microscopically controlled excision of cancer. J Lab Clin Med 1948; 33:392.
8. Lewis P. Frederic Mohs, 92, inventor of cancer surgery technique. The New York Times July 5, 2002. Available at: http://www.nytimes.com/2002/07/05/us/frederic-mohs-92-inventor-of-cancer-surgery-technique.html. Accessed January 28, 2011.
9. Mohs F. Chemosurgery: a microscopically controlled method. Arch Surg 1941;42(2):279–95.
10. Mohs F, Severinghaus E, Schmidt E. Conservative amputation of gangrenous parts by chemosurgery. Ann Surg 1941;114:274–82.
11. Mohs F. Chemosurgical treatment of cancer of the lip: a microscopically controlled method of excision. Arch Surg 1944;48:478–88.
12. Mohs F. Chemosurgical treatment of cancer of the nose: a microscopically controlled method. Arch Surg 1946;53:327–44.
13. Mohs F. Chemosurgical treatment of carcinoma of the ear: a microscopically controlled method of excision. Surgery 1947;21:605–22.
14. Mohs F. Chemosurgical treatment of carcinoma of the face. Arch Dermatol 1947;56:143–56.

15. Mohs F. Chemosurgery in cutaneous malignancy. Calif Med 1949;71:173–6.
16. Bennet R. Mohs surgery, new concepts and applications. Dermatol Clin 1987;5:409–28.
17. Greenway H, Maggio K. Mohs micrographic surgery and cutaneous oncology. In: Robinson J, Sengelmann R, Hanke C, et al, editors. Surgery of the skin, procedural dermatology. St Louis (MO): Elsevier; 2005. p. 777–800.
18. Mohs F. The chemosurgical method for the microscopically controlled excision of cutaneous cancer. In: Epstein E, editor. Skin surgery. Philadelphia: Lea & Febiger; 1956. p. 171–89.
19. Mohs F. Cancer of the eyelids. Bull Am Coll Chemosurg 1970;3:10–1.
20. Tromovitch T, Stegman S. Microscopically controlled excision of skin tumors: chemosurgery (Mohs) fresh tissue technique. Arch Dermatol 1974;110:231–2.
21. James W, Berger T, Elston D. Andrews' diseases of the skin, clinical dermatology. 10th edition. Philadelphia (PA): Saunders Elsevier; 2006. p. 881–2.
22. Swanson N. Mohs surgery. Arch Dermatol 1983;119: 761–73.
23. Mohs F. Chemosurgery for skin cancer. Fixed tissue and fresh tissue techniques. Arch Dermatol 1976; 112:211–5.
24. Picoto A, Camacho F, Walker N, et al. Mohs micrographic surgery: european experience. In: Roenigk R, Noenigk H, editors. Surgical dermatology. St Louis (MO): Mosby; 1993. p. 125–261.
25. Gonzalez A. Practice of Mohs surgery in Argentina. In: Snow S, Mikhail G, editors. Mohs micrographic surgery. Madison (WI): University of Wisconsin Press; 2004. p. 301–6.
26. Vinciullo C, Paver R. Practice of Mohs surgery in Australia. In: Snow S, Mikhail G, editors. Mohs micrographic surgery. Madison (WI): University of Wisconsin Press; 2004. p. 307–11.
27. Briggs P. Practice of Mohs surgery in Brazil. In: Snow S, Mikhail G, editors. Mohs micrographic surgery. Madison (WI): University of Wisconsin Press; 2004. p. 313–7.
28. Kohn T, Stone M. Practice of Mohs surgery in Canada. In: Snow S, Mikhail G, editors. Mohs micrographic surgery. Madison (WI): University of Wisconsin Press; 2004. p. 319–22.
29. Picoto A. Practice of Mohs surgery in Portugal. In: Snow S, Mikhail G, editors. Mohs micrographic surgery. Madison (WI): University of Wisconsin Press; 2004. p. 323–5.
30. Davis J, Randle H, Zalla M, et al. A comparison of Mohs micrographic surgery with wide excision for the treatment of atypical fibroxanthoma. Dermatol Surg 1997;23:105–10.
31. Snow S, Gordon E, Larson P, et al. Dermatofibrosarcoma protuberans: a report on 29 patients treated by Mohs micrographic surgery with long-term follow-up and review of the literature. Cancer 2004; 101:28–38.
32. Leibovitch I, Huilgol S, Selva D. Microcystic adnexal carcinoma: treatment with Mohs micrographic surgery. J Am Acad Dermatol 2005;52:295–300.
33. Spencer J, Nossa R, Tse DT. Sebaceous carcinoma of the eyelid treated with Mohs micrographic surgery. J Am Acad Dermatol 2001;44:1004–9.
34. O'Connor W, Roenigk R, Brodland D. Merkel cell carcinoma: comparison of Mohs micrographic surgery and wide excision in eighty-six patients. Dermatol Surg 1997;23:929–33.
35. O'Connor W, Lim K, Zalla M, et al. Comparison of Mohs micrographic surgery and wide excision for extramammary Paget's disease. Dermatol Surg 2003;29:723–7.
36. Bernstein S, Roenigk R. Leiomyosarcoma of the skin: treatment of 34 cases. Dermatol Surg 1996; 22:631–5.
37. Cook J, Zitelli J. Mohs micrographic surgery: a cost analysis. J Am Acad Dermatol 1998;39:698–703.
38. Hanke C. Frederic E. Mohs, MD - the first Mohs micrographic surgeon. Dermatol Surg 2002;28:1.

Mohs Micrographic Surgery Technique

Paul X. Benedetto, MD[a],*, Christine Poblete-Lopez, MD[b]

KEYWORDS

- Mohs micrographic surgery • Surgical technique
- Tissue sparing • Margin control

Mohs micrographic surgery (MMS) consists of a standardized series of steps in cutaneous surgery for the purpose of extirpation of skin cancers. The advantages of MMS over standard excision are precise and thorough histologic margin control, superior cure rates, and maximal preservation of normal tissue. It is a technique developed for the management of cutaneous tumors that grow in predictably contiguous fashion, such that once the excision has been observed histologically to be carried out beyond the boundary of the tumor, a surgeon can feel confident that a true negative margin has been achieved. This fact is reflected in the superior cure rates of MMS compared with traditional surgical excision.[1,2] The beauty of the technique lies in the simplicity of its individual steps, but the elegance and synergy of those steps in aggregate. Furthermore, when MMS is the chosen method for tumor clearance in accordance with the generally accepted indications for the procedure, the average cost to patients and the health care system as a whole is at least equal to, if not less than, traditional surgical excision.[3] This article provides a protocol for the systematic approach to skin cancer excision and tissue mapping, transportation and processing of the surgical specimen, histopathology interpretation, and wound closure and management.

INDICATIONS FOR MOHS MICROGRAPHIC SURGERY

Prior to performing MMS on a given tumor, it must be determined if the technique is indicated for the particular lesion in question. There is general acceptance of most indications for MMS, which are based on tumor size and histology as well as anatomic location and previous treatments (**Box 1** and **Fig. 1**).[4] As the discipline of MMS continues to evolve, new applications for the technique draw support and criticism. There have been attempts to utilize MMS in the treatment of other types of skin cancer that have traditionally been excised with wide local excision. There are reports of utilizing MMS for lentigo maligna melanoma, invasive malignant melanoma, Merkel cell carcinoma, dermatofibrosarcoma protuberans, sebaceous carcinoma, extramammary Paget disease, and microcystic adnexal carcinoma, among other skin cancers, with varying success rates. Some investigators now consider these tumor types to be reasonable indications for MMS.[5–9]

PREOPERATIVE EVALUATION

Once establishing that a patient's skin cancer is an appropriate candidate for extirpation utilizing MMS, a series of preoperative evaluations is important to prepare the patient for surgery. A review of medications, allergies, previous infections and hospitalizations, artificial implants, need for preoperative imaging or consultation with other surgical specialists, and history of smoking and alcohol consumption and a discussion of the patient's expectations of the surgical outcome are all necessary components of a preoperative evaluation. A thorough perusal of these components of the patient's history can prevent, or at least alert a clinician to, potential adverse

The authors have nothing to disclose.
[a] Department of Dermatology, Cleveland Clinic Foundation, 9500 Euclid Avenue, Suite A60, Cleveland, OH 44195, USA
[b] Section of Dermatologic Surgery and Cutaneous Oncology, Department of Dermatology, Cleveland Clinic Foundation, 9500 Euclid Avenue, Suite A60, Cleveland, OH 44195, USA
* Corresponding author.
E-mail address: benedep@ccf.org

Dermatol Clin 29 (2011) 141–151
doi:10.1016/j.det.2011.02.002

Box 1
Indications for MMS

Nonmelanoma skin cancers (basal cell carcinoma and squamous cell carcinoma) greater than 0.4 cm in high-risk location (H zone of face)

Large tumors (>1 cm on the face; >2 cm on the trunk and extremities)

Recurrent and/or incompletely excised tumors

Tumors with aggressive histologic subtypes or indistinct clinical borders (infiltrative, micronodular, and morpheaform basal cell carcinoma; basal cell carcinoma and squamous cell carcinoma with perineural or perivascular invasion)

Tumors in cosmetically sensitive or functionally important locations (genital, anal, hand, and foot locations)

Nonmelanoma skin cancer arising in an immunosuppressed patient

Tumors arising in sites of chronic inflammation, long-standing wounds, burns, or scars

Genetic conditions predisposing to many skin cancers (eg, basal cell nevus syndrome, xeroderma pigmentosa, and Muir-Torre syndrome)

events. Furthermore, patients should be informed of the benefits of MMS as well as alternatives to the procedure and be made aware of the steps involved and the time required to perform those steps. Patients should be prepared to spend at least one half-day in the clinic and should also be instructed to bring someone with them to the office who can assist in transporting them home after surgery.

A medication and allergy history is important to determine both potential interactions that have an impact on the surgery and potential complications of the topical surgical preparation and perioperative medical management. Medications to review include anticoagulants (eg, warfarin, heparin, and heparin derivatives, such as fondaparinux), antiplatelet agents (eg, aspirin, clopidogrel, ticlopidine, and dipyrimadole), herbal blood-thinning medications (eg, garlic and ginkgo),[10] immunosuppressants (which may raise a patient's risk for postoperative infection and poor wound healing, in the case of systemic corticosteroids), and chronic antibiotics that may alter normal skin flora and raise the risk of postoperative infection with resistant organisms. Allergy history is important in case a patient requires perioperative antibiotics or is allergic to local anesthetics. A history of topical allergies may be elicited by asking patients about adverse reactions to preparation soaps, surgical gloves, dermal adhesives, and tape during previous procedures.

A history of previous skin infections may clue in clinicians to nasal colonization with methicillin-resistant *Staphylococcus aureus* (MRSA) or predisposition to infections due to chronic diseases, such as diabetes mellitus. Furthermore, chronic antibiotic use can increase a patient's chances of harboring resistant bacteria on the skin. In patients known to harbor methicillin-resistant *S aureus* intranasally, some data have suggested that decolonizing the anterior nares with mupirocin ointment and oral antibiotics prior to MMS can reduce the risk of postoperative wound infection, although the clinical practicality and the cost-effectiveness of such measures has yet to be determined.[11] Despite the paucity of randomized controlled trials guiding the use of antimicrobial prophylaxis in cutaneous surgery, it is important to keep in mind which summary data do exist when prescribing perioperative antibiotics.

In a 2008 advisory statement released by the American Academy of Dermatology,[12] the role of prophylactic antibiotics in dermatologic surgery was addressed. For the most part, MMS is considered a clean procedure and rarely requires the use of prophylactic antibiotics. When surgical site infections do occur, however, they can lead to infective endocarditis and prosthetic joint infection, so they must be treated early and aggressively.

In 2008, the American Heart Association (AHA) revised its guidelines for the prevention of infective endocarditis and advocated for limited use of antibiotics in high-risk situations.[13] Although the AHA guidelines do not specifically address MMS, it is possible to extrapolate a protocol for cutaneous

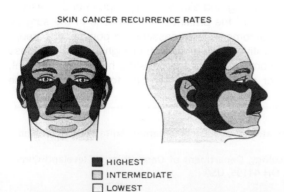

SKIN CANCER RECURRENCE RATES

■ HIGHEST
□ INTERMEDIATE
□ LOWEST

Fig. 1. H zone of the face indicates areas of high risk for tumor recurrence.

surgery. According to the panel, the only situations in which antibiotic prophylaxis is indicated for the prevention of infective endocarditis during routine minor surgery are those that occur on clean contaminated sites, such as oral, nasal, or ano-genital mucosa or axillary skin, as well as during surgery on infected or inflamed tissue in patients who are at a high risk for a poor outcome from bacterial endocarditis. Those high-risk patients are defined as people with prosthetic heart valves, congenital heart disease, or a history of infectious endocarditis and transplant recipients who have developed heart valve disease.

Similarly, in 2003, the American Dental Association (ADA) in conjunction with the American Academy of Orthopaedic Surgeons (AAOS) revised the groups' 1997 advisory statement recommending the use of prophylactic antibiotics for patients undergoing oral procedures in which bleeding is expected or for patients at high risk for prosthetic joint infection.[14] The latter group is defined as those with a prosthetic joint replacement within the preceding 2 years, those with a history of previous prosthetic joint infection, and those with comorbidities, such as diabetes mellitus, HIV, malignancy, and other forms of immunosuppression. Certain cases, such as those in which a wound is open for many hours, may be considered extenuating circumstances and require less strict adherence to the AHA and ADA/AAOS guidelines.[12]

Depending on size, location, and duration of a tumor, consideration must be given to the need for preoperative imaging and consultation with other surgical specialists. In the case of a tumor that feels fixed to underlying tissue and bone, preoperative, high-resolution images, such as CT scans and MRI, should be considered. In certain cases of aggressive tumors with clinically indistinct margins, such as dermatofibrosarcoma protuberans in a pediatric population, the use of preoperative MRI has been shown useful and, in some cases, can even alter surgical planning and outcomes.[15] If a tumor appears sizeable enough that it may leave a defect too large to repair under local anesthesia or without the use of composite grafts, enlisting the help of plastic surgery, otolaryngology, and ophthalmology colleagues is advisable. Also, tumors that border structures, such the eyelid margins, lips, nasal ala, ears, and urethral and vaginal meati, may require assistance for the repair.

More advanced imaging modalities have been studied for their potential utility in the preoperative evaluation of tumors in dermatologic surgery. A recent review was conducted of several techniques, such as CT, MRI, positron emission tomography, Doppler ultrasonography, and confocal microscopy, and all were found to have mixed results in terms of their clinical utility.[16] Several investigators have attempted to use high-frequency, high-resolution ultrasonography to delineate tumor boundaries prior to MMS but found no advantage over clinical assessment.[17,18] Other investigators have attempted to use photodynamic diagnosis, a process that makes use of 5-aminolevulinic acid and a Wood light, to determine tumor margins, but again no true advantage has been reported over standard preoperative clinical assessment.[19,20]

A social history is an important component of the preoperative evaluation, because steady, long-term alcohol consumption can increase intraoperative bleeding and smoking can lead to worse surgical outcomes due to poor wound healing and decreased tissue oxygenation. It is also paramount to assess patients' understanding of the Mohs procedure and what they expect in terms of aesthetic outcome. This helps prevent patient dissatisfaction with the surgical scar, especially if a complex repair is required.

SURGICAL TECHNIQUE OF THE FIRST MOHS STAGE (A-LAYER)

Once the preoperative assessment (described previously) is completed and a patient is ready for surgery, the area is cleaned with alcohol and the visible area of tumor is marked with a surgical marking pen. Any important natural skin tension lines, anatomic cosmetic subunits, or functional margins should also be marked prior to infiltration of the area with local anesthetic (Fig. 2).

Next the area is anesthetized with a mixture of 1% lidocaine and epinephrine, the latter typically in a 1:100,000 dilution. The solution can be buffered with sodium bicarbonate in a ratio of 1:9 with lidocaine, in order to decrease the pain of injection caused by the acidic pH of lidocaine.[21,22] Very slow injection of the anesthetic also helps decrease the stinging sensation caused during infiltration of the tissue. Cases of true allergy to the amide class of local anesthetics are rare, and most instances of adverse reactions are more likely to be caused by sensitivity to the epinephrine. Symptoms of epinephrine sensitivity include giddiness, palpitations, and anxiety. If a patient reports a true allergy to lidocaine, an ester anesthetic, such as tetracaine, may be substituted, although the ester class of local anesthetics is more likely to be allergenic.[23]

Next the tumor may be debulked with a curette (Fig. 3). This helps the surgeon delineate subclinical boundaries of the tumor that were not visible

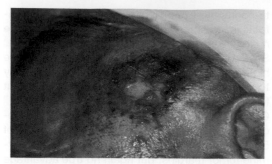

Fig. 2. The clinically observed tumor margins are marked with ink and the site is then anesthetized and prepared for surgery with surgical soap. (*From* Vidimos A, Ammirati CT, Poblete-Lopez C. Dermatologic Surgery. In: Elston DM, ed. Requisites in Dermatology. Philadelphia: Saunders Elsevier, 2009; with permission.)

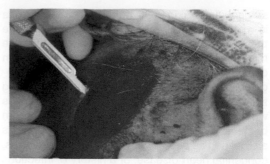

Fig. 4. The excision is carried out with a 1-mm to 2-mm margin of normal appearing skin around the curetted site with the scalpel angled at a 45° bevel. (*From* Vidimos A, Ammirati CT, Poblete-Lopez C. Dermatologic Surgery. In: Elston DM, ed. Requisites in Dermatology. Philadelphia: Saunders Elsevier, 2009; with permission.)

to the naked eye and can actually decrease the number of required Mohs layers.[24,25] Tumor curettage tends to be more helpful in cases of basal cell carcinoma, rather than squamous cell carcinoma, because the tissue is much more friable, thus more easily distinguished from normal tissue. If it appears that the tumor extends beyond the pen markings, the initially planned excision should be altered accordingly. It is important to start the excision with a small margin of epidermis outside the curetted area so that the epidermis can help orient the specimen during review of the histopathology (**Fig. 4**). If the excision is carried out over the area of curettage and no epidermis is visible once the tissue from the first layer is processed, it may be necessary to take a second layer to confirm the margins are indeed negative, thus sacrificing a greater amount of normal tissue.

The first layer is then excised with the scalpel blade positioned at a 45° angle to the skin surface

so that the periphery of the specimen lies down easily in the same plane as the deep margin during processing (see **Fig. 4**). Other techniques to ensure that the epidermal margins lie down flush with the deep plane of section include using curved scalpel blades or excising the specimen at a 90° angle followed by incising it with circumferential and radial partial-thickness slits to facilitate tissue manipulation.[26,27]

Once a scoring incision is made circumferentially around the tumor, some type of marking nick must be made extending onto the surrounding tissue in order to orient the specimen. Traditionally, two nicks are made at the 12-o'clock and 6-o'clock positions for smaller specimens and also at the 3-o'clock and 9-o'clock positions for larger specimens, although individual cases may require alteration in this technique (**Fig. 5**). In cases of piriform or fusiform excisions, it is best to make one or both of the marking nicks at the acute angle of the specimen to make processing the tissue easier.

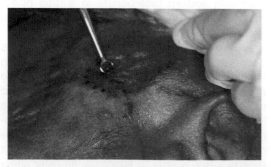

Fig. 3. Preoperative curettage is performed to debulk the tumor and assess the accuracy of the marking made of the clinically observable tumor margins. (*From* Vidimos A, Ammirati CT, Poblete-Lopez C. Dermatologic Surgery. In: Elston DM, ed. Requisites in Dermatology. Philadelphia: Saunders Elsevier, 2009; with permission.)

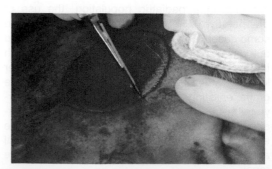

Fig. 5. Hash marks are placed in the surrounding skin and specimen to be excised for orientation purposes. (*From* Vidimos A, Ammirati CT, Poblete-Lopez C. Dermatologic Surgery. In: Elston DM, ed. Requisites in Dermatology. Philadelphia: Saunders Elsevier, 2009; with permission.)

The specimen is typically taken with a 1-mm to 2-mm margin and carried down to the level of subcutaneous fat. The tumor may then be removed from the normal surrounding skin using the scalpel or scissors to cut through the fat. Care must be taken to excise the tissue in the same plane of dissection for ease of processing and interpreting the histopathology.

MOHS MAPPING

Once the specimen is obtained, it should be placed carefully on a piece of blotting paper that has a drawing of the patient's tumor site until the tissue can be marked for processing with ink (**Fig. 6**). The Mohs map, a larger schematic drawing of the excision site, ultimately provides proper orientation to the specimen, containing information, such as site, size, specimen orientation, number of pieces, and ink markings.[28]

The next step, if tumor size or a histotechnician should require, is to section the specimen. Some histotechnicians may be comfortable processing the specimen in toto if it fits on the slide. Other histotechnicians may prefer that it be at least bisected in order to orient the specimen properly on a slide.[28,29] Once a decision is made as to how the specimen is to be processed and sectioned, color-coding is necessary to orient the specimen to the map and body location.

Color inks are used to stain specific segments of the surgical specimen. In bisected samples (or samples with a greater number of sections depending on tumor size), ink is applied to the cut medial edges and numbers are given to tissue pieces (**Fig. 7**). Often one color marks the medial or superior edge and another color is used to mark the lateral or inferior edge. In smaller specimens that are processed in toto, the ink is applied to the lateral edges and the color markings are drawn in relation to the hash marks on the specimen. It makes no difference which color is chosen for which margin because the color-coding is drawn on the Mohs map as well in order to preserve the orientation after sectioning.[30] Maintaining the same color coordination each time (such as blue for superior and medial and red for inferior and lateral), however, reduces the chances of a processing error and disorienting the specimen. Furthermore, the Mohs surgeon should be responsible for each step in the process to reduce the potential for error in delegating key steps to assistants.[31]

TISSUE TRANSPORT AND PROCESSING

Once a surgical specimen has been transected, if necessary, and color-coded, it is ready to be processed for microscopic examination. The tissue pieces are moved from the blotting paper to a piece of gauze in a specimen dish for transport to the laboratory. By convention, an ink dot is placed in the upper left corner of the gauze, and the piece placed closest to it is designated piece number 1. Successive pieces are placed in columns below piece number 1 and to the right of it, and all pieces of the surgical specimen are oriented with their cut edge facing up towards the dot (**Fig. 8**). Whatever the orientation method used, it is imperative that the numbering is transferred to the Mohs map to preserve the orientation of the tumor after processing.

Once histotechnicians receive the samples, the processing begins. First, the tissue sample must

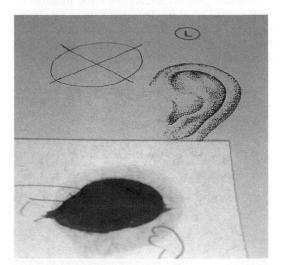

Fig. 6. The anatomic position of the specimen, its orientation at that site, and the location of the hash marks are transferred to the Mohs map. (*From* Vidimos A, Ammirati CT, Poblete-Lopez C. Dermatologic Surgery. In: Elston DM, ed. Requisites in Dermatology. Philadelphia: Saunders Elsevier, 2009; with permission.)

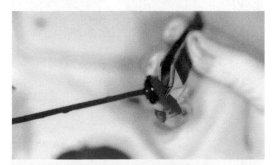

Fig. 7. The specimen is marked with ink on its cut edge and deep margin. (*From* Vidimos A, Ammirati CT, Poblete-Lopez C. Dermatologic Surgery. In: Elston DM, ed. Requisites in Dermatology. Philadelphia: Saunders Elsevier, 2009; with permission.)

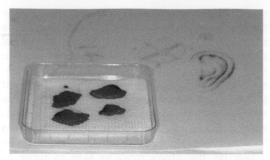

Fig. 8. Note the successive pieces of the surgical specimen oriented in relation to the ink dot in the upper left corner of the transfer gauze. (*From* Vidimos A, Ammirati CT, Poblete-Lopez C. Dermatologic Surgery. In: Elston DM, ed. Requisites in Dermatology. Philadelphia: Saunders Elsevier, 2009; with permission.)

be grossed or flattened out so that the epidermis is laid down in the same plane as the deeper margin. For specimens that are beveled at less than 45° or come from anatomic sites with relatively thick dermis and are not very pliable, relaxing cuts may be made with a scalpel to ensure that the epidermis lies down in the same plane as the subcutaneous fat. This ensures that once samples of the frozen section are cut and placed on slides the surgeon is able to examine 100% of the specimen's margin (**Fig. 9**).

Next, the flattened specimen must be preserved in this orientation by placing it into the embedding medium and attaching it to a specimen-holder button or chuck, which is used to hold the specimen during sectioning.[32] Many varieties of embedding media exist, but they are all generally composed of some combination of polyvinyl

alcohol and polyethylene glycol and function optimally in a temperature range between approximately −15°C and −30°C. Freezing the specimen should be done as rapidly as possible to reduce the formation of ice crystals in the tissue, a complication of slow freezing.[33]

Once the specimen is embedded and frozen in the medium and mounted on the stage, it is sectioned in the microtome and placed on the slide (**Fig. 10**). The number of slices cut per piece of processed tissue and the average thickness of each slice vary depending on the preferences of the surgeon. A recent survey of practicing Mohs surgeons revealed that most preferred between 3 and 6 slices for review, with the numbers ranging between 1 and 9. The surgeons also preferred an average thickness of 5 μm to 6 μm, with the range between 4 μm and 9 μm.[28] This same survey found that most laboratories used hematoxylin-eosin as the routine staining method, but approximately 6% of the respondents used toluidine blue in the microscopic evaluation of basal cell carcinomas.

Because the processing of frozen sections (described previously) is rapid, reliable, and reproducible, MMS has become the standard of care for basal cell and squamous cell carcinomas that meet the appropriate criteria. As the scope of practice expands to include other tumor types, however, novel processing methods and staining techniques are being developed to quickly provide adequate specimens for histologic review in the outpatient setting. One such new method of tissue processing is microwave preparation of permanent paraffin sections for the treatment of melanoma in situ. The microwave technique requires 2 hours to process each layer, double the time of conventional frozen section, but substantially less than the 24 hours required to

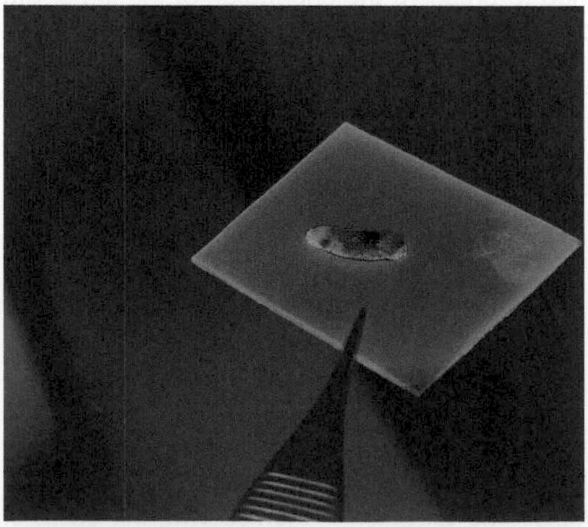

Fig. 9. The inked specimen is flattened using a frozen glass slide so the epidermis, dermis, and subcutaneous fat lie in the same plane. (*Courtesy of* Christie T. Ammirati.)

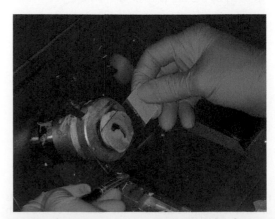

Fig. 10. The specimen is embedded in the freezing medium, mounted on the stage, sectioned on the microtome, and placed on a glass slide. (*Courtesy of* Christie T. Ammirati.)

process permanent paraffin-embedded sections. A recent prospective clinical trial found that the quality of slides produced via this method, hence its utility in the treatment of melanoma in situ, was comparable to conventional permanent tissue processing and superior to standard frozen section as well as frozen section with immunostains.[34] Advanced staining techniques and immunostaining are discussed by Miller and colleagues elsewhere in this issue.

HISTOPATHOLOGY INTERPRETATION

As discussed previously, the main advantage of the MMS technique is achieving the highest possible cure rate by microscopically examining 100% of the surgical margin while preserving the maximum amount of normal skin. The ability to examine the entire margin is made possible by the processing of the tissue in the histology laboratory, but the interpretation and localization of residual tumor requires an understanding of the embedding technique and careful attention to the specimen's orientation.

Each mounted slide should contain epidermis, dermis, and subcutaneous fat, but the successive layers of skin and subcutis on the slide do not overlie one another in a 2-D plane. As the specimen progresses from more superficial to deep skin structures on the slide (ie, from epidermis to subcutis), it also moves from the periphery to the center in the corresponding surgical defect; that is, residual tumor in the epidermis and dermis requires extending the periphery of the surgical defect laterally in the second layer whereas residual tumor in the subcutaneous fat, especially portions well separated from the overlying dermis, may only require removal of a second layer from the base of the surgical defect. In the latter case, sometimes it may be necessary to excise a small adjacent section of epidermis and dermis in order to orient the successive layer, in case more Mohs layers are required.

SURGICAL TECHNIQUE OF THE SECOND (AND SUBSEQUENT) MOHS LAYER(S)

In order to ensure true tumor clearance, it is important that the excision achieves some margin of normal skin beyond the observable boundary of the neoplasm. Depending on the thickness of specimens cut from the microtome, with the standard approximately 5 µm to 6 µm, at least 3 to 4 successive sections should be observed to be free of tumor to be satisfied that true negative margins have been achieved.

In the event that residual tumor persists at deep or lateral margins of the specimen, more Mohs layers are required (Fig. 11). The location of the residual tumor observed under the microscope and localized based on the ink markings should be drawn on the Mohs map for reference in the operating room (Fig. 12). Utilizing the hash marks on the skin, an estimation of where the residual tumor resides can be made and the next layer can be taken from a specific point in the surgical wound (Fig. 13).[35] An attempt should be made to take a small (1–2 mm) margin of normal skin around the site of presumed involvement where the residual tumor lies. As stated previously, foci of cancer that persist in the epidermis and dermis require extending the defect laterally whereas persistent neoplasm in the subcutaneous fat or underlying structures may only require extending the excision in a deeper plane. Once clear margins are confirmed histologically, the reconstruction may be planned (Figs. 14 and 15).

MANAGEMENT OF THE SURGICAL DEFECT

Many options for repair of the surgical defect exist, and the proper choice of technique relies on

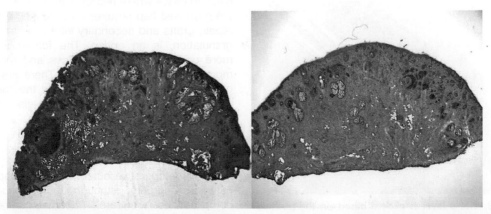

Fig. 11. Residual basal cell carcinoma persists at the peripheral margin approaching on both sides of the cut edge.

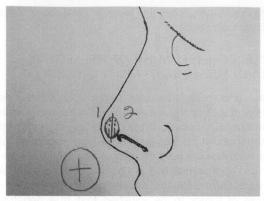

Fig. 12. The positive margins as seen on histology are marked on the Mohs map for reference in the operating room.

a multifactorial approach to achieve the best possible functional and cosmetic outcome. As a rule, function is paramount when planning a repair and should be the first and most important consideration. Factors, such as eyelid and lip margin integrity and mobility and nasal cavity and external auditory meatus patency, are important functions for everyday life and must be preserved when a surgical repair is undertaken.

Provided that the intended repair achieves this goal, the next consideration should be attempting to approximate anatomic form. Regardless of where suture lines, and ultimately scars, fall, texture, contour, shadowing, concavities, and convexities impart the underlying form to a repair and have a greater effect on cosmetic outcome than the suture line itself. Wide regional variation of skin color, texture, thickness, suppleness, and pliability as well as density of pilosebaceous units exists even on apparently close anatomic sites. The skin of the nose, for example, has different qualities from the skin on the malar cheek, despite

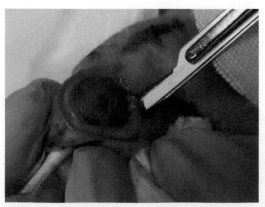

Fig. 13. The B-layer is excised based on the positive margins as drawn on the Mohs map.

separated by a distance of only a few millimeters. In general, it is best to use adjacent skin to repair a surgical defect whenever possible, in order to maintain similar qualities and appearance of the skin. When this is not possible, consideration should be given to the factors listed previously when choosing a donor site for skin to match.

Once these minimum requirements are achieved, attention may be focused on the surgical scar itself. Certain basic principals govern the planning of scar placement. Respect should be paid to anatomic cosmetic units and, whenever possible, the scar should be oriented in the natural dividing lines between these units. Furthermore, angled and curved scars are often less noticeable to the observer than straight lines. Suture marks and tram tracking can make even a well-performed repair less than optimal, and the duration of time sutures are left in to give the new wound strength and stability should be weighed against the expected cosmetic outcome of track marking.[36]

When choosing a closure method, it is recommended that a stepwise approach is taken in order at achieve optimal cosmetic outcome. In general, primary closure is considered the best option, whenever possible. If the wound is too large to close primarily or if doing so will likely cause a functional impairment, using a flap is often the next best option. A flap is a segment of tissue that is moved to a recipient site but maintains its vascular supply from a partially attached segment. Most often in cutaneous surgery local or regional flaps are used, which maintain nearby attachments for their blood supply, as opposed to free flaps, which are fully detached from distant sites and anastamosed microvascularly. There are many types of flaps, which are classified by their location in relation to the surgical defect, how they move into position, their shape or configuration, and their blood supply, whether random, axial, or microvascular. In cases where nearby skin is unavailable or the proposed flap requires a burdensome staged repair, grafts and secondary intention healing, or granulation, is an option. The former is often more useful on convex surfaces and the latter more so on concave surfaces. There are many options from which to choose and they are discussed further by Zhang and Meine elsewhere in this issue.

POSTOPERATIVE COURSE

Certain postoperative outcomes are expected in cutaneous surgery, although true postoperative complications are rare. Patients can expect some degree of pain, swelling, erythema, and

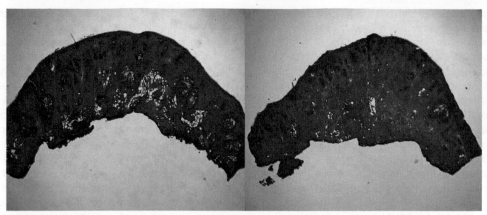

Fig. 14. Negative margins are observed on examination of the histopathology from the B-layer.

bruising. Healing times can be variable, depending on factors, such as patient age and health status, defect size, type of repair, anatomic location, decreased tissue vascularization due to peripheral vascular disease and smoking status, and concomitant use of medications that inhibit wound repair, such as systemic corticosteroids and anticoagulants.

Postoperative complications, when they occur, include events, such as infection, bleeding, hematoma formation, wound dehiscence, scar contracture, and less than optimal cosmetic outcome. These risks can be mitigated by instructing patients on proper wound care and maintaining overall optimal conditions for wound healing. Wounds should be cleaned once to twice daily with hydrogen peroxide and covered with petrolatum or a similar ointment-based topical antiseptic. Some studies have demonstrated that the intraincisional injection of nafcillin or, in penicillin-allergic patients, clindamycin prior to surgical reconstruction can statistically significantly reduce

risk of postoperative infection.[37,38] If blood-thinning medications, such as aspirin or herbal supplements, can be temporarily halted without negative impact on patient health, that is advisable to prevent bleeding and hematoma formation. If bleeding or hematoma formation occurs, early intervention and vessel cauterization or ligation improves the final outcome. If patients have been taking long-term systemic steroids, certain suture techniques, such as the horizontal mattress and pulley techniques, can be used to give added strength to the closure and prevent wound dehiscence. Scar contracture and hypertrophy can be addressed by immobilizing the underlying muscles as best as possible and frequently massaging the scar beginning several weeks after the repair is completed.

SUMMARY

In summary, MMS should be considered an excellent option and, in fact, the treatment of choice for nonmelanoma skin cancer removal for situations in which the criteria (discussed previously) are met. In such cases, MMS offers cure rates superior to all other treatment modalities with the added benefit of being the most conservative option in regards to tissue-sparing potential. Maximum normal tissue preservation leads to surgical defects of the smallest possible size, thus optimal reconstructive results, as well as minimal risk of poor surgical outcomes. Overall, the risks of the procedure are few, the benefits numerous and great, and the outcomes well worth the time and effort spent.

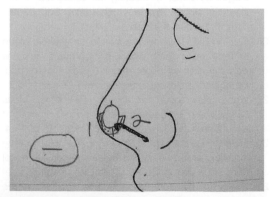

Fig. 15. The negative B-layer is drawn on the corresponding Mohs map.

REFERENCES

1. Rowe DE, Carroll RJ, Day CL Jr. Prognostic factors for local recurrence, metastasis, and survival rates

in squamous cell carcinoma of the skin, ear, and lip. Implications for treatment modality selection. J Am Acad Dermatol 1992;26(6):976–90.

2. Rowe DE, Carroll RJ, Day CL Jr. Long-term recurrence rates in previously untreated (primary) basal cell carcinoma: implications for patient follow-up. J Dermatol Surg Oncol 1989;15(3):315–28.

3. Bialy TL, Whalen J, Veledar E, et al. Mohs micrographic surgery vs traditional surgical excision: a cost comparison analysis. Arch Dermatol 2004; 140(6):736–42.

4. Swanson NA. Mohs surgery. Technique, indications, applications, and the future. Arch Dermatol 1983; 119(9):761–73.

5. Levy RM, Hanke CW. Mohs micrographic surgery: facts and controversies. Clin Dermatol 2010;28(3): 269–74.

6. O'Connor WJ, Roenigk RK, Brodland DG. Merkel cell carcinoma. Comparison of Mohs micrographic surgery and wide excision in eighty-six patients. Dermatol Surg 1997;23(10):929–33.

7. Tan WP, Barlow RJ, Robson A, et al. Dermatofibrosarcoma protuberans: 35 patients treated with Mohs micrographic surgery using paraffin sections. Br J Dermatol 2011;164(2):363–6.

8. Thomas CJ, Wood GC, Marks VJ. Mohs micrographic surgery in the treatment of rare aggressive cutaneous tumors: the Geisinger experience. Dermatol Surg 2007;33(3):333–9.

9. Zitelli JA, Moy RL, Abell E. The reliability of frozen sections in the evaluation of surgical margins for melanoma. J Am Acad Dermatol 1991;24(1):102–6.

10. Dinehart SM, Henry L. Dietary supplements: altered coagulation and effects on bruising. Dermatol Surg 2005;31(7 Pt 2):819–26 [discussion: 826].

11. Cordova KB, Grenier N, Chang KH, et al. Preoperative methicillin-resistant Staphylococcus aureus screening in Mohs surgery appears to decrease postoperative infections. Dermatol Surg 2010; 36(10):1537–40.

12. Wright TI, Baddour LM, Berbari EF, et al. Antibiotic prophylaxis in dermatologic surgery: advisory statement 2008. J Am Acad Dermatol 2008;59(3):464–73.

13. Wilson W, Taubert KA, Gewitz M, et al. Prevention of infective endocarditis: guidelines from the American Heart Association: a guideline from the American Heart Association Rheumatic Fever, Endocarditis and Kawasaki Disease Committee, Council on Cardiovascular Disease in the Young, and the Council on Clinical Cardiology, Council on Cardiovascular Surgery and Anesthesia, and the Quality of Care and Outcomes Research Interdisciplinary Working Group. J Am Dent Assoc 2008;139(Suppl):3S–24S.

14. American Dental Association, American Academy of Orthopedic Surgeons. Antibiotic prophylaxis for dental patients with total joint replacements. J Am Dent Assoc 2003;134(7):895–9.

15. Thornton SL, Reid J, Papay FA, et al. Childhood dermatofibrosarcoma protuberans: role of preoperative imaging. J Am Acad Dermatol 2005;53(1):76–83.

16. Mogensen M, Jemec GB. Diagnosis of nonmelanoma skin cancer/keratinocyte carcinoma: a review of diagnostic accuracy of nonmelanoma skin cancer diagnostic tests and technologies. Dermatol Surg 2007; 33(10):1158–74.

17. Marmur ES, Berkowitz EZ, Fuchs BS, et al. Use of high-frequency, high-resolution ultrasound before Mohs surgery. Dermatol Surg 2010;36(6):841–7.

18. Bobadilla F, Wortsman X, Munoz C, et al. Presurgical high resolution ultrasound of facial basal cell carcinoma: correlation with histology. Cancer Imaging 2008;8:163–72.

19. Lee CY, Kim KH, Kim YH. The efficacy of photodynamic diagnosis in defining the lateral border between a tumor and a tumor-free area during Mohs micrographic surgery. Dermatol Surg 2010; 36(11):1704–10.

20. Redondo P, Marquina M, Pretel M, et al. Methyl-ALA-induced fluorescence in photodynamic diagnosis of basal cell carcinoma prior to Mohs micrographic surgery. Arch Dermatol 2008;144(1):115–7.

21. Stewart JH, Cole GW, Klein JA. Neutralized lidocaine with epinephrine for local anesthesia. J Dermatol Surg Oncol 1989;15(10):1081–3.

22. Stewart JH, Chinn SE, Cole GW, et al. Neutralized lidocaine with epinephrine for local anesthesia–II. J Dermatol Surg Oncol 1990;16(9):842–5.

23. Eggleston ST, Lush LW. Understanding allergic reactions to local anesthetics. Ann Pharmacother 1996;30(7–8):851–7.

24. Ratner D, Bagiella E. The efficacy of curettage in delineating margins of basal cell carcinoma before Mohs micrographic surgery. Dermatol Surg 2003; 29(9):899–903.

25. Chung VQ, Bernardo L, Jiang SB. Presurgical curettage appropriately reduces the number of Mohs stages by better delineating the subclinical extensions of tumor margins. Dermatol Surg 2005; 31(9 Pt 1):1094–9 [discussion: 1100].

26. Shelton RM. The use of a curved ophthalmic blade to facilitate incising Mohs micrographic sections with the desired bevel despite anatomic obstructions. Dermatol Surg 1998;24(8):897–9.

27. Weber PJ, Moody BR, Dryden RM, et al. Mohs surgery and processing: novel optimizations and enhancements. Dermatol Surg 2000;26(10):909–14.

28. Silapunt S, Peterson SR, Alcalay J, et al. Mohs tissue mapping and processing: a survey study. Dermatol Surg 2003;29(11):1109–12 [discussion: 1112].

29. Chen TM, Wanitphakdeedecha R, Whittemore DE, et al. Laboratory assistive personnel in Mohs

micrographic surgery: a survey of training and laboratory practice. Dermatol Surg 2009;35(11):1746–56.

30. Robins P, Albom MJ. Mohs' surgery—fresh tissue technique. J Dermatol Surg 1975;1(2):37–41.

31. Cottel WI, Bailin PL, Albom MJ, et al. Essentials of Mohs micrographic surgery. J Dermatol Surg Oncol 1988;14(1):11–3.

32. Fish Frederick S III, editor. Manual of frozen section processing for Mohs micrographic surgery. Milwaukee (WI): American College of Mohs Surgery; 2008.

33. Cocco C, Melis GV, Ferri GL. Embedding media for cryomicrotomy: an applicative reappraisal. Appl Immunohistochem Mol Morphol 2003;11(3):274–80.

34. Mallipeddi R, Stark J, Xie XJ, et al. A novel 2-hour method for rapid preparation of permanent paraffin sections when treating melanoma in situ with Mohs micrographic surgery. Dermatol Surg 2008;34(11): 1520–6.

35. Zitelli JA. Mohs surgery. Concepts and misconceptions. Int J Dermatol 1985;24(9):541–8.

36. Robinson JK, Sengelmann RD, Hanke CWilliam, et al, editors. Surgery of the skin: procedural dermatology. St Louis (MO): Elsevier Mosby; 2005.

37. Griego RD, Zitelli JA. Intra-incisional prophylactic antibiotics for dermatologic surgery. Arch Dermatol 1998;134(6):688–92.

38. Huether MJ, Griego RD, Brodland DG, et al. Clindamycin for intraincisional antibiotic prophylaxis in dermatologic surgery. Arch Dermatol 2002;138(9): 1145–8.

An Overview of Mohs Micrographic Surgery for the Treatment of Basal Cell Carcinoma

Lance D. Wood, MD*, Christie T. Ammirati, MD

KEYWORDS

- Basal cell carcinoma • Mohs micrographic surgery
- Skin cancer

MOHS MICROGRAPHIC SURGERY IN THE MANAGEMENT OF BASAL CELL CARCINOMA
Basal Cell Carcinoma

Basal cell carcinoma (BCC) makes up about 80% of all skin cancers, and it has been estimated that approximately 1 in 4 Americans will develop BCC during their lifetime.[1] BCC is highly associated with ultraviolet radiation exposure, and as such, the most common locations for it to develop are the head and neck (**Box 1**).[2] Although BCCs are usually asymptomatic and only rarely metastasize, if left untreated, they can lead to significant functional and cosmetic morbidity (**Figs. 1** and **2**).[3]

In general, treatment of this slow-growing and rarely metastasizing type of skin cancer is simple and straightforward, particularly for lesions on the trunk and extremities. In these locations, techniques such as curettage (often in combination with electrodesiccation or cryosurgery) or simple surgical excision can provide high cure rates.[4] However, treatment can be more challenging in cosmetically sensitive locations such as the head, neck, and genital area. In these regions, it is particularly crucial to both completely remove the neoplasm, thus limiting recurrence, and preserve function and appearance as much as possible. These requirements have led to the development of Mohs micrographic surgery (MMS) as the most widely accepted treatment of BCC in areas with the greatest demand for tissue preservation and those at greatest risk for recurrence.[5–8]

MMS

As it is practiced today, MMS has evolved significantly from its first description as chemosurgery by Dr Frederic Mohs in 1941.[9] Initially, his technique involved direct injections of zinc chloride solution into the tumor and surrounding area for in vivo tissue fixation. After 12 to 24 hours, the involved tissue was removed from an often bloodless field for microscopic examination. However, instead of traditional vertical sections, the tissue was oriented into tangential sections, which examined the entire peripheral and deep margins and led to cure rates approaching 99%.[9–11]

Over time, Dr Mohs and others contributed to advancement in the field by introducing the removal of fresh tissue under local anesthesia for evaluation.[12,13] In 1970, Dr Theodore Tromovitch presented the first series of patients using the fresh tissue technique. This series was followed by another supporting study by Tromovitch and Stegman[14] in 1974. Both these studies illustrated success rates that were comparable to the previously described fixed tissue technique, opening the door to all of the potential benefits of using the fresh tissue technique without sacrificing the excellent outcomes that were achieved with the

The authors have nothing to disclose.
Penn State Hershey Department of Dermatology, Penn State Milton S. Hershey Medical Center, 500 University Drive, PO Box 850, Hershey, PA 17033-0850, USA
* Corresponding author.
E-mail address: lwood@hmc.psu.edu

Dermatol Clin 29 (2011) 153–160
doi:10.1016/j.det.2011.02.005
0733-8635/11/$ – see front matter © 2011 Elsevier Inc. All rights reserved.

derm.theclinics.com

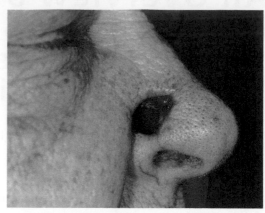

Fig. 2. An advanced BCC that has ulcerated entirely through the nasal wall resulting in significant morbidity.

older method. These benefits included the following:

1. Decreased pain for the patient. The previously used chemosurgical technique with in vivo tissue fixation was associated with significant presurgical and postsurgical patient discomfort, often requiring hospital admission for narcotic analgesia. This discomfort was caused by the significant pain and edema within and around the surgical wound from the chemical fixative.[15,16]

2. Increased efficiency for both the surgeon and the patient. Rapid freezing of the tissue could be used for microscopic evaluation within a matter of minutes instead of the slower zinc chloride fixation that took hours to complete.

3. Vastly improved cosmetic outcomes and decreased wound healing time. Following complete eradication of the tumor with the fresh tissue technique, the surgeon was now able to immediately reconstruct and close the associated defect. With the former in vivo fixed tissue technique, a rim of devitalized tissue was created, which could not be repaired until it had sloughed spontaneously, often taking weeks. This delay in reconstruction resulted in allowing many wounds to heal by secondary intention, leading to much slower healing and, in some instances, poorer cosmetic outcomes for the patient.

Improvements in systems and equipment associated with the MMS procedure have continued to advance since the 1970s; nevertheless, the concept of complete margin control through tangential sections of excised tumor, as first reported by Dr Frederic Mohs, still prevails in the procedure as it is practiced today.

What makes MMS different from surgical excision with standard pathologic evaluation

Tumors treated by standard excision with vertical histologic sectioning are traditionally removed with margins large enough to have a statistically satisfactory high cure rate without recurrence (usually 3–4 mm for low-risk BCCs and larger margins for higher-risk tumors) (**Box 2**). To achieve an acceptable rate of success, a significant amount of normal tissue has to be removed. However, when the Mohs technique is used,

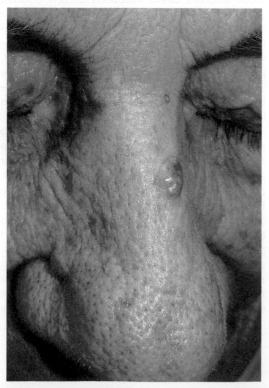

Fig. 1. A common "pearly papule with telangiectasias" presentation of 2 uncomplicated BCCs on the right medial upper nose near the canthus and nasal bridge.

> **Box 2**
> **Histologic types of BCC frequently treated with MMS**
>
> - BCC with poorly defined clinical margins (**Fig. 3**)
> - Multiple BCCs associated with syndromes (**Fig. 4**)
> - Large and deeply penetrating BCC (**Fig. 5**)
> - Morphea-like, sclerotic, micronodular BCC (**Fig. 6**)
> - Superficial multicentric BCC (**Fig. 7**)
> - Metatypical (basosquamous) BCC (**Fig. 8**)
> - BCC arising within a scar (**Fig. 9**)
> - BCC within an existing lesion (**Fig. 10**)
> - BCCs with perichondral, perivascular, periosteal, and perineural invasion (**Fig. 11**)

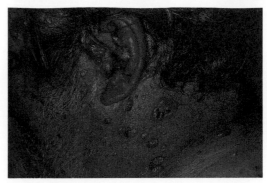

Fig. 4. Multiple BCCs associated with basal cell nevus (Gorlin) syndrome.

minimal margins can be obtained as the entire peripheral and deep margins of the lesion are examined histologically, removing the need for taking extra tissue to allow for a margin of error.

What differentiates MMS from standard surgical excision is illustrated by the term micrographic, which describes the first critical component of the technique. Once the lesion is excised, it is mapped or graphed and then examined microscopically by the surgeon. This procedure is covered in detail in the article on Mohs Technique elsewhere in this issue.

Why MMS works well in treating BCCs

There are 2 key characteristics that define the tumors, which are treated most successfully by MMS.

Contiguity of tumor cells As the Mohs procedure is based on identifying tumor cells at the entire margin of the excised tissue microscopically, breaks within the tumor, or intervening islands of normal tissue, can make MMS less effective. As long as the tumor is contiguous, the Mohs surgeon can continue to follow whatever path it may take until complete removal is confirmed. Previous surgeries, other antitumor therapies, or atypical natural growth of the tumor resulting in skip areas or tumor noncontiguity may cause the Mohs surgeon to stop short of removing the entire lesion and ultimately lead to recurrence or persistence of the neoplasm.

Tumor cells identifiable with frozen section processing techniques Because the turnaround time for tissue processing during MMS is so

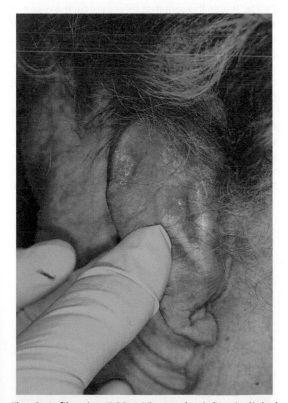

Fig. 3. Infiltrative BCC with poorly defined clinical margins on the posterior helix.

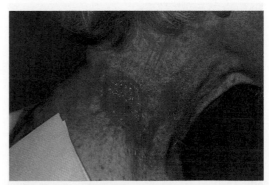

Fig. 5. Large and deeply penetrating BCC, which eroded into the trapezius muscle.

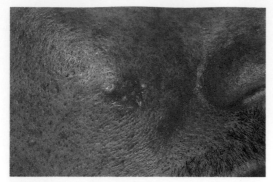

Fig. 6. Morphea-like, sclerotic BCC on the right medial cheek.

much shorter than that required for standard histologic preparation techniques, the Mohs surgeon has comparatively limited number of available methods of preparing the tissue for histopathologic evaluation. Therefore, tumor types that can easily be identified on hematoxylin and eosin or toluidine blue staining are more amenable to treatment by MMS than other tumor types that can be more difficult to visualize microscopically without the aid of additional immunostains and cell markers. Although many advances are being made with regard to immunostains and tissue markers available to Mohs surgeons, in most cases, use of permanent section processing is still preferred. For further discussion, see article on special stains elsewhere in this issue.

Indications for MMS in the Treatment of BCC

Illustrating the challenge surrounding the decision of whether or not a particular BCC warrants treatment with MMS are the results of a recent study comparing the evolving characteristics of the BCCs of patients referred for MMS at a single institution in 1996 versus 2004.[17] The investigators

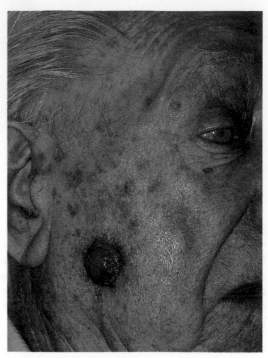

Fig. 8. Metatypical (basosquamous) BCC.

found that referral patterns shifted toward a preference for MMS for the treatment of smaller, primary BCCs. It was thought that this "may be the result of increased awareness by the dermatologic and medical community of the numerous advantages of MMS and a greater appreciation of its tissue-sparing properties, which may result in less complex and more successful aesthetic reconstructions."

As it is impossible to consider the infinite number of different patient scenarios and variables with which the clinician may be presented, it is also impossible to provide an exact outline of the correct way to proceed in every case. However, there are general principles that can guide the

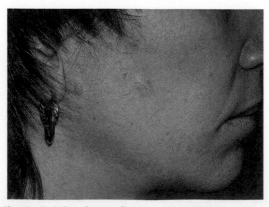

Fig. 7. Ill-defined superficial multicentric BCC.

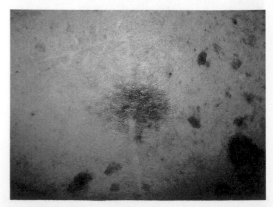

Fig. 9. BCC arising within a scar on the superior back.

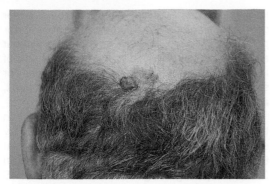

Fig. 10. BCC arising within a nevus sebaceous.

decision of whether or not MMS is the preferred treatment. Making the decision to treat BCC with MMS is based on 3 variables: (1) location and size, (2) histology with margin definition, and (3) whether or not the tumor has been previously treated.[8]

Location

In choosing a treatment modality for BCC in various locations, the foremost considerations are cure rate, form, and function. As discussed earlier, MMS is currently the most effective method of completely eradicating BCC and also maximizing tissue preservation. The most common indication for MMS is for BCC located on the head and neck. This area is not only the

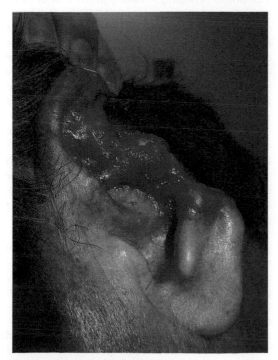

Fig. 11. BCC with perichondral invasion.

most common site that patients develop BCC but also generally the most cosmetically sensitive part of the body and carries a significant rate of recurrence. In the surgical removal of BCCs around the eyes, lips, nose, and ears, preservation of normal, healthy skin is paramount, and as larger surgical margins are often required to approach the cure rate of MMS in these sites, standard excision is often less desirable in these locations. MMS considerations in the eyelids, nose, lips, fingers, ears, and genitalia (**Fig. 12**) are discussed elsewhere in this issue.

A final important point regarding the location of BCCs that are generally best treated by MMS has to do with particular regions where the recurrence rate after standard surgical excision has been shown to be higher than expected. Although the propensity of BCCs to spread in the dermis, fascial planes, nerve sheaths, lymphatic channels, and blood vessels has been noted,[7] attention has also been paid to embryonic fusion planes. Embryonic fusion planes form as tissues come together in embryogenesis and are regions that offer decreased resistance to perpendicular spread of tumor cells.[8] Because of this decreased resistance, tumors in these locations are associated with higher recurrence rates than BCCs in other areas. Embryonic fusion planes include the inner canthus, the nasolabial fold, the preauricular area, the retroauricular sulcus, the mental crease, and the philtrum.[18]

In addition to regions associated with embryonic fusion planes, structurally complex structures, particularly on the face (nasal ala, periocular area, ear, scalp, and temple), have also been associated with increased risk of BCC recurrence.[19–21] This increased risk for recurrence is likely because of the tendency of unpredictable spread in these

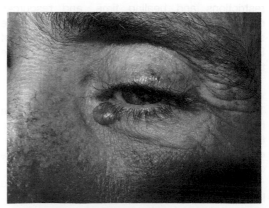

Fig. 12. BCC on the lower eyelid near the medial canthus where tumor extirpation along with preservation of normal tissue are exceedingly important.

locations and the increased difficulty of performing tissue-preserving surgical excision of BCCs in these cosmetically critical locations.

Histology

As mentioned earlier, one of the key components of the MMS procedure is the histologic evaluation of 100% of the deep and peripheral borders of the excised lesion. The importance of this evaluation is easily appreciated when considering the vast number of ways that tumors spread and grow. Although most BCCs can be categorized into 3 primary subtypes (nodular, superficial, and morpheaform/infiltrative),[22] dermatopathologists have described a multitude of different variations of each of these subtypes, and many different classification schemes for BCC have been described.

The most important consideration regarding the type of BCC is the ability of the practitioner to clinically and histopathologically identify the extent of the neoplasm, resulting in complete removal of the lesion. The difficulty associated with this identification varies from the simplest and most straightforward nodular BCC with clearly apparent margins to the recurrent morpheaform BCC that stealthily courses through tissues and spreads deceptively through various fascial planes and along vasculature.

Consistent with the myriad patterns of BCC, there are numerous forms of treatment used. The effectiveness of each treatment, to varying degrees, depends on the type of BCC being treated. Although techniques such as cryosurgery, curettage alone, or in combination with cryosurgery or electrodessication, simple excision, imiquimod, 5-fluorouracil cream, photodynamic therapy, and radiation have all been shown to be relatively effective[4] and possibly preferred in certain situations (depending on multiple variables such as available practitioner training, decreased patient restrictions and healing time, and resources needed for many of these procedures), there are several well-recognized histologic subtypes of BCC for which MMS has been shown to be the treatment of choice (see **Box 2**).

Previously treated BCC

The most obvious explanation of BCC recurrence is failure to completely eradicate the tumor in the first place. Tumor may persist because of greater complexity of tumor growth and subtlety of the clinical and/or histologic tumor margins.

Treatment failures may create BCCs that are histologically and clinically more aggressive. Inadequate treatment, either by surgical or by medical therapy, can further disguise BCCs by disrupting the contiguity of the tumor with scar tissue, leading to more difficult histopathologic tumor cell identification. Sukal and colleagues[23] reported 3 cases of deeply recurrent BCCs without superficial involvement following off-label use of imiquimod 5% cream and advise its use for superficial, nonfacial BCCs on the trunk, neck, and extremities.

Studies comparing MMS with other methods in the treatment of BCC have illustrated statistically significant greater success in treating recurrent BCCs.[7] A recent prospective study published in 2008 comparing surgical excision with MMS demonstrated recurrence rates of 12.1% and 2.4%, respectively, for recurrent BCCs.[24]

SUMMARY AND FUTURE CONSIDERATIONS

MMS has come a long way since Dr Frederic Mohs first developed this method in the 1930s. The largest step forward since that time was the development of the fresh tissue technique. Contributors to the field have continued to refine and improve the technique. Advancements in tissue preparation and developments in tumor cell markers have helped to make MMS faster and more effective.

Various modalities to visualize tumor extent before surgery are currently being evaluated. These efforts include studies in the fields of high-resolution ultrasonography, confocal microscopy,[25] fluorescence imaging,[26] and quantitative multiphoton imaging.[27] Although the role of high-resolution ultrasonography in MMS for the treatment of BCC is still debatable, it shows promise as a potentially useful and noninvasive tool for determining presurgical and intraoperative tumor extent.[28,29] In this way, ultrasonography may prove to help decrease both the time requirement and cost of MMS by decreasing the number of stages required for tumor eradication.

Tissue staining and tumor marking methods continue to become faster and more precise.[30] Decreased tissue preparation time along with increased reliability of markers and probes for BCC will also serve to make MMS more cost-effective and more convenient for the Mohs surgeon and the patient.

Some investigators have performed cost analysis studies comparing MMS with other surgical modalities for BCC and other cutaneous neoplasms and have illustrated that it is continually becoming closer to and more competitive with the cost associated with other treatment modalities.[31,32] As a result of its increasingly competitive cost, its generally accepted decreased rate of recurrence, and tissue-sparing cosmesis,[6] use of MMS will most surely increase.[17]

Despite the current prominent role of MMS in the treatment of BCC, Mohs surgeons continue to team with other physicians and scientists in seeking other ways to help cure and/or improve the lives of those who suffer from this most common of all human cancers.[2] Multiple nonsurgical treatments continue to be studied. These include methods of protection from ultraviolet radiation, retinoids, photodynamic therapy, and lasers, in addition to newer medical agents such as hedgehog signaling pathway inhibitors, hormone analogues, epidermal growth factor inhibitors, and anti–epidermal growth factor receptor monoclonal antibodies.[33]

Other medicines, procedures, and modalities will surely come. Progress in treating BCC and other cancers will continue until some future point when our modern method of MMS will likely become obsolete. Until that time, efforts to improve the techniques and the availability of this method, first described by Dr Frederic Mohs nearly 70 years ago, will continue to move forth as it serves in its role as the current optimal treatment for BCC.

REFERENCES

1. Nseir A, Estève E. Basal cell carcinoma. Presse Med 2008;37(10):1466–73.
2. Kyrgidis A, Vahtsevanos K, Tzellos TG, et al. Clinical, histological and demographic predictors for recurrence and second primary tumours of head and neck basal cell carcinoma. A 1062 patient cohort study from a tertiary cancer referral hospital. Eur J Dermatol 2010;20(3):276–82.
3. Ozgediz D, Smith EB, Zheng J, et al. Basal cell carcinoma does metastasize. Dermatol Online J 2008;14(8):5.
4. Bath-Hextall FJ, Perkins W, Bong J, et al. Intervention for basal cell carcinoma of the skin. Cochrane Database Syst Rev 2007;1:CD003412.
5. Smeets NW, Kuijpers DI, Nelemans P, et al. Mohs' micrographic surgery for treatment of basal cell carcinoma of the face—results of a retrospective study and review of the literature. Br J Dermatol 2004;151(1):141–7.
6. Muller FM, Dawe RS, Mosely H, et al. Randomized comparison of Mohs micrographic surgery and surgical excision for small nodular basal cell carcinoma: tissue-sparing outcome. Dermatol Surg 2009;35(9):1349–54.
7. Swanson NA. Mohs surgery: technique, indications, applications, and the future. Arch Dermatol 1983;119(9):761–73.
8. Lang PG. Mohs micrographic surgery for basal cell carcinoma. Facial Plast Surg Clin North Am 1998;6:275–95.
9. Mohs F. Chemosurgery: a microscopically controlled method of cancer excision. Arch Surg 1941;42:279–95.
10. Tromovitch TA, Beirne GA, Beire CG. Cancer chemosurgery. Cutis 1965;1:523–9.
11. Phelan JT, Milgrom H. The use of the Mohs' chemosurgery technique of the treatment of skin cancers. Surg Gynecol Obstet 1967;125:549–60.
12. Mohs FE. Cancer of the eyelids. Bull Am Coll Chemosurg 1970;3:10–1.
13. Henkind P, Menn H, Mohs FE. Chemosurgery in treatment of cancer of the periorbital area. Trans Am Acad Ophthalmol Otolaryngol 1971;75:1228–35.
14. Tromovitch TA, Stegman SJ. Microscopic-controlled excision. Dermatol Digest 1976;15:12–9.
15. Dinehart SM, Pollack SV. Mohs micrographic surgery for skin cancer. Cancer Treat Rev 1989;16(4):257–65.
16. Shriner DL, McCoy DK, Goldberg DJ, et al. Mohs micrographic surgery. J Am Acad Dermatol 1998;39(1):79–97.
17. Kaplan AL, Weitzul SB, Taylor RS. Longitudinal diminution of tumor size for basal cell carcinoma suggests shifting referral patterns for Mohs surgery. Dermatol Surg 2008;34(1):15–9.
18. Granstrom G, Aldenbrug F, Jeppson PG. Influence of embryonal fusion line for recurrence of basal cell carcinomas in the head and neck. Otolaryngol Head Neck Surg 1986;95(1):76–82.
19. Mora RG, Robins P. Basal cell carcinoma in the center of the face: Special diagnostic, prognostic, and therapeutic considerations. J Dermatol Surg Oncol 1978;4:315.
20. Binstock JH, Stegman SJ, Tromovitch TA. Large aggressive basal cell carcinomas of the scalp. J Dermatol Surg Oncol 1981;7:565.
21. Carruthers JA, Stegman SJ, Tromovitch TA, et al. Basal cell carcinomas of the temple. J Dermatol Surg Oncol 1983;9:759.
22. Scrivener Y, Grosshans E, Cribier B. Variations of basal cell carcinomas according to gender, age, location and histopathological subtype. Br J Dermatol 2002;147(1):41–7.
23. Sukal SA, Mahlberg MJ, Brightman L, et al. What lies beneath? A lesson for the clinician. Intraoperative frozen section appearance of persistent basal cell carcinoma after apparent cure with imiquimod 5% cream. Dermatol Surg 2009;35:1831–4.
24. Mosterd K, Krekels GA, Nieman FH, et al. Surgical excision versus Mohs' micrographic surgery for primary and recurrent basal-cell carcinoma of the face: a prospective randomized controlled trial with 5-years' follow-up. Lancet Oncol 2008;9(12):1149–56.
25. Chung VQ, Dwyer PJ, Nehal KS, et al. Use of ex vivo confocal scanning microscopy during Mohs surgery for nonmelanoma skin cancers. Dermatol Surg 2004;30(12 Pt 1):1470–8.

26. Alkalay R, Alcalay J, Maly A, et al. Fluorescence imaging for the demarcation of basal cell carcinoma tumor borders. J Drugs Dermatol 2008; 7(11):1033–7.

27. Lin SJ, Jee SH. Discrimination of basal cell carcinoma from normal dermal stroma by quantitative multiphoton imaging. Opt Lett 2006;31(18):2756–8.

28. Bobadilla F, Wortsman X, Munoz C, et al. Presurgical high resolution ultrasound of facial basal cell carcinoma: correlation with histology. Cancer Imaging 2008;8:163–72.

29. Marmur ES, Berkowitz EZ, Fuchs BS, et al. Use of high-frequency, high-resolution ultrasound before Mohs surgery. Dermatol Surg 2010;36(6):841–7.

30. Stranahan D, Cherpelis B, Glass F, et al. Immunohistochemical stains in Mohs surgery: a review. Dermatol Surg 2009;35(7):1023–34.

31. Rogers HW, Coldiron BM. A relative value unit-based cost comparison of treatment modalities for nonmelanoma skin cancer: effect of the loss of the Mohs multiple surgery reduction exemption. J Am Acad Dermatol 2009;61(1):96–103.

32. Tierney EP, Hanke CW. Cost effectiveness of Mohs micrographic surgery: review of the literature. J Drugs Dermatol 2009;8(10):914–22.

33. Amini S, Viera MH, Valins W, et al. Nonsurgical innovations in the treatment of nonmelanoma skin cancer. J Clin Aesthet Dermatol 2010;3(6):20–34.

Mohs Surgery for Squamous Cell Carcinoma

Daniel Belkin[a], John A. Carucci, MD, PhD[b,c],*

KEYWORDS

- Mohs surgery • Cutaneous squamous cell carcinoma
- Micrographic surgery • Cancer

Cutaneous squamous cell carcinoma (SCC) is a neoplasm of keratinizing cells that shows malignant characteristics, including anaplasia, rapid growth, local invasion, and metastatic potential (**Fig. 1**).[1,2] More than 250,000 cases of SCC are diagnosed in the United States each year, making it the second most common human cancer after basal cell carcinoma (BCC). The biologic behavior of SCC is determined by several variables.[3–5] The overall invasiveness and depth of the neoplasm is significant when determining the risk of recurrence after treatment. SCCs that invade the reticular dermis and subcutis tend to recur if not properly treated. Immerman and coworkers[6] observed a 20% incidence of recurrence in 86 subjects with invasive SCC. Degree of cellular differentiation is also important, with poorly differentiated neoplasms showing increased rates of recurrence. SCC that is incompletely treated or neglected can result in metastases (**Fig. 2**).

Squamous cell carcinoma in situ tends to arise in association with preexisting actinic keratosis, most commonly on sun-damaged skin. Although SCC in situ is considered to have little to no risk of metastasis, invasive SCC can metastasize[3–5] and can originate in neglected SCC in situ. The incidence of metastasis of invasive SCC is 3% to 5%. A higher incidence (10%–30%) is associated with SCC arising on mucosal surfaces (lip, genitalia) and on sites of prior injury (scars, chronic ulcers).

In a review of studies of SCCs treated over a 30-year period, Rowe and colleagues[3] correlated risk for local recurrence and metastasis with treatment modality, prior treatment, location, size, depth, histologic differentiation, evidence of perineural involvement, precipitating factors other than ultraviolet light, and immunosuppression. They found that with tumors greater than 2 cm, recurrence rates doubled from 7.4% to 15.2%. In addition, they demonstrated that tumors less than 4 mm in depth were at low risk for metastasis (6.7%) compared with tumors greater than 4 mm in depth (45.7%). Locally recurrent SCCs showed an overall metastatic rate of 30% with high rates of metastasis in the context of local recurrence in skin (25.0%), lip (31.5%), and ear (45.0%). Poorly differentiated SCC metastasized more frequently (32.9%) than well-differentiated SCC (9.2%). SCC arising on sun-exposed skin recurred at a rate of 7.9% and metastasized at a rate of 5.2%. Recurrence rates were increased in SCC on the lip (10.5%) and ear (18.7%), as were metastatic rates from the lip (13.7%) and ear (11%). SCCs with perineural invasion (PNI) recurred in almost one-half of cases (47.2%) and showed a similar rate of metastasis (47.3%).

Patients who are immunosuppressed are a special high-risk group and are thought to have a 5- to 20-fold increase in the incidence of SCC compared with the general population, with a reversal of the SCC/BCC ratio from 0.25:1 to

[a] Department of Dermatology, Weill Cornell Medical College, 1305 York Avenue, New York, NY 10021, USA
[b] Mohs Micrographic and Dermatologic Surgery, Weill Cornell Medical College, 1305 York Avenue, New York, NY 10021, USA
[c] Department of Dermatology, New York University Langone Medical Center, 530 First Avenue, New York, NY 10016, USA
* Corresponding author. Department of Dermatology, New York University Langone Medical Center, 530 First Avenue, Suite 7H New York, NY 10016.
E-mail address: john.carucci@nyumc.org

Dermatol Clin 29 (2011) 161–174
doi:10.1016/j.det.2011.02.006
0733-8635/11/$ – see front matter © 2011 Elsevier Inc. All rights reserved.

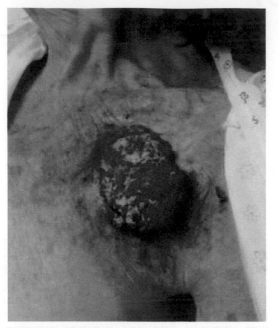

Fig. 1. SCC is a cancer of the keratinizing cells of the epidermis and has the potential to behave aggressively.

3.0:1.[3] The number of SCCs per patient is increased and the age at initial presentation is decreased[3] (see later discussion of SCC in organ transplant recipients). Rowe and colleagues[3] found that in patients who are immunosuppressed, the overall rate of metastasis was 12.9%.

Therapy for SCC should be selected on the basis of the size of the lesion, anatomic location, depth of invasion, degree of cellular differentiation, and history of previous treatment.[7] There are 3 general approaches to the treatment of SCC: (1) removal by traditional excisional surgery or Mohs micrographic surgery (MMS), (2) destruction by curettage and electrodesiccation, and (3) radiation therapy. In this article the authors review the use of Mohs micrographic surgery for cutaneous squamous cell carcinoma and discuss its role as the treatment of choice for select squamous cell cancers.

MOHS MICROGRAPHIC SURGERY

Mohs micrographic surgery facilitates optimal margin control and conservation of normal tissue in the management of nonmelanoma skin cancer. Individuals specially trained in the technique perform MMS in an office setting under local anesthesia. Briefly, following gentle curettage,

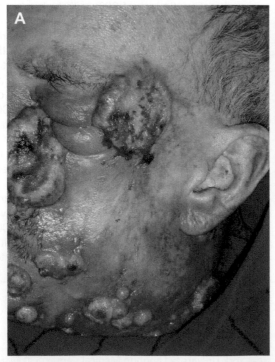

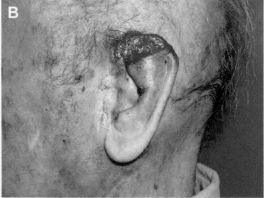

Fig. 2. SCC may eventuate in local recurrence and metastasis. (*A*) Metastatic SCC in a patient with chronic lymphocytic leukemia. The primary lesion was an SCC on the temple that recurred and subsequently metastasized. (*B*) Patient with untreated SCC that continued to invade locally and subsequently metastasized to regional lymph nodes.

a tangential specimen of tumor with a minimal margin of clinically normal-appearing tissue is obtained, precisely mapped, and processed immediately by frozen section for microscopic examination. Optimal margin control is obtained by examination of the entire perimeter of the specimen and contiguous deep margin. Meticulous mapping allows for directed extirpation of any remaining tumor. A key defining feature of MMS is that the surgeon excises, maps, and reviews the specimen personally, minimizing the chance of error in tissue interpretation and orientation. MMS has gained acceptance as the treatment of choice for recurrent skin cancers as well as primary skin cancers located on anatomic sites requiring maximal tissue conservation for preservation of function and cosmesis.

MMS is indicated in cases of primary or recurrent SCC because this modality allows conservation of normal tissue with preservation of function and enhanced cosmesis. MMS is also superior to other forms of treatment with regard to local recurrence.[7,8] Recurrence rates with MMS are superior to those obtained with traditional excisional surgery in primary SCC of the ear (3.1% vs 10.9%), primary SCC of the lip (5.8% vs 18.7%), recurrent SCC (10.0% vs 23.3%), SCC with PNI (0% vs 47%), SCC greater than 2 cm (25.2% vs 41.7%), and poorly differentiated SCC (32.6% vs 53.6%).[3] MMS has proven useful in SCC involving the nail unit,[9] and has been used as a limb-sparing procedure in cases of SCC arising in osteomyelitis.[10] MMS is indicated for invasive lesions, poorly differentiated lesions, and for lesions occurring on high-risk anatomic sites or sites where conservation of normal tissue is essential for preservation of function or cosmesis.

In addition to providing the highest cure rates for the most aggressive SCCs, MMS remains cost effective when compared with other modalities. For example, the overall cost for MMS and immediate reconstruction by a fellowship-trained Mohs micrographic and reconstructive surgeon may be 3-fold less than that performed by a colleague from an allied surgical subspecialty in an ambulatory surgical center.[11] Five-year recurrence rates also remain lower for patients treated using the Mohs technique.

Pugliano-Mauro and Goldman[12] reviewed 215 subjects with 260 high-risk cutaneous SCCs treated with MMS in a single-center retrospective study, and considered rates of recurrence, metastasis, and death. A total of 77% of the subjects were men and 23% were women. The average age was 70.6 years. Twenty percent of the subjects were immunosuppressed. Mean follow-up was 3.9 years. There were 3 local recurrences

(1.2%). Six (2.3%) tumors metastasized, with one fatality from disease. In general, prompt recognition of metastatic disease allowed for curative therapy. Twelve (4.6%) tumors involved named nerve trunks and in 8 of these cases, adjuvant radiation therapy was employed (adjuvant radiotherapy was reserved for large-nerve perineural disease). A total of 75% of the subjects went on to develop another cutaneous SCC, and 7.7% developed subsequent malignant melanoma, suggesting that once a patient has one high-risk SCC they are likely to develop secondary primary SCC and melanoma. The investigators concluded that MMS is an effective treatment for high-risk cutaneous SCC, providing a low recurrence rate and a low disease-specific mortality. This study is the largest single-center study of high-risk SCC supporting the use of MMS.

Jumbusaria and colleagues[13] reported variation in perioperative management in patients with PNI or otherwise high-risk SCC. The authors at this time do not routinely recommend sentinel lymph node biopsy for cutaneous SCC. However, the authors do refer patients with PNI for evaluation for radiation therapy and recommend evaluation of patients with PNI by a radiation oncologist with expertise and experience treating cutaneous SCC (see later discussion of perineural invasion).

SCC IN ORGAN TRANSPLANT RECIPIENTS

It has been well documented that cutaneous malignancies are more frequent in patients on immunosuppressive medication following solid organ transplant. Just as in the general population, skin cancers, particularly nonmelanoma skin cancers (NMSC), are the most common malignancies in this group.[14–18] In fair-skinned people, cutaneous squamous cell carcinoma is the most common post-transplantation malignancy.[19] Although in the general population, basal cell carcinomas are more frequent than SCC, this is reversed in organ transplant recipients (OTR).[20] Together, SCC and BCC make up more than 90% of cutaneous malignancies in this group.[15,17,21,22]

In OTR, not only is NMSC more frequent but it is also often more devastating. Tumors in this group tend to be more histologically aggressive[23] and more likely to recur, metastasize, and be lethal.[14,20,24–27] For example, in an Australian cohort, 4 years after heart transplant, 27% of 41 subjects died of skin cancer.[25] In the Cincinnati Tumor Registry, 5.2% of patients who received a transplant died of skin malignancies.[28] OTR tend to be diagnosed with skin cancer at younger ages than their immune-competent counterparts.[29] A subset of OTR may be particularly affected, with the possibility of more than 100 NMSC in a year in a few high-risk individuals.[20] Adequate treatment of OTR with cutaneous malignancies often involves a multimodality approach and can greatly impact morbidity and mortality in this group.

According to guidelines established by the International Transplant Skin Cancer Collaborative (ITSCC), MMS may be used in this group with low-risk to moderate-risk SCC where tissue conservation is desired as well as with high-risk, or aggressive, SCC.[30] Alternatives in low-risk lesions include destructive techniques, such as cryosurgery and electrodesiccation and curettage, as well as excision with postoperative margin assessment.[30] For OTR, this requires margins of at least 6 mm beyond surrounding erythema, as reported by Brodland and Zitelli,[31] based on subclinical tumor extension (up to 4 mm in 95% of low-risk SCC and up to 6 mm in 95% of high-risk SCC). In high-risk lesions, ideally, the only alternative is standard excision with intraoperative frozen-section control. If neither this nor MMS is available, excision with postoperative margin assessment is an option,[30] which would require margins of at least 6 to 10 mm beyond surrounding erythema as well as resection into subcutaneous fat.[3,30] Many investigators agree that in high-risk lesions, margin-controlled excision with MMS is the treatment of choice in this group.[3,32] This point is especially true given that subclinical tumor extension of SCC is greater in OTR than in immune-competent counterparts.[33]

OTHER RISK FACTORS

The ITSCC outlined what constitutes high-risk SCC. Factors conferring high risk are the presence of multiple SCC; indistinct clinical borders; rapid growth; ulceration; location on genitalia, digits, or mask areas of the face (central face, eyelids, eyebrows, periorbital, nose, lips, chin, mandible, preauricular and postauricular areas, temple, and ear); location in a scar, in a bed of chronic inflammation, or in a prior radiation field; recurrence; presence of satellite lesions; large size (more than 0.6 cm on hands, feet, genitalia, and mask areas of the face; more than 1.0 cm on cheeks, forehead, neck, and scalp; and more than 2.0 cm on trunk and extremities); depth greater than 4 mm; and aggressive histology (including deep extension into subcutaneous fat, perineural invasion/inflammation, perivascular or intravascular invasion, and poor differentiation).[3,24,30] Some investigators think location on the scalp should be included, given particular surgical difficulties in this area (see later discussion of SCC on the

scalp).[32,34] Poor outcomes may also be influenced by older age,[24] presence of extracutaneous tumors,[35] and history of occupational sun exposure.[14] Lee and colleagues[36] found with head and neck NMSC that the 3 most important factors predicting poor outcomes were recurrent lesions, lesions involving nerve, and lesions involving bone.

DIFFICULT ANATOMIC SITES

MMS is particularly useful in patients who are both immunosuppressed and immune competent for higher-risk anatomic sites.

SCC of the Scalp

Scalp SCC may be particularly aggressive (Fig. 3).[34] for 2 reasons. The first is that the scalp, especially in some male transplant recipients, is more likely to have field disease (see later discussion of extensive field disease) with extensive, confluent actinic keratoses and intervening SCC.[20] Field dysplasia and follicular involvement may lead to higher-than-expected recurrence rates for superficially destructive measures.[20] Berg and Otley[20] suggest repetitive 5-fluorouracil treatments can result in improvement, but that with extensive carcinoma, a wide excision with skin graft may be necessary.

The second reason is that the scalp has unique anatomic features that make eradication difficult, such as extensive vasculature and lymphatic drainage patterns that allow easier penetration and spread of the tumor.[32,34] In the scalp, loose connective tissue separates the fronto-occipital aponeurosis from the pericranium, and tumor may spread easily along this plane, especially if it

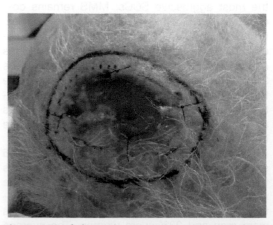

Fig. 3. SCC of the scalp may behave aggressively. CT scan may be necessary to exclude bony involvement. In this case, SCC extended to periosteum necessitating removal of outer table in the operating room.

was previously undermined in surgery.[32] Neubauer and colleagues[32] described a patient with 3 recurrences of SCC on the scalp and ultimately central nervous system (CNS) involvement. The patient had had 2 previous MMS procedures with undermining of this plane and primary closure.[32] These investigators questioned whether undermining should be used on the scalp because it may serve to seed tumor cells into a deeper location.[32] They also noted that on the scalp, deep surgical margins are difficult to determine without seeing clear evidence of involvement of bone, like pitting.[32] They suggested that subclinical bone disease could act as a reservoir for recurrence and CNS invasion.[32] If there is involvement of the periosteum, some investigators suggest a computed tomography (CT) scan or microscopic evaluation of bone chips to determine if there is bone involvement.[37] Even with microscopic evaluation, cells may still escape detection.[37] Skin grafting may be necessary to treat field disease on the scalp, but decorticating bone in preparation for skin grafting is not adequate to eradicate subclinical bone disease.[37] Neubauer and colleagues[32] even wonder whether vertical in-transit metastases may be possible (see later discussion of in-transit metastasis), in this case to involve bone subclinically and explain their difficulty in eradicating the lesion in question. In short, subclinical extension may be quite extensive in these cases, and the Mohs surgeon must be wary of the difficulty in eradicating these lesions as well as the poor prognosis they hold.

SCC of the Lip

SCC of the lip may behave aggressively with increased rates of recurrence and metastasis.[3] In one study by Altynollar and colleagues,[38] sentinel lymph nodes were identified in 18 of 20 subjects (90%) with T2, N0 SCC of the lip. A total of 3 of these 18 subjects (16.6%) had positive sentinel lymph nodes by intraoperative or postoperative histologic examination. Histopathologic examination of the remaining 15 subjects whose sentinel lymph nodes were free of metastasis, showed no metastasis in the nonsentinel lymph nodes. In 2 of the 3 subjects with metastatic sentinel lymph nodes, nonsentinel lymph nodes were free of metastases.

The incidence of SCC of the lip is 20-fold higher in OTR than in the general population.[22] Lip cancer tends to be more frequent in pediatric OTR compared with adult OTR, 23% vs 12% in one study.[39] Many who have SCC of the lower lip also have actinic cheilitis that involves the surrounding mucosal skin.[20] Some surgeons have used MMS to remove SCC of the lip along with a carbon dioxide laser vermilionectomy for surrounding actinic cheilitis.[40]

Follow-up in patients with a history of lip SCC should include a bimanual submental lymph node examination to detect metastases to this basin.[20] Based on margin control, preservation of function, and conservation of normal tissue, MMS remains the treatment of choice for these potentially aggressive tumors (**Fig. 4**).

SCC of the Ear

SCC involving the ear can behave aggressively with metastases in up to 11% of cases.[3] Silapunt and colleagues[41] reviewed 117 subjects with 144 invasive SCCs of the ear. Average follow-up was 35 months with a range of 6 to 67 months after treatment by MMS. Age of patients ranged from 34 to 90 years (mean = 71) with a male-to-female ratio of 22:1. The helix was the most common site of occurrence (50.7%). Local recurrence after MMS was found in 5 of 144 tumors. MMS was performed on these 5 recurrent tumors, with no further recurrences. The 2-year local recurrence rate was 5.7% (5 of 87 tumors) after MMS. The average size of these 87 tumors was 3.5 cm.[2] The authors routinely treat aggressive SCC on the ear (**Fig. 5**) with MMS.

SCC of the Nail Unit

SCC is the most common malignancy of the nail unit and can behave aggressively (**Fig. 6**). Nail-unit SCC is often associated with human papillomavirus (HPV) type 16, HPV26, HPV33, HPV51, HPV56, and HPV73. Zaiac and colleagues[42] reviewed the use of MMS for removal of periungual SCC and supported it as the treatment of choice. The authors recommend preoperative imaging (radiograph or CT scan) to exclude bony involvement in fixed lesions. Peterson and colleagues[43] reported a multidisciplinary approach involving both a Mohs surgeon and hand surgeon for tumors extending to bone. In their series, the SCC was cleared peripherally by the Mohs surgeon followed by referral to the hand surgeon for amputation of the distal phalanx and subsequent reconstruction. They reported no recurrences in 3 subjects treated with this approach at 15-, 17-, and 38-months follow-up.

Penile SCC

SCC involving the penis may evade mimic inflammatory dermatoses, resulting in delayed diagnosis. SCC of the penis can invade deeply and result in extensive local tissue damage (**Fig. 7**). In one study, Brown and colleagues[44] evaluated

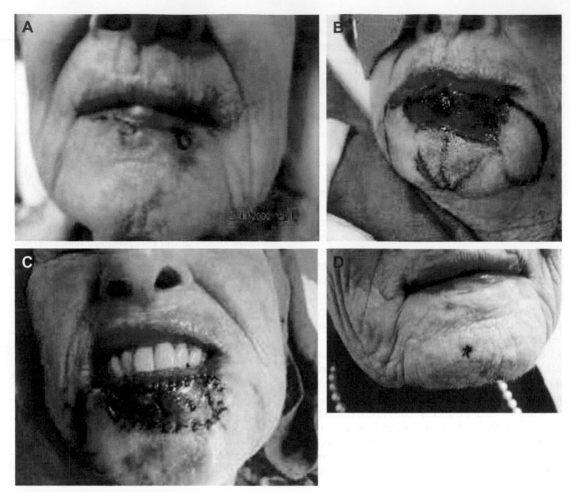

Fig. 4. Mohs was used to treat this SCC involving the lower cutaneous and mucosal with complete tumor removal along with excellent functional and cosmetic results. (*A*) Preoperative view. (*B*) Defect after Mohs surgery. (*C*) Repair. (*D*) At 11-month follow-up.

a series of 20 subjects with SCC on the penis for extent of surgery required for clearance of tumor, local recurrence, metastasis, and disease-specific mortality. Subjects were followed for 6 years. Squamous cell cancers were cleared in an average of 2 stages and most defects were allowed to heal secondarily. One of 20 subjects developed a local recurrence (5%) and 4 of 20 (20%) developed regional nodal metastases with 1 death from metastatic disease (5%).

SPECIAL CONSIDERATIONS
Perineural Invasion

Perineural invasion is a histologic or clinical feature that confers high risk of aggressiveness in SCC (**Fig. 8**).[45] The National Comprehensive Cancer Network says that tumors causing neurologic symptoms, such as pain, burning, paresthesia, diplopia, and so forth, should be considered to

have PNI.[45] However, tumors with PNI are symptomatic only 40% of the time.[45,46] Tumors with this feature are associated with greater morbidity and mortality, as they tend to be larger, have subclinical extension, require more MMS stages for clearance, and metastasize.[47] There is even a case study of SCC that metastasized in a devastating dermatomal zosteriform distribution on the chest of an OTR.[48]

Perineural invasion is associated with moderately to poorly differentiated tumor histology.[47] In a large series, Smith and colleagues[23] found that PNI was more common in OTR than in the general population, along with other features associated with aggressive course, including acantholytic changes, early dermal invasion, desmoplastic changes, and angiogenic components. A smaller series showed no increased frequency of PNI in renal transplant recipients against subjects who were immune competent.[49] They did, however,

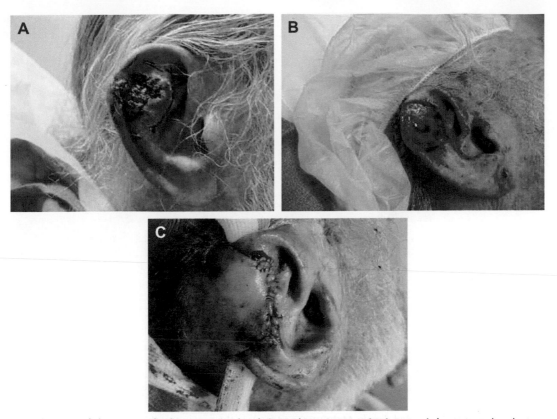

Fig. 5. This SCC of the ear resulted in extensive local tissue damage necessitating repair by a staged scalp-to-ear retroauricular interpolation flap. (*A*) SCC involving the ear. (*B*) After Mohs defect. (*C*) Initial stage of reconstruction. Pedicle was subsequently divided 2 weeks later.

confirm the increased frequency of aggressive tumor histology in OTR, identifying an aggressive spindle cell subtype of SCC particular to OTR and occurring in 20%.[49]

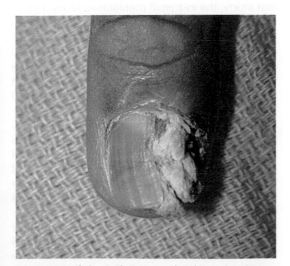

Fig. 6. SCC of the nail unit may be driven by HPV.

The surgeon should note that lesions with PNI are associated with recurrence after previous surgical excision or cryotherapy.[47] Perineurally invasive tumors should be treated as high-risk SCC. Adjuvant radiation therapy is recommended when tumors involve multiple or large nerves or when a tumor extends into a craniofacial foramen.[30,45,47]

When faced with PNI, the authors make every attempt to clear the perineural disease by Mohs. Based on the high rates of local recurrence and potential for metastasis, the authors refer patients for evaluation for postoperative radiation therapy by a radiation oncologist with expertise and experience in the treatment of skin cancers.

In-Transit Metastasis

In-transit metastases are foci of cutaneous SCC within dermal or subcutaneous tissue that are distinct from the primary tumor but occur within the area of the closest regional lymph nodes and are thought to represent local lymphatic metastases (**Fig. 9**).[50] They appear as pinkish gray, nondescript papules, 2 to 8 mm in diameter.[20] It

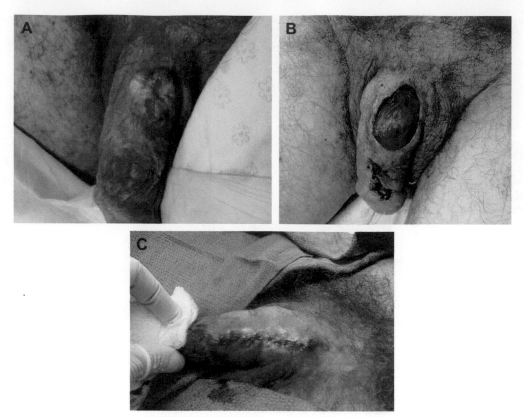

Fig. 7. This penile SCC extended deeply. Mohs was used to clear the tumor and this was followed by immediate repair. (*A*) SCC involving the penis. (*B*) Defect. (*C*) Repair.

should be noted that the definition of in-transit metastasis differs in melanoma, where in-transit metastases are defined by the American Joint Committee on Cancer staging criteria as occurring more than 2 cm from primary tumor; whereas,

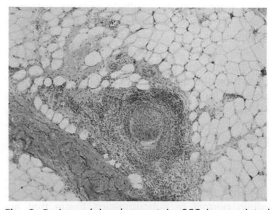

Fig. 8. Perineural involvement in SCC is associated with increased rates of recurrence and metastasis. This example is a perineural invasion discovered on the first stage of Mohs surgery. Two additional stages were required to clear the perineural component of this cancer.

those within 2 cm are termed *satellites*; however, satellites are thought to carry similar prognosis.[51] In a series by Martinez and colleagues,[52] in-transit metastasis comprised about a quarter of skin cancer metastatic events in OTR.

A series of 21 subjects with in-transit metastasis from primary cutaneous SCC were studied.[50] In that study, the in-transit metastases tended to be less than 8.0 mm in size with mean distance of 2.5 cm from the primary tumor.[50] Most (15 of 22) of the primary tumors were located on the head and face; although, in 3 of 22 subjects, the primary tumor site could not be determined.[50] In-transit metastases were discovered an average of 10 weeks after treatment of the primary tumor.[50] In-transit metastases were more common in OTR and associated with increased morbidity and mortality. Most of the tumors were managed with either MMS or standard excision, with subsequent radiation, although in a few, radiotherapy was used alone. This series suggested that in-transit metastasis is an extremely poor prognostic indicator in OTR: at 2 years, disease-specific mortality in OTR was 33%, with another third having nodal or distant metastases, vs 0% in subjects who were immune competent, 5 of 6 of whom had no

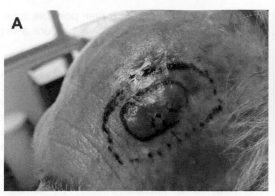

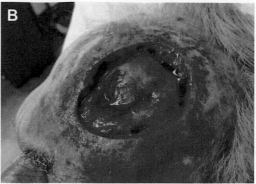

Fig. 9. In-transit metastasis from primary cutaneous SCC. (*A*) In-transit metastasis from SCC in a transplant recipient. (*B*) Intraoperative view of removal before achieving complete clearance.

evidence of disease.[50] Because in-transit metastasis represents lymphatic spread, these patients are at higher risk for regional and distant metastasis.[50] These patients, in addition to being evaluated for nodal and distant metastases, should undergo removal of in-transit metastases with clear margins by either standard excision or MMS, followed by postoperative radiation therapy. Because margins are inherently unreliable in this case, radiation therapy is the critical therapeutic modality in this condition.[20] MMS may be particularly useful in cases where there is difficulty distinguishing solitary in-transit metastasis from deep marginal recurrence.

Radiation Therapy

Postoperative radiation therapy for aggressive SCC is common in practice, despite there not being much data from controlled studies.[50] Radiation therapy can be a primary treatment for inoperable tumors or in patients who cannot or will not undergo surgery.[30,53] Adjunctive radiation therapy should be considered with suspected nodal involvement.[30,45] It should also be considered in invasive SCC in certain situations, such as when margins cannot be considered clear of invasive tumor after surgery or when there is substantial PNI.[30] In in-transit metastasis, surgical margins are inherently compromised and radiotherapy is critical for eradicating residual SCC.[50] In this case, it is appropriate to irradiate a field extending 1 to 5 cm in all directions beyond the furthest histologic or clinical evidence of the disease, with sentinel lymph node biopsy or radiation to regional nodes determined by case.[50] Barring these indications, this modality should be avoided when possible, especially in OTR, given concerns about radiation-induced carcinogenesis.[54] Radiation therapy should not be used as a modality in SCC in situ or field cancerization.[54] It should be noted that radiation

therapy is not as effective in tumors that invade bone.[32]

Extensive Field Disease

Extensive field disease or field cancerization accounts for the majority of NMSC-related morbidity and mortality (**Fig. 10**).[55] The "field effect" as interpreted by Braakhuis and colleagues[56] provides an explanation for multiple recurrence despite adequate treatment. The field effect refers to the presence of multiple foci of

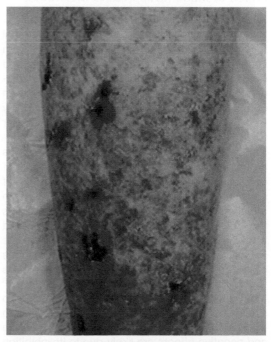

Fig. 10. Extensive field disease may prevent the surgeon from obtaining a true negative margin. This situation would necessitate close follow-up with adjunctive treatment for surrounding remaining dysplasia.

genetically altered cells that may appear clinically to be normal but have the capacity to become invasive.[56] This widespread cutaneous dysplasia is common in fair-skinned, chronically sun-exposed OTR. These patches are of course often left behind during excision of a principle lesion.[56] For this reason, Braakhuis and colleagues[56] thought that it was difficult to determine whether a second tumor was recurrent or primary and decided that a good term to describe either would be a "second-field tumor." Patients with extensive field disease often have high numbers of warts, actinic keratoses, SCC in situ, and invasive SCC. Sometimes, it is difficult to determine where one lesion ends and another begins, a phenomenon that when occurring on the hand has been called "transplant hand". An important implication of extensive field disease is that destructive therapies of primary lesions do not prevent the occurrence of new cancers or local recurrences.[57] These patients require multimodal treatment, including topical agents, destruction, shave excision, and photodynamic therapy. MMS may be useful as an initial step in clearing invasive carcinoma but should be followed by appropriate field treatments to reduce risk of recurrences and second primary tumors.

Effects of Immunosuppressive Medication on Wound Healing

Reports have linked sirolimus, used in many renal transplant recipients (and other OTR), with impaired wound healing[58,59] and an increased incidence of wound complications, such as dehiscence, infections, and hernias.[60,61] Its effects in dermatologic surgery have been explored by Brewer and colleagues,[62] who reported a similar trend that did not, however, reach statistical significance. Postoperative infection in the sirolimus group occurred in 19.2% of subjects vs 5.4% of controls and dehiscence occurred in 7.7% of subjects using sirolimus vs none in controls.[62] In addition, 19.2% of subjects using sirolimus thought the wound was slow to heal compared with 5.4% in controls.[62] Ironically, sirolimus is actually associated with lower rates of cutaneous carcinoma and is thought to inhibit carcinogenesis where other immunosuppressants increase it.[62,63] Many investigator actually suggest switching to sirolimus from other immunosuppressants in high-risk OTR.[54,64] Interestingly, both its positive and negative effects are likely due to its inhibition of fibroblasts and angiogenesis.[62] Although mTOR inhibitors, such as sirolimus, may be good choices of immunosuppressant for OTR at high risk for cutaneous malignancies or recurrences,

the surgeon must consider their possible adverse effect on wound healing, at least before a larger study becomes available.[62]

Organ transplant recipients are also often maintained on corticosteroids, which are well known to impair wound healing. These inhibit all phases of wound healing.[65,66] They are associated with higher incidence of wound infections, dehiscence, and delayed healing.[66] Wound closures in areas of high tension or high mobility, such as the hand and back, tend to have increased incidence of dehiscence in general, and this effect may be enhanced in patients on corticosteroids.[67] By stimulating epithelialization, fibroplasia, and tensile strength, systemic retinoids may actually counteract some of the negative effects or corticosteroids (see later discussion of effects of retinoids on wound healing).[66]

Effects of Retinoids on Wound Healing

The effect of systemic retinoids on wound healing has been in debate because of conflicting results of various observational human and interventional animal studies.[67] Delayed wound healing and keloid formation after dermabrasion has been reported in patients on systemic isotretinoin[68]; whereas, other case series have shown no effect after dermabrasion.[69] There have also been clinical observations that patients on isotretinoin or etretinate have excessive granulation tissue after trauma.[70,71] A more relevant observational study of 29 OTR undergoing excision with reconstruction found no statistically significant effect of acitretin on wound healing.[67] There was, however, a small nonsignificant trend toward increased dehiscence in the acitretin group.[67] Hypertrophic scarring and granulation tissue, the effects reported previously, were not only equal between groups but also not the most common or significant complications.[67] Furthermore, in OTR, oral retinoids have a theoretical benefit of counteracting the adverse effects of corticosteroids on wound healing.[67] Corticosteroids inhibit collagen deposition; whereas, retinoids stimulate collagen production.[65,72] When applied before full-thickness wounding, topical tretinoin accelerated wound healing.[73] The surgeon may wish to keep in mind that hypertrophic scarring and granulation tissue may or may not be a risk in patients on systemic retinoids.

Preventing Surgical Site Infection

Patients who are immunosuppressed must be monitored closely for infections, which may progress rapidly and without the usual signs and symptoms.[67] Because of altered immunity, they may also have higher incidences of sepsis and death from surgical-site infections.[74] Data is lacking on antibiotic prophylaxis in dermatologic surgery. Guidelines by Maragh and colleagues[75] based on a review of the literature and multi-disciplinary consultation suggest that antibiotic prophylaxis for prevention of surgical-site infection may be appropriate in some OTR despite the low rate of infection in dermatologic surgery. Antibiotics should not be administered for class I, or clean, wounds, based on the CDC wound classification.[75,76] However, according to these investigators, prophylactic antibiotics may be administered for class II, or clean-contaminated, wounds in patients for whom a surgical-site infection would be particularly severe, and they include immunocompromised OTR in this group.[75] Technically, MMS is considered clean-contaminated because of delayed closure, but most Mohs surgeons do not administer prophylactic antibiotics.[75] Occasional exceptions may be flap and graft reconstructions on the nose or ear, and procedures that have prolonged operative times.[75] The infection rate with MMS is low and evidence is insufficient to warrant the categorical use of prophylactic antibiotics in OTR. Surgical sites that are inflamed or clearly infected require antibiotics.[75]

Follow-up

Invasive SCC can be a potentially lethal neoplasm and warrants close follow-up. In one study, approximately 30% of subjects with SCC developed a subsequent SCC, with more than half of these occurring within the first year of follow-up.[77] In-transit metastases for the most part occur within 1 year after treatment of primary or recurrent SCC, with most presenting in 3 to 6 months.[50] In another study, the median time to recurrence was 15 months.[78] Thus, it is recommended that patients with SCC be examined every 3 months during the first year following treatment, every 6 months during the second year following treatment, and annually thereafter. Evaluation should include total-body cutaneous examination and palpation of draining lymph nodes. There is currently no role for radiograph, magnetic resonance imaging, or CT in the routine work-up of uncomplicated cutaneous SCC.

For OTR, continued follow-up is essential, as recurrence may be more common and may be rapid in these patients. Patients who have had 1 cutaneous malignancy are at high risk for developing new lesions. Skin examinations must be done as frequently as lesions may develop.[20,45] Examinations should be every 3 to 6 months in patients who have had 1 SCC or BCC, every 3

months in patients who have had multiple NMSC or 1 high-risk SCC, and every 1 to 3 months in patients who have had metastatic SCC.[30,79] The dermatologist must keep in mind the increased prevalence in this group of field disease, in-transit metastasis, and nodal metastasis, and should look for cutaneous satellite lesions and palpate draining lymph nodes.[30]

Patients should be encouraged to perform self skin examinations monthly, looking for new or changing growths.[54] Patients with a history of melanoma, high-risk SCC, or metastatic disease, or who are otherwise high risk, should also be encouraged to self examine lymph nodes every month.[20] Patient education on sun-protective behavior recommendations is also crucial.[80]

SUMMARY

SCC has the potential to behave aggressively. Mohs micrographic surgery offers the highest cure rates and allows for optimal conservation of normal tissue. It is particularly useful in SCCs that occur on high-risk anatomic sites, including scalp, ear, and lip, as well as for SCCs that occur in patients that are immune compromised secondary to solid organ transplantation. In addition to being effective, MMS is safe and convenient for patients, in many cases allowing for tumor removal with clear margins obtained and repair performed in an office setting under local anesthesia. Thus, fellowship-trained Mohs surgeons can offer the highest level of care for patients with cutaneous SCC.

REFERENCES

1. Kibarian MA, Hruza GJ. Nonmelanoma skin cancer. Risks, treatment options, and tips on prevention. Postgrad Med 1995;98:39–40, 45–8, 55–6 passim.
2. Katz MH. Nonmelanoma skin cancer. Md Med J 1997;46:239–42.
3. Rowe DE, Carroll RJ, Day CL Jr. Prognostic factors for local recurrence, metastasis, and survival rates in squamous cell carcinoma of the skin, ear, and lip. Implications for treatment modality selection. J Am Acad Dermatol 1992;26:976–90.
4. Barksdale SK, O'Connor N, Barnhill R. Prognostic factors for cutaneous squamous cell and basal cell carcinoma. Determinants of risk of recurrence, metastasis, and development of subsequent skin cancers. Surg Oncol Clin N Am 1997;6:625–38.
5. Brodland DG, Zitelli JA. Mechanisms of metastasis. J Am Acad Dermatol 1992;27:1–8.
6. Immerman SC, Scanlon EF, Christ M, et al. Recurrent squamous cell carcinoma of the skin. Cancer 1983; 51:1537–40.

7. Goldman GD. Squamous cell cancer: a practical approach. Semin Cutan Med Surg 1998;17:80–95.

8. Leslie DF, Greenway HT. Mohs micrographic surgery for skin cancer. Australas J Dermatol 1991;32:159–64.

9. Goldminz D, Bennett RG. Mohs micrographic surgery of the nail unit. J Dermatol Surg Oncol 1992;18:721–6.

10. Kirsner RS, Spencer J, Falanga V, et al. Squamous cell carcinoma arising in osteomyelitis and chronic wounds. Treatment with Mohs micrographic surgery vs amputation. Dermatol Surg 1996;22:1015–8.

11. Tierney EP, Hanke CW. Cost effectiveness of Mohs micrographic surgery: review of the literature. J Drugs Dermatol 2009;8:914–22.

12. Pugliano-Mauro M, Goldman G. Mohs surgery is effective for high-risk cutaneous squamous cell carcinoma. Dermatol Surg 2010;36:1544–53.

13. Jambusaria-Pahlajani A, Hess SD, Katz KA, et al. Uncertainty in the perioperative management of high-risk cutaneous squamous cell carcinoma among Mohs surgeons. Arch Dermatol 2010;146:1225–31.

14. Euvrard S, Kanitakis J, Claudy A. Skin cancers after organ transplantation. N Engl J Med 2003;348:1681–91.

15. Webb MC, Compton F, Andrews PA, et al. Skin tumours posttransplantation: a retrospective analysis of 28 years' experience at a single centre. Transplant Proc 1997;29:828–30.

16. Hiesse C, Rieu P, Kriaa F, et al. Malignancy after renal transplantation: analysis of incidence and risk factors in 1700 patients followed during a 25-year period. Transplant Proc 1997;29:831–3.

17. Winkelhorst JT, Brokelman WJ, Tiggeler RG, et al. Incidence and clinical course of de-novo malignancies in renal allograft recipients. Eur J Surg Oncol 2001;27:409–13.

18. Sanchez EQ, Marubashi S, Jung G, et al. De novo tumors after liver transplantation: a single-institution experience. Liver Transpl 2002;8:285–91.

19. Sheil AG, Disney AP, Mathew TH, et al. De novo malignancy emerges as a major cause of morbidity and late failure in renal transplantation. Transplant Proc 1993;25:1383–4.

20. Berg D, Otley CC. Skin cancer in organ transplant recipients: epidemiology, pathogenesis, and management. J Am Acad Dermatol 2002;47:1–17 [quiz: 18–20].

21. Bouwes Bavinck JN, Hardie DR, Green A, et al. The risk of skin cancer in renal transplant recipients in Queensland, Australia. A follow-up study. Transplantation 1996;61:715–21.

22. Jensen P, Hansen S, Møller B, et al. Skin cancer in kidney and heart transplant recipients and different long-term immunosuppressive therapy regimens. J Am Acad Dermatol 1999;40:177–86.

23. Smith KJ, Hamza S, Skelton H. Histologic features in primary cutaneous squamous cell carcinomas in immunocompromised patients focusing on organ transplant patients. Dermatol Surg 2004;30:634–41.

24. Euvrard S, Kanitakis J, Pouteil-Noble C, et al. Aggressive squamous cell carcinomas in organ transplant recipients. Transplant Proc 1995;27:1767–8.

25. Ong C, Keogh AM, Kossard S, et al. Skin cancer in Australian heart transplant recipients. J Am Acad Dermatol 1999;40:27–34.

26. Penn I, First MR. Merkel's skin carcinoma in organ recipients: report of 41 cases. Transplantation 1999;68(11):1717–21.

27. Glover MT, Niranjan N, Kwan JT, et al. Non-melanoma skin cancer in renal transplant recipients: the extent of the problem and a strategy for management. Br J Plast Surg 1994;47:86–9.

28. Penn I. Tumors after renal and cardiac transplantation. Hematol Oncol Clin North Am 1993;7:431–45.

29. Harwood CA, Proby CM. Human papillomaviruses and non-melanoma skin cancer. Curr Opin Infect Dis 2002;15:101–14.

30. Stasko T, Brown MD, Carucci JA, et al. Guidelines for the management of squamous cell carcinoma in organ transplant recipients. Dermatol Surg 2004;30:642–50.

31. Brodland DG, Zitelli JA. Surgical margins for excision of primary cutaneous squamous cell carcinoma. J Am Acad Dermatol 1992;27:241–8.

32. Neubauer K, Goldstein GD, Plumb SJ. Squamous cell carcinoma of the scalp in organ transplant recipients: exploring mechanisms for recurrence and treatment guidelines. Dermatol Surg 2010;36:185–93.

33. Mehrany K, Byrd DR, Roenigk RK, et al. Lymphocytic infiltrates and subclinical epithelial tumor extension in patients with chronic leukemia and solid-organ transplantation. Dermatol Surg 2003;29:129–34.

34. Cooper JZ, Brown MD. Special concern about squamous cell carcinoma of the scalp in organ transplant recipients. Arch Dermatol 2006;142:755–8.

35. Adamson R, Obispo E, Dychter S, et al. High incidence and clinical course of aggressive skin cancer in heart transplant patients: a single-center study. Transplant Proc 1998;30:1124–6.

36. Lee WR, Mendenhall WM, Parsons JT, et al. Radical radiotherapy for T4 carcinoma of the skin of the head and neck: a multivariate analysis. Head Neck 1993;15:320–4.

37. Lang PG Jr, Braun MA, Kwatra R. Aggressive squamous carcinomas of the scalp. Dermatol Surg 2006;32:1163–70.

38. Altinyollar H, Berberoglu U, Celen O. Lymphatic mapping and sentinel lymph node biopsy in squamous cell carcinoma of the lower lip. Eur J Surg Oncol 2002;28:72–4.

39. Penn I. De novo malignances in pediatric organ transplant recipients. Pediatr Transplant 1998;2:56–63.

40. Holmkvist KA, Roenigk RK. Squamous cell carcinoma of the lip treated with Mohs micrographic surgery: outcome at 5 years. J Am Acad Dermatol 1998;38:960–6.
41. Silapunt S, Peterson SR, Goldberg LH. Squamous cell carcinoma of the auricle and Mohs micrographic surgery. Dermatol Surg 2005;31:1423–7.
42. Zaiac MN, Weiss E. Mohs micrographic surgery of the nail unit and squamous cell carcinoma. Dermatol Surg 2001;27:246–51.
43. Peterson SR, Layton EG, Joseph AK. Squamous cell carcinoma of the nail unit with evidence of bony involvement: a multidisciplinary approach to resection and reconstruction. Dermatol Surg 2004;30:218–21.
44. Brown MD, Zachary CB, Grekin RC, et al. Penile tumors: their management by Mohs micrographic surgery. J Dermatol Surg Oncol 1987;13:1163–7.
45. National Comprehensive Cancer Network Basal Cell and Squamous Cell Skin Cancers. Basal cell and squamous cell skin cancers. Clinical practice guidelines in oncology. J Natl Compr Canc Netw 2004;2:6–27.
46. Johnson IM, Rowe DE, Nelson BR, et al. Squamous cell carcinoma of the skin (excluding lip and oral mucosa). J Am Acad Dermatol 1992;26:467–84.
47. Leibovitch I, Huilgol SC, Selva D, et al. Cutaneous squamous cell carcinoma treated with Mohs micrographic surgery in Australia II. Perineural invasion. J Am Acad Dermatol 2005;53:261–6.
48. Shafqat A, Viehman GE, Myers SA. Cutaneous squamous cell carcinoma with zosteriform metastasis in a transplant recipient. J Am Acad Dermatol 1997;37:1008–9.
49. Harwood CA, Proby CM, McGregor JM, et al. Clinicopathologic features of skin cancer in organ transplant recipients: a retrospective case-control series. J Am Acad Dermatol 2006;54:290–300.
50. Carucci JA, Martinez JC, Zeitouni NC, et al. In-transit metastasis from primary cutaneous squamous cell carcinoma in organ transplant recipients and nonimmunosuppressed patients: clinical characteristics, management, and outcome in a series of 21 patients. Dermatol Surg 2004;30:651–5.
51. Balch CM, Buzaid AC, Soong SJ, et al. Final version of the American Joint Committee on Cancer staging system for cutaneous melanoma. J Clin Oncol 2001;19:3635–48.
52. Martinez JC, Otley CC, Stasko T, et al. Defining the clinical course of metastatic skin cancer in organ transplant recipients: a multicenter collaborative study. Arch Dermatol 2003;139:301–6.
53. Morrison WH, Garden AS, Ang KK. Radiation therapy for nonmelanoma skin carcinomas. Clin Plast Surg 1997;24:719–29.
54. Hofbauer GF, Anliker M, Arnold A, et al. Swiss clinical practice guidelines for skin cancer in organ transplant recipients. Swiss Med Wkly 2009;139:407–15.
55. Ulrich C, Hackethal M, Ulrich M, et al. Treatment of multiple actinic keratoses with topical diclofenac 3% gel in organ transplant recipients: a series of six cases. Br J Dermatol 2007;156(Suppl 3):40–2.
56. Braakhuis BJ, Tabor MP, Kummer JA, et al. A genetic explanation of Slaughter's concept of field cancerization: evidence and clinical implications. Cancer Res 2003;63:1727–30.
57. Ulrich C, Kanitakis J, Stockfleth E, et al. Skin cancer in organ transplant recipients–where do we stand today? Am J Transplant 2008;8:2192–8.
58. Troppmann C, Pierce JL, Gandhi MM, et al. Higher surgical wound complication rates with sirolimus immunosuppression after kidney transplantation: a matched-pair pilot study. Transplantation 2003;76:426–9.
59. Langer RM, Kahan BD. Incidence, therapy, and consequences of lymphocele after sirolimus-cyclosporine-prednisone immunosuppression in renal transplant recipients. Transplantation 2002;74:804–8.
60. Watson CJ, Friend PJ, Jamieson NV, et al. Sirolimus: a potent new immunosuppressant for liver transplantation. Transplantation 1999;67:505–9.
61. Dean PG, Lund WJ, Larson TS, et al. Wound-healing complications after kidney transplantation: a prospective, randomized comparison of sirolimus and tacrolimus. Transplantation 2004;77:1555–61.
62. Brewer JD, Otley CC, Christenson LJ, et al. The effects of sirolimus on wound healing in dermatologic surgery. Dermatol Surg 2008;34:216–23.
63. Euvrard S, Ulrich C, Lefrancois N. Immunosuppressants and skin cancer in transplant patients: focus on rapamycin. Dermatol Surg 2004;30:628–33.
64. Mathew T, Kreis H, Friend P. Two-year incidence of malignancy in sirolimus-treated renal transplant recipients: results from five multicenter studies. Clin Transplant 2004;18:446–9.
65. Karukonda SR, Flynn TC, Boh EE, et al. The effects of drugs on wound healing–part II. Specific classes of drugs and their effect on healing wounds. Int J Dermatol 2000;39:321–33.
66. Anstead GM. Steroids, retinoids, and wound healing. Adv Wound Care 1998;11:277–85.
67. Tan SR, Tope WD. Effect of acitretin on wound healing in organ transplant recipients. Dermatol Surg 2004;30:667–73.
68. Zachariae H. Delayed wound healing and keloid formation following argon laser treatment or dermabrasion during isotretinoin treatment. Br J Dermatol 1988;118:703–6.
69. Mandy SH. Tretinoin in the preoperative and postoperative management of dermabrasion. J Am Acad Dermatol 1986;15:878–9 888–9.

70. Katayama H, Okabe N, Kano T, et al. Granulation tissue that developed after a minor trauma in a psoriatic patient on long-term etretinate therapy. J Dermatol 1990;17:187–90.

71. Spear KL, Muller SA. Nonhealing erosions with granulation tissue in the treatment of acne lesions during isotretinoin therapy. Arch Dermatol 1984; 120:1142.

72. Wicke C, Halliday B, Allen D, et al. Effects of steroids and retinoids on wound healing. Arch Surg 2000; 135:1265–70.

73. Popp C, Kligman A, Stoudemayer T. Pretreatment of photoaged forearm skin with topical tretinoin accelerates healing of full-thickness wounds. Br J Dermatol 1995;132:46–53.

74. Bumpous JM, Johnson JT. The infected wound and its management. Otolaryngol Clin North Am 1995; 28:987–1001.

75. Maragh SL, Otley CC, Roenigk RK, et al. Antibiotic prophylaxis in dermatologic surgery: updated guidelines. Dermatol Surg 2005;31:83–91.

76. Garner JS. CDC guideline for prevention of surgical wound infections, 1985. Supersedes guideline for prevention of surgical wound infections published in 1982. (Originally published in November 1985). Revised. Infect Control 1986;7:193–200.

77. Frankel DH, Hanusa BH, Zitelli JA. New primary nonmelanoma skin cancer in patients with a history of squamous cell carcinoma of the skin. Implications and recommendations for follow-up. J Am Acad Dermatol 1992;26:720–6.

78. Eroglu A, Camlibel S. Risk factors for locoregional recurrence of scar carcinoma. Br J Surg 1997;84: 1744–6.

79. Otley C. Organization of a specialty clinic to optimize the care of organ transplant recipients at risk for skin cancer. Dermatol Surg 2000;26(7):709–12.

80. Clowers-Webb HE, Christenson LJ, Phillips PK, et al. Educational outcomes regarding skin cancer in organ transplant recipients: randomized intervention of intensive vs standard education. Arch Dermatol 2006;142:712–8.

Mohs Surgery for Melanoma in Situ

Soon-You Kwon, MD[a], Stanley J. Miller, MD[b],*

KEYWORDS

- Mohs micrographic surgery • Melanoma in situ
- Lentigo maligna • Immunostaining • Fresh frozen section
- Permanent paraffin section • Peripheral margin control

Mohs micrographic surgery (MMS) was first described as a treatment for melanoma by Frederick Mohs in 1950, as a method to achieve complete peripheral margin examination (CPME) of a tumor using the "fixed tissue" zinc chloride chemical fixation technique.[1] His method was tissue-sparing and had a 5-year cure rate of 35%, similar to that obtained by radical surgery. Twenty cases were described, spanning different subtypes and stages of melanoma, some of which already had clinical lymph node involvement. In a later article, Mohs showed that when comparing melanomas of a similar Clark level, MMS actually had superior 5-year cure rates compared with radical surgery.[2] Of note, in both studies Mohs removed an additional 1- to 3-cm margin after a microscopic melanoma-free plane was obtained, to mitigate the effects of satellite and lymphatic spread. However, even with these extra margins, the MMS approach was still considered relatively tissue-sparing at a time when margins of 5 cm or more were routinely employed in melanoma surgery.[3]

MMS depends on several principles for its success. These factors include: (1) the existence of a contiguous tumor growth pattern to avoid a false-negative margin; (2) tumor cells must be easily mapped and identifiable in the sections and be differentiated from nontumor cells; and (3) total processing time for excision, CPME, and defect repair should be within a reasonable time frame. Therefore, with the goal of achieving a local cure, the authors review how MMS is currently applied in the treatment of melanoma in situ (MIS).

There are several variations in techniques and application of CPME for MIS. While the use of MMS for nonmelanoma skin cancer has been well established, its use for MIS is less universally practiced. The challenges of histologic examination of atypical melanocytes at the margin make interpretation by frozen section difficult, especially on chronically sun-damaged skin. The current gold standard for interpretation of atypical melanocytes is by paraffin permanent sections, and therapeutic success is ultimately determined by recurrence rates based on long-term clinical follow-up.

RATIONALE FOR SURGERY

Lentigo maligna (LM) is the most prevalent subtype of MIS (>75%), and its incidence is increasing, especially in the elderly white male population.[4] Lentigo maligna melanoma (LMM), the invasive counterpart to LM, comprises 12% of all melanomas. LM and LMM present clinically as an asymmetric and irregularly pigmented patch located on chronically sun-damaged skin. Margins can be poorly defined, with extensive subclinical disease beyond the area of pigmentation. The majority of LMs occur on cosmetically sensitive areas such as the head and neck region, especially on the cheeks, where tissue conservation of normal skin is a priority. LM can often involve important functional areas such as the eyelids,

The authors have nothing to disclose.

a Department of Dermatology, University of Maryland, 419 West Redwood Street, Suite 240, Baltimore, MD 21201, USA
b Dermatology and Otolaryngology/Head and Neck Surgery, Johns Hopkins Hospital, Baltimore, MD, USA
* Corresponding author. 1104 Kenilworth Drive, Suite 201, Towson, MD 21204.
E-mail address: smiller@stanleyjmiller.com

Dermatol Clin 29 (2011) 175–183
doi:10.1016/j.det.2011.01.001
0733-8635/11/$ – see front matter © 2011 Elsevier Inc. All rights reserved.

and individual tumors may cover large surface areas of the face. Lesions often present clinically as variations of tan, dark brown, or black colors within a large patch, and it is the darker regions or an area with thickening that is usually sampled by biopsy for diagnosis. LM typically undergoes a prolonged centrifugal horizontal growth phase along the dermal-epidermal junction, which can at some point progress to LMM, with the development of invasive foci. LM is treated to prevent this progression to LMM, which occurs in a range of 2% to 50% of cases.[5–7] Once LMM develops, prognosis is similar to other melanomas of the same depth and staging.[8]

Although there may be times when surgery is contraindicated, complete surgical excision is the standard of care for biopsy-proven LM. It is especially important to examine the entire lesion by histopathology to rule out an invasive component. A review of the literature finds that a range of 5% to 67% of lesions initially determined to be LM by biopsy examination turn out to contain foci of invasive disease when the remainder of the lesion is examined after therapeutic excision (**Table 1**).[6,9–22] The potential for missing an invasive component in these instances averages 21%. Although not yet formally studied, it seems reasonable that larger tumors are more likely to contain an unseen invasive focus, because the initial biopsy represents a smaller percentage of the entire lesion.

Al-Niaimi and colleagues.[9] reviewed 65 cases and reported that 3-mm or 4-mm punch biopsies were the most commonly used method to diagnose LM. While their recommendation to use incisional biopsies or larger punch biopsies would lower the incidence of missing an invasive component, the emphasis should still be placed on complete excision and histologic examination of the entire specimen to rule out invasive disease.

The type of histologic analysis of biopsy and excisional specimens may be important as well. Prompted by a patient with a diagnosis of MIS who subsequently developed metastatic disease, Megahed and colleagues[16] recently studied the utility of Melan-A compared with traditional hematoxylin and eosin staining in making a diagnosis of in situ versus invasive melanocytic disease. In 104 cases initially diagnosed as MIS by hematoxylin and eosin staining, an additional 30 (29%) were shown to contain foci of invasive disease when the tissue was examined using Melan-A. In the latter group, 2 patients subsequently developed local recurrences or metastases during an average of 23 months' follow-up.

Finally, preliminary studies describe how confocal microscopy may help guide physicians in the future to determine where to take sampling biopsies within a given lesion of suspected LM/LMM. Its use, however, is currently limited to research centers, and limitations include size, affordability, and accessibility.[23]

Table 1
Upstaging of MIS to invasive melanoma after complete histopathologic examination of the entire lesion

Study	Total Number of Specimens with Initial Biopsy Diagnosis as MIS	Number Found to have an Invasive Component After Complete Histopathologic Examination of the Lesion	% MIS Upstaged to Malignant Melanoma
Bosbous et al,[10] 2009	49	6	12
Al-Niaimi et al,[9] 2009	37	5	14
Möller et al,[17] 2008	49	6	12
Hazan et al,[13] 2008	91	15	16
Mahoney et al,[15] 2005	11	2	18
Huilgol et al,[14] 2004	36	24	67
Bub et al,[11] 2004	58	3	5
Megahed et al,[16] 2002	104	30	29
Osborne and Hutchinson,[18] 2002	89	5	6
Zalla et al,[20] 2000	46	3	7
Cohen et al,[12] 1998	29	3	10
Somach et al,[19] 1996	46	9	20
Weedon,[21] 1982	66	8	12
Wayte and Helwig,[6] 1968	85	45	53
Total	796	164	21

NONSURGICAL TREATMENT

Nonsurgical treatment for LM, such as imiquimod and cryotherapy, is a cosmetically appealing option especially in the presence of extensive disease. However, these therapies carry a higher potential for incomplete treatment, and with it, the risk of progression to invasive melanoma. In addition, as already noted, a significant percentage of biopsy-proven MIS lesions already contain foci of invasive disease at the time of initial treatment. Radiation and laser therapy have also been used for LM in patients not amenable to surgical treatment.

Imiquimod is a topical synthetic imidazoquinoline amine that exhibits antiviral and antitumor effects through stimulation of both the innate and cell-mediated immune system by activation of toll-like receptors 7 and 8, which induce transcription factor NΓ-κB and Th1 cytokines such as interferon-α, interferon-γ, and interleukin-12.[24–26] Further, imiquimod can induce FasR-mediated apoptosis. It is currently approved by the Food and Drug Administration for treatment of superficial basal cell carcinomas, actinic keratosis, and warts. In 2000, Ahmed and Berth-Jones[24] first reported the use of imiquimod 5% cream as a treatment for LM on the scalp in a patient who refused surgical treatment. Because systemic interferon-α is used for metastatic melanoma, they chose to try imiquimod for its potential to stimulate interferon-α locally. In a review of the literature in 2006, Rajpar and Marsden[27] reported that the overall composite clinical clearance rate for LM treated with topical imiquimod was 88%. However, they noted that many of the case reports and small series presented did not confirm complete histologic clearance of tumor, and follow-up times for the majority of studies were less than 3 years, shorter than the cancer standard of 5 years. In a well-designed study in 2007, Cotter and colleagues[28] treated 40 patients with imiquimod 5% cream 5 times a week for 3 months and followed this with a complete staged excision of the area 2 months later. These investigators found an initial complete clinical response rate of 83% (33/40). However, following complete staged excision of all sites, 2 patients were found to have residual LM and a third was found to have an invasive component. Thus, the actual clearance rate was 75%. In 2009, Powell and colleagues[29] reported results from 48 patients treated with imiquimod 5% cream for 6 weeks and then followed for a mean duration of 49 months. The study showed a 77% (37/49) clinical response rate. Punch biopsies were obtained at 3 months' follow-up in all clinical responders and no recurrences were found. In the 11 clinical nonresponders, one patient was found to have invasive melanoma following complete excision. Finally, in 2010 Van Meurs and colleagues[30] reported a 44% (4/9) recurrence rate in a small case series of LM treated with imiquimod followed for an average of 31 months.

One of the difficulties with imiquimod therapy for LM is that it can provide a false sense of clinical improvement by removing pigmentation, while in fact the area may still harbor atypical melanocytes or malignancy. These lesions require close histologic monitoring posttreatment for potential recurrence and malignant change. In toto, imiquimod is best considered as a therapy for patients with disease involvement and/or comorbidities that preclude surgical removal and reconstruction.

EXCISIONAL SURGERY

Surgical excision with 5-mm margins around the clinically visible lesion is the current "standard of care" treatment recommendation for MIS. It was established by a National Institutes of Health consensus conference in 1992.[31] Soon afterwards, however, data begin to show a need for wider margins to achieve complete clearance in selected cases, especially with larger diameter lesions and those of the LM subtype located in the head and neck area. In 1994, Robinson reported that a 6-mm margin cleared only 23% of MIS cases and that the recurrence rate after 8 years was 6% (1/16).[32] In 1997, Zitelli and colleagues[3] showed that 9-mm margins were required to clear 95% of MIS cases during Mohs surgery. Based on their data, the investigators recommended the following margins for traditional excisional surgery: 1-cm margins for lesions smaller than 2 cm in diameter located on the trunk and 1.5-cm margins for lesions larger than 2 cm in diameter on the trunk and those located on the head and neck. Zalla and colleagues[20] confirmed these findings and noted that 1.5-cm margins cleared 96% of MIS located primarily on the head and neck. Finally, in 2008 Hazan and colleagues[13] analyzed 117 cases, and again noted a correlation between lesion diameter and the surgical margin necessary for tumor clearance. In a recent review of the literature, 3- to 5-year recurrence rates following surgical excision with 5-mm margins are in the range of 6% to 20%.[33] In about half of these instances the pathology will return with positive margins.[20,34] Thus, the National Comprehensive Cancer Network guidelines of care for melanoma currently recommend a 5-mm excisional margin for MIS, but a footnote states: "For large melanoma in situ, lentigo maligna type, surgical margins >0.5 cm may be necessary to achieve histologically negative margins; techniques for more exhaustive histologic assessment of margins should be considered."[31] Therefore, when MIS is being surgically excised, consideration of the lesion's subtype, location, and diameter can help a surgeon to decide if margins greater than 0.5 cm may be necessary.

The discovery of positive margins on permanent section assessment a week after a surgical excision can be anxiety provoking for many patients, especially if multiple reexcisions are subsequently needed to clear the MIS. When performing a reexcision the location of the positive margin is usually unknown, and therefore an additional layer is often taken from all sides of the lesion, usually around a linear scar. Subclinical spread is usually the reason for the initial incomplete excision, and re-excision is performed without a clear picture of the borders. This situation occurs more often than not because of the ill-defined nature of LM. Furthermore, these lesions occur frequently on cosmetically sensitive areas such as the head and neck, where a tissue-sparing technique would be valuable to both maximize cure rate and minimize final defect size.

Mohs Micrographic Surgery

MMS achieves the goals of maximizing cure rate and minimizing defect size by employing CPME during excision. Although challenges exist in interpreting frozen sections of melanocytes, the literature indicates that MMS is a successful therapy for LM, with much lower recurrence rates than nonsurgical methods and standard 5-mm margin surgical excisions (**Table 2**).[22,30,33–37] There is a range of MIS recurrences rates after MMS, and it is likely an operator-dependent and technique-dependent process (**Table 3**). Several forms of CPME are described in the literature for LM including traditional frozen sections, frozen sections with a final layer sent for permanent

sections, frozen sections with immunostaining, and staged excision with rush permanent sections.

With all the forms of CPME, several common steps occur. A complete skin examination (if not already done) and regional lymph node assessment are performed, and the LM lesion is then examined under bright lights and usually a Wood lamp as well, to carefully ascertain the full extent of clinical involvement. The clinical borders of the lesion are then carefully marked. Some practitioners draw in an additional margin around this as well. The tissue is then excised down to the subcutaneous layer, to include all epithelial appendageal structures, and the lateral margins are processed and examined in one of several approaches (see later discussion). The central portion of the specimen is sent for permanent section assessment to rule out occult invasion.

Traditional frozen section

In traditional frozen section CPME, the tissue is processed into frozen sections in en face sectioning starting from the outer side with 2- to 4-μm thickness cuts, and stained with hematoxylin and eosin.[3] Quick freezing of the tissue helps to reduce vacuolization freeze artifact. The tissue is then examined for nesting of more than 3 atypical melanocytes, uneven distribution of contiguous basal layer melanocytes, pagetoid spread, and adnexal involvement.[3,8,11,35,38,39] Cohen[8] also mentions observing multinucleated melanocytes with prominent dendritic processes in LM lesions. If any of the aforementioned characteristics are found, another 2- to 3-mm layer is taken at the positive margin, and repeated as necessary until clear. Signs of regression evident by fibrosis, dermal macrophages, or a brisk lymphohistiocytic infiltrate may also indicate the need for another layer of tissue removal at that border.[40]

Difficulties arise when trying to differentiate atypical melanocytic hyperplasia from benign melanocytic hyperplasia and actinic keratinocytic damage. Not infrequently, single atypical melanocytes can extend for a significant distance beyond the LM lesion, especially in chronically sun-damaged skin. Bricca and colleagues,[35] Zitelli and colleagues,[3] and Bene and colleagues[41] do not excise the isolated single atypical melanocytes. These groups consider them part of chronic actinic changes, and show success by maintaining a very low recurrence rate. However, Barlow and colleagues[42] differ in opinion, suggesting that single atypical melanocytes are a sign of early MIS that are better interpreted on permanent paraffin sections and need to be excised. The biological behavior of these single atypical melanocytes is thus a matter of debate. Deciding when to call a margin clear

Table 2 Comparison of recurrence rates of proposed treatments of MIS	
Method	Recurrence Rate (3–5-Year Follow-up) (%)
Cryotherapy[34]	7–34
Imiquimod[30,37]	0–44
Radiation therapy[33,34]	0–19
Excisional surgery[22]	6–20
Mohs surgery[22,36]	0–7.3 (33% outlier)

Table 3
Recurrence rates of different peripheral margin examination methods

Method	Number of MIS Treated and Followed	Average Follow-Up (mo)	Recurrence Rate (%)
Frozen sections Mohs (FS MMS)			
Zitelli et al,[3] 1997	184	60	0.5
Bienert et al,[39] 2003	76	33	0
Bricca et al,[35] 2005	331	58	0.3
(HMB-45 in 33%, otherwise FS)			
Walling et al,[36] 2007	18[a]	118	33
FS MMS with final permanent sections (PS)			
Cohen et al,[12] 1998	38[a]	58	2.6
Bene et al,[41] 2008	110	63	1.8
FS MMS with immunostains			
Bricca et al,[35] 2005	331	58	0.3
(HMB-45 in 33%, otherwise FS)			
Bhardwaj et al,[57] 2006 (Mel-5)	200[a]	38	0.5
Staged excisions with PS for each layer			
Johnson et al,[54] 1997 (square modification)	35[a]	<24	0
Hill and Gramp,[58] 1999 (vertical section)	66	<40	1.5
Clayton et al,[59] 2000 (en face section)	81[d]	22	1.2
Anderson et al,[60] 2001 (square)	150[a]	<60	0.7
Agarwal-Antal et al,[43] 2002 (polygonal modification)	92	<48	0
Bub et al,[11] 2004 (radial section)	55	57	3.6
Huilgol et al,[14] 2004 (bread-loaf/vertical sections)	161[a]	38	2
Mahoney et al,[15] 2005 (vertical section)	9	5	0
Walling et al,[36] 2007 (vertical section)	41[a]	3	7.3
Möller et al,[17] 2008 (en face section)	49	14	0
Then et al,[61] 2009 (en face section)	8	36	0
Bosbous et al,[10] 2009 (en face section)	59[a]	27	1.7

[a] LM and LMM analyzed together.

requires a considerable amount of training, familiarity with pathology and MMS, and high-quality frozen sections to interpret. One technique mentioned in the literature to help assess the LM border is to take a control sample of skin from an equally sun-damaged area that may then be histologically compared with the border of the LM lesion.[43,44] Whereas Zitelli and colleagues[40] reported 100% sensitivity and 90% specificity of fresh frozen sections compared with permanent sections, Barlow and colleagues reported 59% sensitivity and 81% specificity.[42] This difference may be the result of Barlow and colleagues selecting and studying only difficult and equivocal slides from the majority of their samples, or the fact that Zitelli and colleagues excluded from their calculations 4 false-negative frozen sections because they believed the permanent sections were actually "false positives," resulting from deeper cuts in the same tissue block. In any event, some MMS surgeons follow frozen sections with a final permanent section layer, or perform immunostaining on the frozen sections as well.

Frozen sections with permanent sections for final layer

As examined MMS layers get closer to the periphery of a lesion, assessment of the slides can get more difficult because of the interpretation of atypical single-cell melanocytes, which could represent the edge of the MIS lesion, chronic actinic damage without malignant potential, or keratinocytes that are misinterpreted as melanocytes. After a final frozen layer during MMS is determined to be clear, some Mohs surgeons will remove an additional 1- to 3-mm layer and send it for permanent paraffin processing and interpretation by a dermatopathologist. Others will melt the final frozen tissue layer, place it in a formalin bottle, and send it for processing.

With the latter option, the paraffin section will be taken from deeper in the existing block by en face sectioning, increasing the chance that correlation will not occur; for example, a negative margin on frozen section may be read as a positive margin on permanent section. With either approach, the surgeon will usually choose to take another layer from any area found to be positive on permanent section assessment. In a study of 97 cases, Bienert and colleagues[39] reported a 100% correlation between frozen and permanent section assessment of negative margins. There were no cases of recurrence in 92 of the 97 patients who were followed for an average of 33 months. Bene and colleagues[41] treated 167 MIS cases with MMS and reported a 95.1% clearance rate when frozen sections were checked with a final permanent section en face sectioning. Thus, in the latter study, for every 20 cases performed, there was one case in which another layer needed to be taken after the final permanent sections were read. The clinical cure rate was 98.2% (2/110 recurrence) during a mean of 63 months' follow-up. When sending Mohs tissues for permanent section assessment, close communication between the Mohs surgeon and the pathologist is needed. The surgeon will often place a suture in the specimen and provide a map for orientation.

Immunostaining

Immunostains may enhance the recognition of melanocytes on both frozen and paraffin sections. Several melanocytic markers, such as S-100, HMB45, MART-1/Melan-A, Mel-5, and MITF, have been studied and used over the past several years to aid in margin examination of melanoma. These markers serve as an adjunctive method to verify what is seen on hematoxylin and eosin staining, facilitate identification of atypical melanocytes, and may increase the accuracy of interpreting margin status. Immunostains were initially developed and applied to paraffin sections; they have since then been applied to frozen sections in the context of MMS.

Several recent modifications of the immunostaining process have proved useful for MMS. For instance, the traditional immunostaining process takes several hours to complete. Several articles have in the last few years have described rapid and ultra-rapid immunostaining techniques. In 2002, Kelley and Starkus[44] used MART-1 in an 80- to 90-minute protocol on frozen tissue, reduced from 2- to 2.5-hour protocols, with 100% correlation with permanent paraffin sections (PPS). If the slides remain in any way equivocal after immunostaining, they recommended sending tissue for permanent

sections. In 2004 Bricca and colleagues[45] further reduced the time to a 1-hour protocol using a MART-1 polymer-based system that amplified the DAB-chromogen. These investigators were able to eliminate the secondary antibody linking step and shorten the blocking step, reducing the overall time needed for immunostaining. In a study of 40 patients, they showed that MART-1 approached 100% sensitivity for primary cutaneous melanomas, with the exception of spindle cell and desmoplastic melanomas. Also, because MART-1 stains both normal and atypical melanocytes, the sections act as an internal positive control. Further, Bricca and colleagues found that the MART-1 staining helped interpret equivocal slides on frozen hematoxylin and eosin and categorize them as either positive or negative margins. Finally, in 2009 Cherpelis and colleagues[46] reported a 19-minute protocol for MART-1 frozen sections and compared it with MART-1 in permanent sections. This group found no differences in the number and nuclear diameter of melanocytes found. Also, there was no difference in the ability to interpret melanocytic confluence, pagetoid spread, nesting, and atypia in 25 dog ear samples.

Cost effectiveness may be an issue with immunostaining. The reimbursement in 2010 for the Medicare code for immunohistochemistry staining (88342) is around $100 per specimen, whereas the cost per slide in the Cherpelis and colleagues[46] study was $30. Depending on how many slides must be prepared during MMS, immunostaining may or may not be cost effective.

Among the different melanocytic markers S-100 is the most sensitive, and it is useful in identifying spindle cell and desmoplastic melanoma. The other markers, HMB-45, MART-1, and MITF, are more specific than S-100, but are not helpful with spindle and desmoplastic variants.[47] MART-1 has been the preferred immunostain in MMS for MIS because of its intense and diffuse staining of normal and atypical melanocytes.[35] Melan-A, a clone of MART-1, has been criticized for staining keratinocytes, especially in an inflammatory state; the results can mimic melanocytic hyperplasia or the pattern of nesting and pagetoid spread in MIS.[48] Helm and Findeis-Hosey[49] explored this issue, and found that while Melan-A did stain actinic keratoses and lentigines positively, there was a statistically significant increase in its staining of MIS cells. HMB-45, a marker of cytoplasmic premelanosomal glycoprotein gp100, has staining that may be spotty and less intense; therefore, MART-1 is preferred in MMS.[20,50] Mel-5 is a murine IgG antibody against melanosomal glycoprotein 75, and it stains epidermal melanocytes with greater intensity than S-100 but less specificity than HMB-45.[51] MITF is a nuclear stain, which helps to interpret both melanocyte density and nuclear diameter.[52] Specificity of MITF is in a range of 88% to 100%, but it is reported to also stain histiocytes, lymphocytes, fibroblasts, Schwann cells, and smooth muscle cells. Of importance, the aforementioned characterizations of all the immunostains apply to both frozen section and paraffin section slides. Immunostaining can be a useful tool in assessing the margins of MIS during MMS. The frozen slides must, as always, be of high quality. As the immunostaining protocols get shorter in duration and the immunostains themselves become more affordable, more laboratories may be using this tool.

Staged excision by permanent sections

Finally, PPS are considered by many to be the gold standard for the interpretation of melanocytic lesions. In PPS sections, melanocytes retain their pericytoplasmic vacuolization, which is used to help identify them, and freeze artifact is not a confounding factor. Because of this, some investigators advocate using staged excisions with rush PPS for each MMS layer.[11,36,42,53] A variety of names have been used in the literature to describe different forms of this process, including slow Mohs, rush paraffin sections, staged marginal and central excision technique, perimeter technique, square technique, and paraffin sections with tissue mapping before delayed defect closure. Walling and colleagues[36] reviewed the results of staged excision with PPS and compared them to traditional frozen MMS in a single practice site, and found that for that site recurrence rates were higher in the traditional frozen MMS group. One major limitation of PPS is the time needed to process the tissue, which increases the time between stages and before a reconstruction can be performed to one to several days. There are several modifications reported on the margin contour (square, polygonal, round, lesional) and timing of the central lesion removal.[43,54,55] In addition, most paraffin sections of the margins are prepared in one of two ways, either by en face (MMS-like) vertical cuts or perpendicular radial cuts. CPME is typically achieved only with the en face method. However, the advantages of the radial cuts, in the view of some pathologists, include the ability to observe morphologic features of the tumor from its center to its periphery, to obtain a clear view of the distance from the margin edge to the tumor, and to have a direct comparison of the tumor with surrounding chronic sun-damaged skin.[13,53,56] The major disadvantage is that the entire margin is not examined.

SUMMARY

Because of the issues of lower cure rate and possible occult invasive foci within MIS lesions at the time of treatment, topical therapy for MIS is not routinely recommended. It is probably best used when surgical removal of a lesion is not possible. Surgical excision with 5-mm margins is an appropriate approach for many MIS lesions with well-defined clinical borders. In the setting of larger diameter lesions, and those of the ill-defined LM subtype, more extensive surgical margins in the range of 0.5 to 1.5 cm may be indicated. Several different variants of MMS may be used to perform CPME of LM, and there does not appear to be an obviously superior variant in terms of the long-term cure rate (see **Table 3**). ALL CPME approaches appear to provide cure rates superior to traditional surgical excision, and are especially useful for treating ill-defined lesions, larger and recurrent tumors, and those of the LM subtype, because of their ability to assess the complete peripheral margin, to minimize surgical defect size, and to maximize the cure rate. In all instances, the central portion of the CPME specimen should be sent for complete PPS examination to rule out an undetected invasive component.

REFERENCES

1. Mohs FE. Chemosurgical treatment of melanoma; a microscopically controlled method of excision. Arch Derm Syphilol 1950;62(2):269–79.
2. Mohs FE. Chemosurgery for melanoma. Arch Dermatol 1977;113(3):285–91.
3. Zitelli JA, Brown C, Hanusa BH. Mohs micrographic surgery for the treatment of primary cutaneous melanoma. J Am Acad Dermatol 1997;37(2 Pt 1):236–45.
4. Swetter SM, Boldrick JC, Jung SY, et al. Increasing incidence of lentigo maligna melanoma subtypes: northern California and national trends 1990–2000. J Invest Dermatol 2005;125(4):685–91.
5. Rhodes AR. Melanocytic precursors of cutaneous melanoma. Estimated risks and guidelines for management. Med Clin North Am 1986;70(1):3–37.
6. Wayte DM, Helwig EB. Melanotic freckle of Hutchinson. Cancer 1968;21(5):893–911.
7. Weinstock MA, Sober AJ. The risk of progression of lentigo maligna to lentigo maligna melanoma. Br J Dermatol 1987;116(3):303–10.
8. Cohen LM. Lentigo maligna and lentigo maligna melanoma. J Am Acad Dermatol 1995;33(6):923–36 quiz: 37–40.
9. Al-Niaimi F, Jury CS, McLaughlin S, et al. Review of management and outcome in 65 patients with lentigo maligna. Br J Dermatol 2009;160(1):211–3.

10. Bosbous MW, Dzwierzynski WW, Neuburg M. Staged excision of lentigo maligna and lentigo maligna melanoma: a 10-year experience. Plast Reconstr Surg 2009;124(6):1947–55.

11. Bub JL, Berg D, Slee A, et al. Management of lentigo maligna and lentigo maligna melanoma with staged excision: a 5-year follow-up. Arch Dermatol 2004; 140(5):552–8.

12. Cohen LM, McCall MW, Zax RH. Mohs micrographic surgery for lentigo maligna and lentigo maligna melanoma. A follow-up study. Dermatol Surg 1998; 24(6):673–7.

13. Hazan C, Dusza SW, Delgado R, et al. Staged excision for lentigo maligna and lentigo maligna melanoma: a retrospective analysis of 117 cases. J Am Acad Dermatol 2008;58(1):142–8.

14. Huilgol SC, Selva D, Chen C, et al. Surgical margins for lentigo maligna and lentigo maligna melanoma: the technique of mapped serial excision. Arch Dermatol 2004;140(9):1087–92.

15. Mahoney MH, Joseph M, Temple CL. The perimeter technique for lentigo maligna: an alternative to Mohs micrographic surgery. J Surg Oncol 2005;91(2):120–5.

16. Megahed M, Schon M, Selimovic D, et al. Reliability of diagnosis of melanoma in situ. Lancet 2002; 359(9321):1921–2.

17. Möller MG, Pappas-Politis E, Zager JS, et al. Surgical management of melanoma-in-situ using a staged marginal and central excision technique. Ann Surg Oncol 2009;16(6):1526–36.

18. Osborne JE, Hutchinson PE. A follow-up study to investigate the efficacy of initial treatment of lentigo maligna with surgical excision. Br J Plast Surg 2002;55(8):611–5.

19. Somach SC, Taira JW, Pitha JV, et al. Pigmented lesions in actinically damaged skin. Histopathologic comparison of biopsy and excisional specimens. Arch Dermatol 1996;132(11):1297–302.

20. Zalla MJ, Lim KK, Dicaudo DJ, et al. Mohs micrographic excision of melanoma using immunostains. Dermatol Surg 2000;26(8):771–84.

21. Weedon D. A reappraisal of melanoma in situ. J Dermatol Surg Oncol 1982;8:774–5.

22. Dawn ME, Dawn AG, Miller SJ. Mohs surgery for the treatment of melanoma in situ: a review. Dermatol Surg 2007;33(4):395–402.

23. Ahlgrimm-Siess V, Massone C, Scope A, et al. Reflectance confocal microscopy of facial lentigo maligna and lentigo maligna melanoma: a preliminary study. Br J Dermatol 2009;161(6):1307–16.

24. Ahmed I, Berth-Jones J. Imiquimod: a novel treatment for lentigo maligna. Br J Dermatol 2000;143(4):843–5.

25. Bilu D, Sauder DN. Imiquimod: modes of action. Br J Dermatol 2003;149(Suppl 66):5–8.

26. Woodmansee C, Pillow J, Skinner RB Jr. The role of topical immune response modifiers in skin cancer. Drugs 2006;66(13):1657–64.

27. Rajpar SF, Marsden JR. Imiquimod in the treatment of lentigo maligna. Br J Dermatol 2006;155(4):653–6.

28. Cotter MA, McKenna JK, Bowen GM. Treatment of lentigo maligna with imiquimod before staged excision. Dermatol Surg 2008;34:147–51.

29. Powell AM, Robson AM, Russell-Jones R, et al. Imiquimod and lentigo maligna: a search for prognostic features in a clinicopathological study with long-term follow-up. Br J Dermatol 2009;160(5):994–8.

30. Van Meurs T, Van Doorn R, Kirtschig G. Treatment of lentigo maligna with imiquimod cream: a long-term follow-up study of 10 patients. Dermatol Surg 2010;36(6):853–8.

31. National Institutes of Health Consensus Development Conference Statement on Diagnosis and Treatment of Early Melanoma, January 27–29, 1992. Am J Dermatopathol 1993;15:34–43.

32. Robinson JK. Margin control for lentigo maligna. J Am Acad Dermatol 1994;31(1):79–85.

33. Erickson C, Miller SJ. Treatment options in melanoma in situ: topical and radiation therapy, excision and Mohs surgery. Int J Dermatol 2010;49(5):482–91.

34. McKenna JK, Florell SR, Goldman GD, et al. Lentigo maligna/lentigo maligna melanoma: current state of diagnosis and treatment. Dermatol Surg 2006;32(4):493–504.

35. Bricca GM, Brodland DG, Ren D, et al. Cutaneous head and neck melanoma treated with Mohs micrographic surgery. J Am Acad Dermatol 2005;52(1):92–100.

36. Walling HW, Scupham RK, Bean AK, et al. Staged excision versus Mohs micrographic surgery for lentigo maligna and lentigo maligna melanoma. J Am Acad Dermatol 2007;57(4):659–64.

37. Woodmansee CS, McCall MW. Recurrence of lentigo maligna and development of invasive melanoma after treatment of lentigo maligna with imiquimod. Dermatol Surg 2009;35(8):1286–9.

38. Weyers W, Bonczkowitz M, Weyers I, et al. Melanoma in situ versus melanocytic hyperplasia in sun-damaged skin. Assessment of the significance of histopathologic criteria for differential diagnosis. Am J Dermatopathol 1996;18(6):560–6.

39. Bienert TN, Trotter MJ, Arlette JP. Treatment of cutaneous melanoma of the face by Mohs micrographic surgery. J Cutan Med Surg 2003;7(1):25–30.

40. Zitelli JA, Moy RL, Abell E. The reliability of frozen sections in the evaluation of surgical margins for melanoma. J Am Acad Dermatol 1991;24(1):102–6.

41. Bene NI, Healy C, Coldiron BM. Mohs micrographic surgery is accurate 95.1% of the time for melanoma in situ: a prospective study of 167 cases. Dermatol Surg 2008;34(5):660–4.

42. Barlow RJ, White CR, Swanson NA. Mohs' micrographic surgery using frozen sections alone may be unsuitable for detecting single atypical melanocytes at the margins of melanoma in situ. Br J Dermatol 2002;146(2):290–4.

43. Agarwal-Antal N, Bowen GM, Gerwels JW. Histologic evaluation of lentigo maligna with permanent

sections: implications regarding current guidelines. J Am Acad Dermatol 2002;47(5):743–8.

44. Kelley LC, Starkus L. Immunohistochemical staining of lentigo maligna during Mohs micrographic surgery using MART-1. J Am Acad Dermatol 2002;46(1):78–84.

45. Bricca GM, Brodland DG, Zitelli JA. Immunostaining melanoma frozen sections: the 1-hour protocol. Dermatol Surg 2004;30(3):403–8.

46. Cherpelis BS, Moore R, Ladd S, et al. Comparison of MART-1 frozen sections to permanent sections using a rapid 19-minute protocol. Dermatol Surg 2009; 35(2):207–13.

47. Ohsie SJ, Sarantopoulos GP, Cochran AJ, et al. Immunohistochemical characteristics of melanoma. J Cutan Pathol 2008;35(5):433–44.

48. El Shabrawi-Caelen L, Kerl H, Cerroni L. Melan-A: not a helpful marker in distinction between melanoma in situ on sun-damaged skin and pigmented actinic keratosis. Am J Dermatopathol 2004;26(5):364–6.

49. Helm K, Findeis-Hosey J. Immunohistochemistry of pigmented actinic keratoses, actinic keratoses, melanomas in situ and solar lentigines with Melan-A. J Cutan Pathol 2008;35(10):931–4.

50. Albertini JG, Elston DM, Libow LF, et al. Mohs micrographic surgery for melanoma: a case series, a comparative study of immunostains, an informative case report, and a unique mapping technique. Dermatol Surg 2002;28(8):656–65.

51. Gross EA, Andersen WK, Rogers GS. Mohs micrographic excision of lentigo maligna using Mel-5 for margin control. Arch Dermatol 1999;135(1):15–7.

52. Glass LF, Raziano RM, Clark GS, et al. Rapid frozen section immunostaining of melanocytes by microphthalmia-associated transcription factor. Am J Dermatopathol 2010;32(4):319–25.

53. Prieto VG, Argenyi ZB, Barnhill RL, et al. Are en face frozen sections accurate for diagnosing margin status in melanocytic lesions? Am J Clin Pathol 2003;120(2):203–8.

54. Johnson TM, Headington JT, Baker SR, et al. Usefulness of the staged excision for lentigo maligna and lentigo maligna melanoma: the "square" procedure. J Am Acad Dermatol 1997;37(5 Pt 1):758–64.

55. Clark GS, Pappas-Politis EC, Cherpelis BS, et al. Surgical management of melanoma in situ on chronically sun-damaged skin. Cancer Control 2008; 15(3):216–24.

56. Stretch JR, Scolyer RA. Surgical strategies and histopathologic issues in the management of lentigo maligna. Ann Surg Oncol 2009;16(6):1456–8.

57. Bhardwaj SS, Tope WD, Lee PK. Mohs micrographic surgery for lentigo maligna and lentigo maligna melanoma using Mel-5 immunostaining: University of Minnesota experience. Dermatol Surg 2006; 32(5):690–6 [discussion: 696–7].

58. Hill DC, Gramp AA. Surgical treatment of lentigo maligna and lentigo maligna melanoma. Australas J Dermatol 1999;40(1):25–30.

59. Clayton BD, Leshin B, Hitchcock MG, et al. Utility of rush paraffin-embedded tangential sections in the management of cutaneous neoplasms. Dermatol Surg 2000;26(7):671–8.

60. Anderson KW, Baker SR, Lowe L, et al. Treatment of head and neck melanoma, lentigo maligna subtype: a practical surgical technique. Arch Facial Plast Surg 2001;3(3):202–6.

61. Then SY, Malhotra R, Barlow R, et al. Early cure rates with narrow-margin slow-Mohs surgery for periocular malignant melanoma. Dermatol Surg 2009; 35(1):17–23.

Mohs Micrographic Surgery in the Treatment of Microcystic Adnexal Carcinoma

Stephanie A. Diamantis, MD[a], Victor J. Marks, MD[b],*

KEYWORDS

- Microcystic adnexal carcinoma • Mohs surgery
- Sclerosing sweat duct carcinoma • Malignant syringoma
- Syringoid carcinoma

Microcystic adnexal carcinoma (MAC), also known as *sclerosing sweat duct carcinoma*, *malignant syringoma*, and *syringoid carcinoma*, was first described as a distinct clinicopathologic entity in 1982.[1,2] MAC is a tumor with follicular and sweat gland differentiation and overall benign features histologically; however, it exhibits aggressive local behavior.[2] This article describes clinical presentation, pathologic hallmarks, and treatment options.

CLINICAL PRESENTATION

MAC is an uncommon tumor. In a retrospective case series at a Mohs referral center, the mean number of cases per year was 1.63.[3] MAC generally presents a smooth flesh-colored or yellow slow-growing indurated plaque or cystic nodule on the central facial region (**Fig. 1**). The average tumor size at diagnosis is 2 cm.[4] Other rare locations include the scalp, axillae, buttocks, and genitals.[5]

Surveillance, Epidemiology and End Results (SEER) database analysis of 223 patients showed middle-aged to older patients are preferentially affected (median age, 68 years), and the most common site of involvement is the head and neck, including the lips (74%). MAC rarely occurs in children.[6] Women were affected more often than men (57% vs 43%). MAC was noted mostly in whites (90%).[7] A cases have been reported in African Americans, and in Japanese, Puerto Rican, Korean, Spanish, and Jewish people.[8] Similar demographics were described in a large case series from University of California, San Francisco (UCSF). This series also reported left-sided predominance.[9] Another smaller series of patients with MAC referred for Mohs surgery also described 6 of 10 cases occurring on the left side. These investigators postulate a possible role of ultraviolet light in the pathogenesis of this tumor.[10] Radiation may increase the risk of developing MAC.[10–13] Three cases have been associated with immune suppression: two in renal organ transplant recipients (one who also had radiation for acne) and one associated with chronic lymphocytic leukemia.[13,14]

MAC is slow-growing but can be locally aggressive. Generally, the extent of tumor burden is confined to the skin (in 75% of cases according to the SEER database). However, invasion into underlying soft tissue, muscle, and bone is possible. In fact, because of subtle clinical presentation, MAC is often diagnosed at a later stage and

The authors have nothing to disclose.
[a] Procedural Dermatology, Department of Dermatology, Geisinger Health System, 115 Woodbine Lane, Danville, PA 17822, USA
[b] Department of Dermatology, Geisinger Health System, 115 Woodbine Lane, Danville, PA 17822, USA
* Corresponding author.
E-mail address: vmarks@geisinger.edu

Dermatol Clin 29 (2011) 185–190
doi:10.1016/j.det.2011.01.012
0733-8635/11/$ – see front matter © 2011 Published by Elsevier Inc.

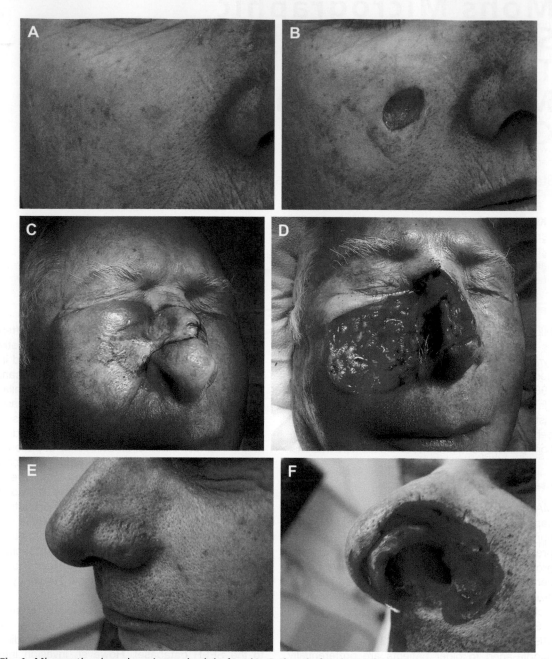

Fig. 1. Microcystic adnexal carcinoma both before (*A, C, E*) and after (*B, D, F*) Mohs surgery. Note the variation in clinically apparent tumor and extent of disease evident after Mohs.

has invaded deep into the dermis or subcutis by diagnosis. One case report describes a patient who presented with an indurated plaque over the chin and was found to have tumor invading the mandibular bone marrow.[15]

MAC is usually asymptomatic, but if perineural involvement is present, patients may report or complain of numbness, paresthesia, or tingling.[12] Yu and colleagues[7] noted lymph node involvement

in 1% of patients, and only 1 case in 223 was metastatic. Although MAC causes high morbidity because of its locally aggressive nature, overall survival is good, and death secondary to MAC is unlikely. Yu and colleagues[7] note a 97% 10-year survival rate, which is similar to patients of similar age without MAC.

Clinical differential diagnosis includes benignadnexal tumors, such as trichoepithelioma, trichoadenoma, and syringoma, and a scar, cyst, basal cell carcinoma (especially the morpheaform subtype), and squamous cell carcinoma.[4]

Histopathology

On initial description, microcystic adnexal carcinoma was believed to originate from an adnexal keratinocyte capable of undergoing follicular or sweat gland differentiation.[2,15] More recently, cases of MAC have been reported with sebaceous or apocrine differentiation.[16,17] Most authors agree that MAC has follicular and eccrine origins.[2,5,12,16]

Pathology is characterized by multiple islands of basaloid epithelial cells, ductal structures, and keratinizing cysts, located intradermally but often extending deep as thin strands of tumor cells intercalating between collagen bundles. Stroma is often fibrotic, and perineural and intramuscular invasion are common. The tumor is not well defined. Tumor cells often appear benign with lack of cytologic atypia, and few if any mitoses.[2]

Histopathologic analysis is necessary for diagnosis. Tissue biopsy must be of adequate depth and size because architectural features are important in diagnosis. In one case series, misdiagnosis occurred in 27% of cases.[9] In another prospective study, MAC was diagnosed intraoperatively during Mohs surgery in 32.5% of cases (these patients had been referred for excision of a different lesion).[4] Often misdiagnosis is secondary to inadequate sampling, because the pathologist cannot see the breadth or depth of the tumor. Also, the bland histologic features with little cytologic atypia or mitoses can make diagnosis difficult.

Differential diagnosis on histopathology is similar to the clinical differential diagnosis, and includes morpheaform basal cell carcinoma,

desmoplastic trichoepithelioma, syringoma, and trichoadenoma.[2] Ductal features differentiate MAC from desmoplastic trichoepithelioma and trichoadenoma. Asymmetry, single-cell strands, and perineural and intramuscular (deep) invasion differentiate MAC from a syringoma (which tend to be symmetric, circular, and well-circumscribed). Squamous cell carcinoma and metastatic breast carcinoma are also diagnostic considerations.[4]

Immunohistochemistry can help distinguish MAC from other tumors, and highlights eccrine and pilar differentiation.[12] Carcinoembryonic antigen (CEA), epithelial membrane antigen (EMA), and cytokeratin stains are most reliable. Broad-spectrum antikeratin antibodies (AE1/AE3) strongly stain epithelial cells in MAC. EMA stains ductal structures.[15,18] CEA (which is positive in MAC) helps differentiate microcystic adnexal carcinoma from desmoplastic trichoepithelioma.[10,11]

Treatment

Surgical modalities are most definitive in the treatment of microcystic adnexal carcinoma. Incompletely excised lesions will recur. Recurrence rates for conventional excision may be as high as 47% (usually within the first 3 years).[12] Mohs micrographic surgery is invaluable for tissue sparing and may increase the chance of cure with fewer procedures. Recurrence rates for Mohs surgery range from 0% to 22% with a 5-year follow-up (Table 1). Currently, most primary tumors are treated with wide local excision (87% of cases in the SEER database), with 10.8% of cases treated with Mohs micrographic surgery.[7] Multiple case series and one prospective study have examined the efficacy of Mohs surgery for treatment of MAC (see Table 1).

Table 1
Treatment of microcystic adnexal carcinoma with Mohs surgery

Author/Year	Study Type	Number of Cases Treated With Mohs	Primary Vs Recurrent at Time of Referral for Mohs	Number of Recurrences (%)	Average Follow-up
Friedman et al, 1999[12]	Retrospective	11	9 vs 2	0 (0%)	5 y
Chiller et al, 2000[9]	Retrospective	25	19 vs 6	2 (8%)	3.2 y
Abbate et al, 2003[10]	Retrospective	6	Not specified	0 (0%)	23.3 mo
Leibovitch et al, 2005[4]	Prospective	44	30 vs 14	1 (5%)	5 y
Thomas et al, 2007[3]	Retrospective	25	19 vs 6	3 (12%)	39 mo
Snow et al, 2001[13]	Retrospective	13	10 vs 3	0 (0%)	5 y
Palamaras et al, 2010[20]	Retrospective	9	6 vs 3	2 (22%)	5.4 y
Hamm et al, 1987[27]	Retrospective	3	1 vs 2	0 (0%)	19 mo
Burns et al, 1994[28]	Retrospective	10	6 vs 4	0 (0%)	25 mo

Only one prospective study evaluating Mohs surgery for the treatment of MAC has been reported. Leibovitch and colleagues[4] reported 44 cases treated with Mohs surgery; tumor recurrence rate was 5% with a 5-year follow-up. In this series, recurrent tumors referred for treatment with Mohs surgery needed more stages to clear, had larger postoperative defects, and were more likely to have perineural invasion.

Other studies detailing Mohs surgery for the treatment of MAC are retrospective in nature. One of the larger retrospective studies at UCSF involved 48 patients treated with either Mohs surgery or conventional excision. Mohs defects were four times larger than clinically evident tumors. An average of 2.6 stages were necessary to clear the tumor (range, 1–4). Notably, 30% of patients with conventional excision had positive margins and needed additional surgery. No patients treated with Mohs surgery needed further treatment. Both groups experienced similar complication rates. Clear margins and therefore fewer procedures were noted in the Mohs treatment group.[9] Another retrospective review of 10 patients compared Mohs surgery with

conventional excision. Six patients were treated with excision, and 33% of those needed additional procedures to clear the tumor. One recurrence was noted (16.7%), with an average follow-up of 32 months. The other four patients were treated with Mohs surgery, and no additional procedures were needed. The average number of stages needed to clear the tumor was 2.5 (range, 1–4). No recurrences were noted in the Mohs group almost 2 years after. In this series, clear margins with fewer procedures were obtained with Mohs surgery.[10]

Another retrospective review of 26 cases of MAC treated with Mohs surgery had a 12% recurrence rate (mean follow-up 39 months). The mean number of stages to clear the tumor in this series was three. Importantly, postoperative defects were larger than expected when compared with the preoperative clinical assessment of tumor margin. Tumors were more likely to recur after Mohs surgery if the tumor at initial presentation was recurrent rather than primary.[3]

Immunostains may highlight tumor cells, further delineating histologic margins during Mohs surgery. Special stains are especially useful in

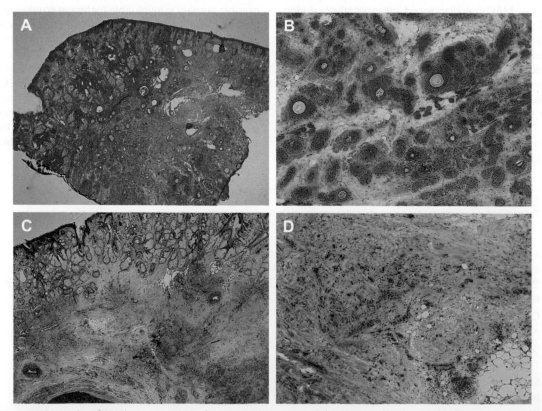

Fig. 2. Microcystic adnexal carcinoma on frozen sections prepared intraoperatively during Mohs surgery using hematoxylin and eosin (*A* at 20×, *B* at 100×) and toluidine blue (*C* at 20×, *D* at 100×). Note the tumor islands are highlighted in a magenta color with toluidine blue stain.

banal-appearing tumors, especially if significant inflammation is present to mask the tumor cells. Immunostains tend to work well on frozen sections because the target antigen is preserved in tissue processing. Unfortunately, immunostains are time-consuming (in processing and interpretation) and costly. Special stains helpful in the evaluation of MAC were discussed in further detail earlier, but in summary include CEA, AE1/AE3, and EMA (positive); other immunostains such as CK20 are negative.[18]

Paraffin sections are occasionally used during staged excisions (also known as *slow Mohs*) to improve tumor detection. The surgeon sends a final layer for paraffin embedding for further margin control. This method is slower than preparing frozen sections, but permanent paraffin sections are often easier to interpret then frozen sections.[12,19] In a retrospective review of nine cases treated with Mohs surgery, two were found to have perineural invasion in tumors located around the eye. Both tumors persisted after Mohs surgery, indicating incomplete histologic clearance. Recurrence may have arguably been prevented had an additional layer been submitted for permanent sectioning. These authors recommend sending an additional layer for permanent sectioning after apparent tumor clearance, especially if the tumor is in a periocular location with involvement of deep ocular fat, or exhibits perineural involvement.[20]

Toluidine blue staining may also be useful in detecting subtle tumor islands in microcystic adnexal carcinoma. Toluidine blue is useful in Mohs surgery because it stains tumor stroma pink, identifying mucopolysaccharides such as hyaluronic acid.[21] Developing a rapid staining technique using toluidine blue makes this stain easy to use in conjunction with frozen sections. For example, when toluidine blue is used to evaluate basal cell carcinoma treated with Mohs, the total time for tissue processing is less than 2.5 minutes when the solution is alkalinized.[22] MAC has many small nests and clusters of tumor cells that can easily be missed, and therefore toluidine blue may be useful because it stains stroma metachromatically, highlighting small nests or strands of cells and perineural involvement (**Fig. 2**).[23]

Long-term follow-up is important in patients with MAC. Cases of local recurrence have been reported 30 years after initial treatment.[24]

Special considerations
Because of the subtle clinical findings and banal appearance histologically, MAC can grow undiagnosed for years. Rarely, the tumor is inoperable because of large size and involvement of vital

structures. One case reports a 58-year-old woman with an MAC on her forehead, nasal root, cheek, and upper lip (area roughly 12 × 12 cm). After consultation with plastic surgery, the patient elected observation, and at 2-year follow-up was doing well without evidence of metastasis.[25]

Reports of radiotherapy for treatment of MAC are inconclusive. Radiotherapy may even be dangerous, converting the tumor to a more aggressive undifferentiated form.[26] Most patients are not treated with adjuvant radiation.[7] Although chemotherapy is not first-line treatment, it may be useful in patients with widespread disease who have no other treatment options.[25]

SUMMARY

MAC is a rare neoplasm with a propensity for slow growth and extensive local invasion. Mohs surgery allows for fewer procedures and increased likelihood of long-term cure and tissue conservation. Mohs surgery is especially useful in recurrent tumors and those with perineural invasion.

REFERENCES

1. Weedon D. Tumors of cutaneous appendages. In: Weedon D, editor. Skin pathology. 2nd edition. Philadelphia: Elsevier; 2002. p. 895–6.
2. Goldstein DJ, Barr RJ, Santa Cruz DJ. Microcystic adnexal carcinoma: a distinct clinicopathologic entity. Cancer 1982;50(3):566–72.
3. Thomas CJ, Wood GC, Marks VJ. Mohs micrographic surgery in the treatment of rare aggressive cutaneous tumors: the Geisinger experience. Dermatol Surg 2007;33(3):333–9.
4. Leibovitch I, Huilgol SC, Selva D, et al. Microcystic adnexal carcinoma: treatment with Mohs micrographic surgery. J Am Acad Dermatol 2005;52(2):295–300.
5. Callahan EF, Vidimos AT, Bergfeld WF. Microcystic adnexal carcinoma (MAC) of the scalp with extensive pilar differentiation. Dermatol Surg 2002;28(6):536–9.
6. McAlvany JP, Stonecipher MR, Leshin B, et al. Sclerosing sweat duct carcinoma in an 11-year-old boy. J Dermatol Surg Oncol 1994;20(11):767–8.
7. Yu JB, Blitzblau RC, Patel SC, et al. Surveillance, epidemiology, and end results (SEER) database analysis of microcystic adnexal carcinoma (sclerosing sweat duct carcinoma) of the skin. Am J Clin Oncol 2010;33(2):125–7.
8. Nadiminti H, Nadiminti U, Washington C. Microcystic adnexal carcinoma in African-Americans. Dermatol Surg 2007;33(11):1384–7.
9. Chiller K, Passaro D, Scheuller M, et al. Microcystic adnexal carcinoma: forty-eight cases, their treatment,

and their outcome. Arch Dermatol 2000;136(11): 1355–9.

10. Abbate M, Zeitouni NC, Seyler M, et al. Clinical course, risk factors, and treatment of microcystic adnexal carcinoma: a short series report. Dermatol Surg 2003;29(10):1035–8.

11. Antley CA, Carney M, Smoller BR. Microcystic adnexal carcinoma arising in the setting of previous radiation therapy. J Cutan Pathol 1999;26(1):48–50.

12. Friedman PM, Friedman RH, Jiang SB, et al. Microcystic adnexal carcinoma: collaborative series review and update. J Am Acad Dermatol 1999; 41(2 Pt 1):225–31.

13. Snow S, Madjar DD, Hardy S, et al. Microcystic adnexal carcinoma: report of 13 cases and review of the literature. Dermatol Surg 2001;27(4):401–8.

14. Carroll P, Goldstein GD, Brown CW Jr. Metastatic microcystic adnexal carcinoma in an immunocompromised patient. Dermatol Surg 2000;26(6):531–4.

15. Nagatsuka H, Rivera RS, Gunduz M, et al. Microcystic adnexal carcinoma with mandibular bone marrow involvement: a case report with immunohistochemistry. Am J Dermatopathol 2006;28(6):518–22.

16. LeBoit PE, Sexton M. Microcystic adnexal carcinoma of the skin. A reappraisal of the differentiation and differential diagnosis of an underrecognized neoplasm. J Am Acad Dermatol 1993;29(4):609–18.

17. Pujol RM, LeBoit PE, Su WP. Microcystic adnexal carcinoma with extensive sebaceous differentiation. Am J Dermatopathol 1997;19(4):358–62.

18. Thosani MK, Marghoob A, Chen CS. Current progress of immunostains in Mohs micrographic surgery: a review. Dermatol Surg 2008;34(12):1621–36.

19. Barlow RJ, Ramnarain N, Smith N, et al. Excision of selected skin tumours using Mohs' micrographic surgery with horizontal paraffin-embedded sections. Br J Dermatol 1996;135(6):911–7.

20. Palamaras I, McKenna JD, Robson A, et al. Microcystic adnexal carcinoma: a case series treated with Mohs micrographic surgery and identification of patients in whom paraffin sections may be preferable. Dermatol Surg 2010;36(4):446–52.

21. Humphreys TR, Nemeth A, McCrevey S, et al. A pilot study comparing toluidine blue and hematoxylin and eosin staining of basal cell and squamous cell carcinoma during Mohs surgery. Dermatol Surg 1996;22(8):693–7.

22. Todd MM, Lee JW, Marks VJ. Rapid toluidine blue stain for Mohs' micrographic surgery. Dermatol Surg 2005;31(2):244–5.

23. Wang SQ, Goldberg LH, Nemeth A. The merits of adding toluidine blue-stained slides in Mohs surgery in the treatment of a microcystic adnexal carcinoma. J Am Acad Dermatol 2007;56(6):1067–9.

24. Lupton GP, McMarlin SL. Microcystic adnexal carcinoma. report of a case with 30-year follow-up. Arch Dermatol 1986;122(3):286–9.

25. Eisen DB, Zloty D. Microcystic adnexal carcinoma involving a large portion of the face: when is surgery not reasonable? Dermatol Surg 2005;31(11 Pt 1): 1472–7 [discussion: 1478].

26. Stein JM, Ormsby A, Esclamado R, et al. The effect of radiation therapy on microcystic adnexal carcinoma: a case report. Head Neck 2003;25(3):251–4.

27. Hamm JC, Argenta LC, Swanson NA. Microcystic adnexal carcinoma: an unpredictable aggressive neoplasm. Ann Plast Surg 1987;19(2):173–80.

28. Burns MK, Chen SP, Goldberg LH. Microcystic adnexal carcinoma. Ten cases treated by Mohs micrographic surgery. J Dermatol Surg Oncol 1994;20(7):429–34.

Advances in Management of Dermatofibrosarcoma Protuberans

Hillary Johnson-Jahangir, MD, PhD*, Désirée Ratner, MD

KEYWORDS

- Dermatofibrosarcoma protuberans • Skin sarcoma
- Mohs micrographic surgery • Wide local excision
- Complete circumferential peripheral and deep
margin assessment • Platelet-derived growth factor
- Targeted therapy

Dermatofibrosarcoma protuberans (DFSP) is an uncommon, low-grade soft tissue neoplasm accounting for less than approximately 0.1% of all cancers and 1% of all soft tissue sarcomas. The overall annual incidence of DFSP is 4.2 per million of all cancers as reported in the Surveillance, Epidemiology, and End Results (SEER) cancer registries. The incidence rate is higher among blacks compared with other groups (6.5 cases per million population), but the incidence among whites has been slowly increasing over the past 30 years, in part due to improved diagnostic immunohistochemical techniques. DFSP develops at approximately equal rates between women and men except in older individuals (>70 years), in whom men have a higher incidence.[1,2]

CLINICAL PRESENTATION

DFSP growth is characteristically indolent. These tumors enlarge gradually over a period of years, but may present with extensive subclinical invasion into underlying subcutaneous tissue, fascia, muscle, or even bone. The broadly infiltrative nature of DFSP contributes to its high rate of local recurrence following treatment with standard surgical excision.

Although DFSP can occur congenitally or in childhood, it most commonly presents in adults between the ages of 30 and 50.[2] Fewer than 10% of DFSPs are diagnosed before the age of 20, and the incidence of this tumor in childhood may in fact be underestimated, since the diagnosis is often delayed. Congenital DFSP can have a variable presentation and may be challenging to definitively remove if the diagnosis is not made early or if scarring from incomplete excision is present.[3]

DFSP classically appears as a violaceous or erythematous nodular plaque (Fig. 1) but can also feature skin-colored, erythematous, brown-tinged, or yellow-tinged areas within patches, nodules, or plaques. Areas of induration, telangiectasia, or atrophy may be evident at presentation or may appear over time. Its clinical appearance can vary from indistinct small plaques to large, exophytic tumors that can bleed or ulcerate. Early lesions tend to be asymptomatic but can become painful over months to years due to deeper tissue invasion or accelerated growth.[4] Development of DFSP or acceleration of its growth has been associated with trauma and scars, including sites of vaccination, as well as pregnancy.[5–7] While predominantly located on the trunk (42%) and extremities (34%),[8–10] DFSP may also occur on the head and neck, and in these locations it is associated with a greater risk of morbidity and local recurrence.

The authors have nothing to disclose.
Department of Dermatology, Columbia University Medical Center, 161 Fort Washington Avenue, 12th Floor, New York, NY 10032, USA
* Corresponding author.
E-mail address: hillary.johnson@gmail.com

Dermatol Clin 29 (2011) 191–200
doi:10.1016/j.det.2011.02.003

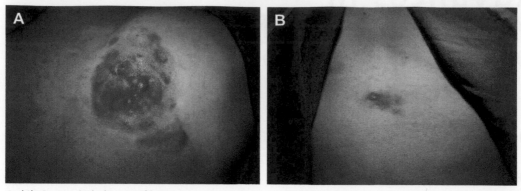

Fig. 1. (*A*) Congenital dermatofibrosarcoma protuberans of the back at presentation in a 16-year-old boy, featuring various morphologic clinical features, including plaques, nodules, atrophy, telangiectasia, and scar-like changes. (*B*) Dermatofibrosarcoma protuberans on the mid-abdomen.

Together with its often-benign clinical appearance, the rare nature of DFSP and its tendency for indolent growth can prompt diagnostic challenges. Clinically, DFSP can be mistaken for hypertrophic or keloidal scarring, morphea, epidermoid cysts, melanoma, or metastatic neoplasms. In congenital DFSP, early lesions may be difficult to distinguish from vascular malformations, infantile fibromatosis or myofibromatosis, fibrosarcoma, or fibrous hamartoma.[3]

STAGING AND PROGNOSIS

A definitive staging system that can assist with prediction of patient outcomes does not yet exist for DFSP. In some cases, the Short German Guidelines or the general American Musculoskeletal Tumor Society Staging System, which take into account high- or low-grade histopathology, local tumor extension, or distant spread, may be helpful,[11,12] but the 5-year survival for classical DFSP is over 99%. Imaging studies for staging purposes are typically not required, since tumor involvement is most frequently limited to local disease. If metastasis occurs, it spreads most frequently to regional lymph nodes. While distant metastasis occurs in less than 5% of cases, it is associated with a poor prognosis, with death from widespread metastatic disease typically occurring within 2 years. In advanced, recurrent, or high-grade variants of DFSP, the risk of hematogenous dissemination is greater and most commonly leads to pulmonary metastases. Imaging of the chest using computed tomography (CT) to evaluate for pulmonary metastasis is therefore indicated in high-risk clinical situations. Other potential sites of hematogenous spread include bone, brain, heart, and other soft tissues.

Distant metastasis and disease-specific mortality are usually consequences of local recurrence after inadequate surgical excision.[2,8,13,14] In some prospective case series, disease-free survival after wide local excision correlated inversely with tumor depth, tumor grade, patient age, positive margin after primary resection, or presence of the high-risk fibrosarcomatous variant on histology.

HISTOPATHOLOGY AND IMMUNOHISTOCHEMISTRY

Clinical suspicion for DFSP following a complete skin examination typically requires an incisional skin biopsy to help confirm the diagnosis. Histological features suggestive of DFSP typically include a dense collection of monomorphous fusiform cells forming focal storiform or cartwheel configurations as demonstrated in **Fig. 2**A. Early lesions may feature an area of dermal sparing, or a Grenz zone, which is clearly seen just beneath the epidermis.[15] Coursing through the dermis and infiltrating the subcutaneous fat (see **Fig. 2**B), an extensive proliferation of spindle cells disrupts the adipose tissue architecture and creates a honeycomb or lace-like appearance. Deeper projections into fascia or muscle can further complicate demarcation of the tumor border and subsequent surgical management.[16] Determination of the precise surgical margin in DFSP can be challenging owing to the tumor's bland histologic appearance and diffuse infiltration, as well as its similarity to other neoplasms. Occasionally DFSP can be difficult to distinguish from dermatofibroma, dermatomyofibroma, fibrosarcoma, leiomyoscarcoma, malignant fibrous histiocytoma (also called pleomorphic scarcoma), or atypical fibroxanthoma. Dermatofibromas have

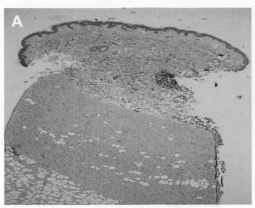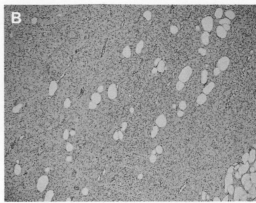

Fig. 2. (A) Biopsy specimen showing bundles of spindle cells in the dermis extending into the subcutaneous fat (hematoxylin–eosin stain; original magnification ×4). (B) Higher-power view (original magnification ×10) demonstrating spindle cells arranged in a storiform pattern and infiltrating the subcutaneous fat.

a tendency to be better demarcated and to have less infiltrative subdermal peripheral extension compared with DFSP. Malignant fibrous histiocytoma and atypical fibroxanthoma display greater mitotic activity and pleomorphism than DFSP.

Approximately 10% of DFSPs transform into a high-grade fibrosarcomatous variant with increased cellularity, mitosis, and pleomorphic spindle cells in a herringbone configuration deep in the dermis.[13,17–20] Other uncommon variants of DFSP include pigmented DFSP, also called Bednar tumor, which occurs in approximately 1% of patients, possibly with a higher incidence among blacks.[2,8] DFSPs with myofibroblastic, myxoid, and neurofibromatous differentiation have been rarely reported.[21–24] The giant cell fibroblastoma variant demonstrates areas with spindle-shaped cells in a myxoid background with characteristic multinucleated giant cells.[25,26]

Additional immunohistochemical markers may be used to improve diagnostic accuracy when required. Besides human hematopoietic progenitor cells, CD34 antigen is expressed by a subpopulation of dermal dendritic cells and has been shown to be selectively expressed in DFSP. Nodular or fibrosarcomatous areas of DFSP may exhibit variable expression of CD34, reducing the sensitivity of this marker.[8] CD34 can help to differentiate DFSP from dermatofibroma. In many cases, DFSP stains positively for CD34 and negatively for factor XIIIa, whereas dermatofibroma is CD34-negative and factor XIIIa-positive.[24] Neural markers (S-100) can help distinguish DFSP from desmoplastic melanoma, neurofibroma, schwannoma, and malignant peripheral nerve sheath tumor. Rarely, DFSP with neurofibromatous changes may be focally positive for immunostaining with S-100.[27] The cytoplasmic histiocyte immunohistochemical marker, CD68, selectively stains for malignant fibrous histiocytoma and atypical fibroxanthoma, but not for DFSP, facilitating the distinction of these other two spindle cell tumors from DFSP.

PATHOGENESIS OF DFSP

DFSP is thought to originate from cutaneous mesenchymal cells. In accordance with the cancer stem cell hypothesis, mutations in multipotent cutaneous mesenchymal stem cells residing in the connective tissue sheath or hair follicle papillae putatively induce formation of DFSP neoplasms.[1,28] Advances in understanding the molecular pathogenesis of DFSP have enabled positive identification of most of these tumors using modern molecular diagnostic techniques. Characteristic cytogenetic chromosomal alterations can now be detected in over 90% of patients with DFSP.[29] Aberrations in chromosomes 17 and 22 were first identified in DFSP in 1990 (Fig. 3A).[30,31] At the cytogenetic level, DFSP harbors either supernumerary ring chromosomes or translocations that are often unbalanced. The supernumerary ring chromosomes combine portions of chromosome 17 with chromosome 22 in a circular formation (see Fig. 3B). Instead of forming rings, t(17;22) translocations connect chromosomes 17 and 22 in a linear manner (see Fig. 3C). Karyotype analysis using fluorescence in situ hybridization (FISH) can detect these chromosomal anomalies within DFSP cells in tissue samples. In case series, supernumerary ring chromosomes are more common in adult DFSP cases

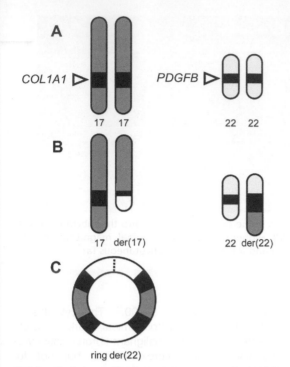

Fig. 3. Chromosomal rearrangements in dermatofibrosarcoma protuberans. (*A*) Schematic representation of normal chromosomes 17 and 22 including the approximate locations of the COL1A1 and PDGFB genes, respectively. (*B*) Diagram of a balanced translocation derived from juxtaposition of the long arms of chromosomes 17 and 22. (*C*) Diagram illustrating the combination of DNA sequences from chromosomes 17 and 22 forming a supernumerary ring chromosome derived from chromosome 22.

while translocations predominate in the pediatric population.[32]

Juxtaposition of chromosomes 17 and 22 in both rings and translocations results in oncogenic fusion of the type 1 alpha I collagen gene (COL1A1) and the beta chain of platelet-derived growth factor (PDGFB) gene. Under normal circumstances, active transcription of the COL1A1 gene produces type 1 collagen, the most abundant protein in the body. Aberrant linkage of the genetic elements that usually drive expression of the COL1A1 gene with that of the PDGFB gene results in amplified expression of PDGFB protein. Overproduction of PDGFB leads to autocrine or paracrine stimulation of its cellular receptor, the PDGF receptor (PDGFR), a cell–surface receptor tyrosine kinase. Since PDGFB serves as a potent cellular growth factor, its overexpression is thought to contribute to tumorigenesis.[33–35] The COL1A1-PDGFB fusion has also been shown to be present in several

uncommon variants including pigmented DFSP (Bednar tumor).[32] The chimeric COL1A1-PDGFB gene fusion can be detected at the DNA level using polymerase chain reaction (PCR) technology, which serves as another diagnostic tool for analyzing tissue samples suspicious for DFSP. Although useful in diagnostic testing, the cytogenetic aberrations in chromosomes 17 and 22 that characterize most DFSP tumors have not been shown to influence or predict clinical outcomes. There is no correlation between COL1A1 breakpoints on chromosome 17 and any particular clinical or histopathologic characteristics.[29,36]

MANAGEMENT OF DFSP: OVERVIEW

Since DFSP tumors exhibit unpredictable and widespread subclinical extension, surgical excision with comprehensive margin evaluation prior to reconstruction is the optimal treatment of choice for DFSP. When a surgical margin is positive or narrow without the possibility of further surgery, use of adjuvant therapies might salvage local control. Alternatives or adjuncts to surgical management include radiation therapy and imatinib (Gleevec) for advanced, recurrent, or metastatic DFSP. Conventional chemotherapy is considered generally ineffective. The uncommon incidence of DFSP precludes development of therapeutic strategies based on clinical evidence from randomized data or comparative studies assessing treatment modalities in parallel. Consensus treatment guidelines developed by the National Comprehensive Cancer Network derive from published case series featuring predominantly retrospective analyses. A basic algorithm for surgical management of DFSP is diagrammed in **Fig. 4**. Because DFSP recurrence after years and

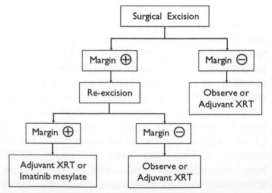

Fig. 4. Therapeutic algorithm for surgical management of dermatofibrosarcoma protuberans.

decades has been a concern, at least semiannual clinical examination for observation is recommended, especially in the first 3 years following surgery, during which 80% of recurrences are thought to occur.[4,37–39]

MANAGEMENT OF DFSP: SURGICAL EXCISION

The deeply infiltrative nature of DFSP necessitates excision at least to the level of the underlying fascia. In addition to physical examination for fixation to deeper structures and the presence or absence of regional lymphadenopathy, presurgical imaging using magnetic resonance imaging (MRI) or CT if bony involvement is suspected can help define the extent of tumor spread.[4,40]

The lowest DFSP recurrence rates have been demonstrated following excision using the Mohs micrographic surgery (MMS) technique or wide local excision (WLE) combined with complete circumferential peripheral and deep margin assessment (CPPDMA).[41–46] Immunostaining with CD34 is sometimes used adjunctively during specimen processing. In the MMS procedure, the excised specimen is uniquely processed for microscopic examination using fresh tissue that is frozen and sliced horizontally or tangentially into serial sections for complete margin evaluation (**Fig. 5**A). The entire peripheral epidermal edge and tissue depth can be visualized in the horizontal plane, since MMS excision allows for relative flattening of the surgical specimen. The process is repeated, often the same day, until the surgical margin is clear. Alternatively, a permanently fixed specimen excised using wide excision can be processed for CPPDMA or full-margin analysis. As depicted in **Fig. 5**B, the perimeter of the specimen undergoes en face tangential sectioning while the residual central portion is sectioned horizontally at the base. Closure of the surgical wound may be delayed if re-excision is needed to remove any residual tumor. These thorough methods for tissue processing yield superior margin assessment, with 5 year recurrence rates as low as 0–1.7%.[42,43,45,47] When wide excision may not be feasible, as in locations on the head and neck or distal extremities (featured in **Fig. 6**A and B, respectively), MMS offers greater tissue-sparing potential in addition to the meticulous margin control, which is critical for minimizing likelihood of recurrence.[48] Wide excision with traditional vertical sectioning or bread loafing (see **Fig. 5**C) produces transverse slices through the excised specimen with the epidermal edge positioned above its adjacent subdermal structures. This approach represents a random sampling in which

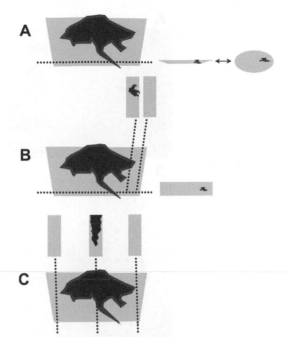

Fig. 5. Options for processing surgical specimens for microscopic examination. (*A*) In Mohs micrographic surgery, fresh tissue is precisely mapped and oriented, flattened, frozen, and sectioned horizontally for visualization of the base and complete peripheral epidermal border. (*B*) En face tangential sectioning combined with horizontal sectioning of the base of a permanently fixed, paraffin-embedded surgical specimen enables complete circumferential peripheral and deep margin assessment following wide local excision. (*C*) Traditional vertical sectioning of a permanently fixed, paraffin-embedded surgical specimen derived from wide local excision featuring transverse bread loaf-style sections with characteristic skip areas that might possess residual tumor.

a minimum of 5% of the surgical margin is examined, leaving a bulk of the margin unchecked, with risk of false-negative interpretation and tumor regrowth.[43,49]

MANAGEMENT OF DFSP: RADIATION THERAPY

In small retrospective case series, field treatment using fractionated radiation therapy for patients with a high risk of residual disease appears to improve local control in some cases. Radiation therapy also may be considered for patients with metastatic or recurrent DFSP in whom surgical excision may not be feasible or effective. Close monitoring is required subsequently, however, since radiation therapy may induce new or more aggressive tumors.[37,50–57]

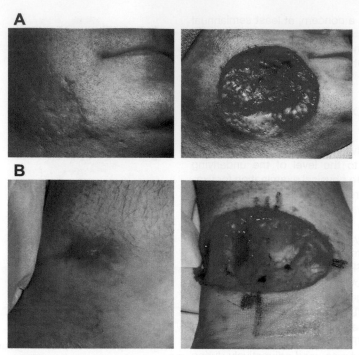

Fig. 6. Recurrent dermatofibrosarcoma protuberans of the (*A*) cheek and (*B*) lateral ankle alongside their respective surgical defects following Mohs micrographic surgical excision.

MANAGEMENT OF DFSP: TARGETED MOLECULAR INHIBITION

Understanding of the molecular pathogenesis of DFSP serves as a basis for targeted molecular therapy to counteract the constitutively active PDGFR.[58] Because over 90% of DFSPs feature detectable chromosomal rearrangements leading to excessive production of the PDGFR ligand, pharmaceutical agents arresting tumor growth by blocking PDGFR activity are beneficial (**Fig. 7**). Imatinib mesylate is a selective tyrosine kinase inhibitor (TKI) with efficacy against the tyrosine kinase receptors PDGFR, KIT, and Abl/Bcr-Abl.[58] Approved by the US Food and Drug Administration (FDA) in 2006, imatinib is indicated as a single agent or adjuvant treatment for patients with unresectable, recurrent, or metastatic DFSP. Imatinib has been shown to induce partial or complete regression of DFSP in approximately one-half to two-thirds of patients treated at a dose of 800 mg daily. It has a favorable safety profile and tolerability, and its generally mild adverse effects tend not to be treatment limiting.[59–64] Long-term outcomes with respect to local margin control and disease-free survival are unknown for this novel drug therapy for DFSP. Also, the ideal drug dosage and duration of therapy have not yet been elucidated. Building on the successful use

of imatinib, it is anticipated that other molecular inhibitors of DFSP may be identified.

Off-label use of imatinib in the months prior to surgery has been shown to reduce preoperative tumor sizes and facilitate effective excision.[65] Several individual reports and small case series have confirmed that neoadjuvant imatinib can reduce tumor burden, thereby limiting postoperative morbidity in difficult cases where complete surgical excision of DFSP might cause deformity or disability.[66–70] Neoadjuvant imatinib alters the histologic appearance of the residual tumor, inducing decreased cellularity plus hyalinization of dermal collagen.[65,71,72] However, these histologic findings have not been shown to affect outcomes in the few patients whose clinical course was monitored over several years.[65,71,72]

Because the pathogenic COL1A1-PDGFB gene fusion is not always detected in DFSP, tumorigenesis may be induced by other genetic aberrations or cryptic molecular arrangements.[32] These tumors, which do not depend on the PDGFR signaling pathway for growth, have been shown not to respond to imatinib.[60,73] Confirming the presence of the COL1A1-PDGFB gene fusion prior to initiation of imatinib, by requesting genetic analysis using FISH or PCR, may help to predict the clinical response.[29,36,74]

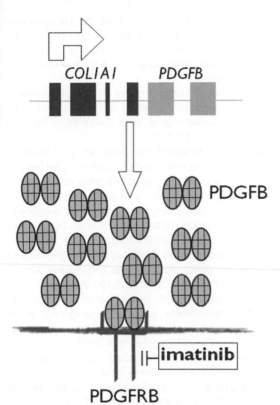

Fig. 7. Illustration depicting the molecular pathogenesis of dermatofibrosarcoma protuberans. The COL1A1-PDGFB fusion gene with the highly active COL1A1 promoter constitutively drives downstream expression of the gene for PDGFB. Excessive production of PDGFB causes concomitant overstimulation of the PDGFR. Imatinib blocks PDGFR activity by selectively inhibiting its receptor tyrosine kinase activity.

SUMMARY

Because DFSP is a rare cutaneous malignancy, the clinical evidence for treatment recommendations is inherently limited. Surgical excision endures as the first-line approach for effective management of DFSP. Advanced tissue processing techniques permitting complete histopathologic assessment of the peripheral and deep surgical margins can reduce risk of local recurrence, particularly for tumors arising in high-risk locations, or locations lacking tissue reserves required for wider excision. A multidisciplinary approach to management is valuable in the event of recurrence, distant metastasis, or consideration of adjuvant therapies for large or difficult tumors. The recent discovery that DFSP is induced by cytogenetic rearrangements resulting in overproduction of PDGFB has served as a foundation for targeted inhibition by imatinib, a selective and potent inhibitor of the PDGFR tyrosine kinase.

Although studies have been limited to small numbers of patients, imatinib induces a partial or complete clinical response in most cases and is well tolerated. Additional experience and clinical investigations will help to delineate parameters for therapeutic usage and applications of imatinib and other novel molecular inhibitors targeted for DFSP.

ACKNOWLEDGMENTS

We thank George Niedt, MD, for expert assistance with dermatopathology.

REFERENCES

1. Mori T, Misago N, Yamamoto O, et al. Expression of nestin in dermatofibrosarcoma protuberans in comparison to dermatofibroma. J Dermatol 2008; 35(7):419–25.
2. Criscione VD, Weinstock MA. Descriptive epidemiology of dermatofibrosarcoma protuberans in the United States, 1973 to 2002. J Am Acad Dermatol 2007;56(6):968–73.
3. Love WE, Keiler SA, Tamburro JE, et al. Surgical management of congenital dermatofibrosarcoma protuberans. J Am Acad Dermatol 2009;61(6): 1014–23.
4. Mendenhall WM, Zlotecki RA, Scarborough MT. Dermatofibrosarcoma protuberans. Cancer 2004; 101(11):2503–8.
5. Elgart GW, Hanly A, Busso M, et al. Bednar tumor (pigmented dermatofibrosarcoma protuberans) occurring in a site of prior immunization: immunochemical findings and therapy. J Am Acad Dermatol 1999;40:315–7.
6. Parlette LE, Smith CK, Germain LM, et al. Accelerated growth of dermatofibrosarcoma protuberans during pregnancy. J Am Acad Dermatol 1999;41: 778–83.
7. Har-Shai Y, Govrin-Yehudain J, Ullmann Y, et al. Dermatofibrosarcoma protuberans appearing during pregnancy. Ann Plast Surg 1993;31(1):91–3.
8. Gloster HM Jr. Dermatofibrosarcoma protuberans. J Am Acad Dermatol 1996;35:355–74 [quiz: 375–6].
9. Weinstein JM, Drolet BA, Esterly NB, et al. Congenital dermatofibrosarcoma protuberans: variability in presentation. Arch Dermatol 2003;139(2):207–11.
10. Maire G, Fraitag S, Galmiche L, et al. A clinical, histologic, and molecular study of 9 cases of congenital dermatofibrosarcoma protuberans. Arch Dermatol 2007;143(2):203–10.
11. Ugurel S, Kortmann RD, Mohr P, et al. Short German guidelines: dermatofibrosarcoma protuberans. J Dtsch Dermatol Ges 2008;6(Suppl 1):S17–8.

12. Enneking Spanier WFSS, Goodman MA. A system for the surgical staging of musculoskeletal sarcoma. Clin Orthop Relat Res 1980;(153):106–20.

13. Mentzel T, Beham A, Katenkamp D, et al. Fibrosarcomatous (high-grade) dermatofibrosarcoma protuberans: clinicopathologic and immunohistochemical study of a series of 41 cases with emphasis on prognostic significance. Am J Surg Pathol 1998;22(5):576–87.

14. Rutgers EJ, Kroon BB, Albus-Lutter CE, et al. Dermatofibrosarcoma protuberans: treatment and prognosis. Eur J Surg Oncol 1992;18(3):241–8.

15. Lindner NJ, Scarborough MT, Powell GJ, et al. Revision surgery in dermatofibrosarcoma protuberans of the trunk and extremities. Eur J Surg Oncol 1999;25(4):392–7.

16. Taylor HB, Helwig EB. Dermatofibrosarcoma protuberans. A study of 115 cases. Cancer 1962;15:717–25.

17. Ohtani N, Fukusato T, Tezuka F. Sarcomatous dermatofibrosarcoma protuberans metastasized to the lung: preservation of CD34 expression in tumor cells. Pathol Int 1998;48(12):989–93.

18. Zelger BW, Ofner D, Zelger BG. Atrophic variants of dermatofibroma and dermatofibrosarcoma protuberans. Histopathology 1995;26(6):519–27.

19. Zelger B, Sidoroff A, Stanzl U, et al. Deep penetrating dermatofibroma versus dermatofibrosarcoma protuberans. A clinicopathologic comparison. Am J Surg Pathol 1994;18(7):677–86.

20. Korkolis DP, Liapakis IE, Vassilopoulos PP. Dermatofibrosarcoma protuberans: clinicopathological aspects of an unusual cutaneous tumor. Anticancer Res 2007;27(3B):1631–4.

21. Calonje E, Fletcher CD. Myoid differentiation in dermatofibrosarcoma protuberans and its fibrosarcomatous variant: clinicopathologic analysis of 5 cases. J Cutan Pathol 1996;23(1):30–6.

22. Frierson HF, Cooper PH. Myxoid variant of dermatofibrosarcoma protuberans. Am J Surg Pathol 1983;7(5):445–50.

23. Reimann JD, Fletcher CD. Myxoid dermatofibrosarcoma protuberans: a rare variant analyzed in a series of 23 cases. Am J Surg Pathol 2007;31(9):1371–7.

24. Mentzel T, Scharer L, Kazakov DV, et al. Myxoid dermatofibrosarcoma protuberans: clinicopathologic, immunohistochemical, and molecular analysis of eight cases. Am J Dermatopathol 2007;29(5):443–8.

25. Shmookler BM, Enzinger FM, Weiss SW. Giant cell fibroblastoma. A juvenile form of dermatofibrosarcoma protuberans. Cancer 1989;64(10):2154–61.

26. Macarenco RS, Zamolyi R, Franco MF, et al. Genomic gains of COL1A1-PDFGB occur in the histologic evolution of giant cell fibroblastoma into dermatofibrosarcoma protuberans. Genes Chromosomes Cancer 2008;47(3):260–5.

27. Kovarik CL, Hsu MY, Cockerell CJ. Neurofibromatous changes in dermatofibrosarcoma protuberans: a potential pitfall in the diagnosis of a serious cutaneous soft tissue neoplasm. J Cutan Pathol 2004;31(7):492–6.

28. Sellheyer K, Nelson P, Krahl D. Dermatofibrosarcoma protuberans: a tumour of nestin-positive cutaneous mesenchymal stem cells? Br J Dermatol 2009;161(6):1317–22.

29. Patel KU, Szabo SS, Hernandez VS, et al. Dermatofibrosarcoma protuberans COL1A1-PDGFB fusion is identified in virtually all dermatofibrosarcoma protuberans cases when investigated by newly developed multiplex reverse transcription polymerase chain reaction and fluorescence in situ hybridization assays. Hum Pathol 2008;39(2):184–93.

30. Bridge JA, Neff JR, Sandberg AA. Cytogenetic analysis of dermatofibrosarcoma protuberans. Cancer Genet Cytogenet 1990;49(2):199–202.

31. Mandahl N, Heim S, Willen H, et al. Supernumerary ring chromosome as the sole cytogenetic abnormality in a dermatofibrosarcoma protuberans. Cancer Genet Cytogenet 1990;49(2):273–5.

32. Sirvent N, Maire G, Pedeutour F. Genetics of dermatofibrosarcoma protuberans family of tumors: from ring chromosomes to tyrosine kinase inhibitor treatment. Genes Chromosomes Cancer 2003;37(1):1–19.

33. Pedeutour F, Coindre JM, Sozzi G, et al. Supernumerary ring chromosomes containing chromosome 17 sequences. A specific feature of dermatofibrosarcoma protuberans? Cancer Genet Cytogenet 1994;76(1):1–9.

34. Naeem R, Lux ML, Huang SF, et al. Ring chromosomes in dermatofibrosarcoma protuberans are composed of interspersed sequences from chromosomes 17 and 22. Am J Pathol 1995;147(6):1553–8.

35. Shimizu A, O'Brien KP, Sjoblom T, et al. The dermatofibrosarcoma protuberans-associated collagen type Ialpha1/platelet-derived growth factor (PDGF) B-chain fusion gene generates a transforming protein that is processed to functional PDGF-BB. Cancer Res 1999;59(15):3719–23.

36. Llombart B, Sanmartin O, Lopez-Guerrero JA, et al. Dermatofibrosarcoma protuberans: clinical, pathological, and genetic (COL1A1-PDGFB) study with therapeutic implications. Histopathology 2009;54(7):860–72.

37. Miller SJ, Alam M, Andersen J, et al. Dermatofibrosarcoma protuberans. J Natl Compr Canc Netw 2007;5(5):550–5.

38. Miller SJ, Alam M, Andersen J, et al. The NCCN dermatofibrosarcoma protuberans guidelines, version 1, 2010. Available at: http://www.nccn.org/professionals/physician_gls/f_guidelines.asp. Accessed September 1, 2010.

39. Bowne WB, Antonescu CR, Leung DH, et al. Dermatofibrosarcoma protuberans: a clinicopathologic

analysis of patients treated and followed at a single institution. Cancer 2000;88(12):2711–20.

40. Thornton SL, Reid J, Papay FA, et al. Childhood dermatofibrosarcoma protuberans: role of preoperative imaging. J Am Acad Dermatol 2005;53(1):76–83.

41. DuBay D, Cimmino V, Lowe L, et al. Low recurrence rate after surgery for dermatofibrosarcoma protuberans: a multidisciplinary approach from a single institution. Cancer 2004;100(5):1008–16.

42. Farma JM, Ammori JB, Zager JS, et al. Dermatofibrosarcoma protuberans: how wide should we resect? Ann Surg Oncol 2010;17(8):2112–8.

43. Ratner D, Thomas CO, Johnson TM, et al. Mohs micrographic surgery for the treatment of dermatofibrosarcoma protuberans. Results of a multiinstitutional series with an analysis of the extent of microscopic spread. J Am Acad Dermatol 1997; 37(4):600–13.

44. Gloster HM Jr, Harris KR, Roenigk RK. A comparison between Mohs micrographic surgery and wide surgical excision for the treatment of dormatofibrosarcoma protuberans. J Am Acad Dermatol 1996; 35(1).82–7.

45. Snow SN, Gordon EM, Larson PO, et al. Dermatofibrosarcoma protuberans: a report on 29 patients treated by Mohs micrographic surgery with long-term follow-up and review of the literature. Cancer 2004;101(1):28–38.

46. Hancox JG, Kelley B, Greenway HT Jr. Treatment of dermatofibroma sarcoma protuberans using modified Mohs micrographic surgery: no recurrences and smaller defects. Dermatol Surg 2008;34(6): 780–4.

47. Wacker J, Khan-Durani B, Hartschuh W. Modified Mohs micrographic surgery in the therapy of dermatofibrosarcoma protuberans: analysis of 22 patients. Ann Surg Oncol 2004;11(4):438–44.

48. Loss L, Zeitouni NC. Management of scalp dermatofibrosarcoma protuberans. Dermatol Surg 2005;31: 1428–33.

49. Rapini RP. Comparison of methods for checking surgical margins. J Am Acad Dermatol 1990;23: 288–94.

50. Dagan R, Morris CG, Zlotecki RA, et al. Radiotherapy in the treatment of dermatofibrosarcoma protuberans. Am J Clin Oncol 2005;28(6):537–9.

51. Heuvel ST, Suurmeijer A, Pras E, et al. Dermatofibrosarcoma protuberans: recurrence is related to the adequacy of surgical margins. Eur J Surg Oncol 2010;36(1):89–94.

52. Sun LM, Wang CJ, Huang CC, et al. Dermatofibrosarcoma protuberans: treatment results of 35 cases. Radiother Oncol 2000;57(2):175–81.

53. Ballo MT, Zagarts GK, Pisters P, et al. The role of radiation therapy in the management of dermatofibrosarcoma protuberans. Int J Radiat Oncol Biol Phys 1998;40(4):823–7.

54. Haas RL, Keus RB, Loftus BM, et al. The role of radiotherapy in the local management of dermatofibrosarcoma protuberans. Soft Tissue Tumours Working Group. Eur J Cancer 1997;33(7):1055–60.

55. Suit H, Spiro I, Mankin HJ, et al. Radiation in management of patients with dermatofibrosarcoma protuberans. J Clin Oncol 1996;14(8):2365–9.

56. Mark RJ, Bailet JW, Tran LM, et al. Dermatofibrosarcoma protuberans of the head and neck. A report of 16 cases. Arch Otolaryngol Head Neck Surg 1993; 119(8):891–6.

57. Marks LB, Suit HD, Rosenberg AE, et al. Dermatofibrosarcoma protuberans treated with radiation therapy. Int J Radiat Oncol Biol Phys 1989;17(2): 379–84.

58. Capdeville R, Silberman S. Imatinib: a targeted clinical drug development. Semin Hematol 2003;40:15–20.

59. Lemm D, Mügge LO, Mentzel T, et al. Current treatment options in dermatofibrosarcoma protuberans. J Cancer Res Clin Oncol 2009;135(5):653–65.

60. McArthur GA. Molecular targeting of dermatofibrosarcoma protuberans: a new approach to a surgical disease. J Natl Compr Canc Netw 2007;5(5): 557–62.

61. McArthur G. Dermatofibrosarcoma protuberans: recent clinical progress. Ann Surg Oncol 2007; 14(10):2876–86.

62. Abrams TA, Schuetze SM. Targeted therapy for dermatofibrosarcoma protuberans. Curr Oncol Rep 2006;8(4):291–6.

63. Rutkowski P, Van Glabbeke M, Rankin CJ, et al. Imatinib mesylate in advanced dermatofibrosarcoma protuberans: pooled analysis of two phase II clinical trials. J Clin Oncol 2010;28(10):1772–9.

64. Food and Drug Administration. Gleevec (Imatinib Mesylate) questions and answers. Available at: http://www.fda.gov/drugs/drugsafety/postmarketdrugsafety informationforpatientsandproviders/ucm110502.htm. Accessed September 1, 2010.

65. Han A, Chen EH, Niedt G, et al. Neoadjuvant imatinib therapy for dermatofibrosarcoma protuberans. Arch Dermatol 2009;145(7):792–6.

66. McArthur GA, Demetri GD, van Oosterom A, et al. Molecular and clinical analysis of locally advanced dermatofibrosarcoma protuberans treated with imatinib: Imatinib Target Exploration Consortium Study B2225. J Clin Oncol 2005;23(4):866–73.

67. Mehrany K, Swanson NA, Heinrich MC, et al. Dermatofibrosarcoma protuberans: a partial response to imatinib therapy. Dermatol Surg 2006;32(3): 456–9.

68. Wright TI, Petersen JE. Treatment of recurrent dermatofibrosarcoma protuberans with imatinib mesylate, followed by Mohs micrographic surgery. Dermatol Surg 2007;33(6):741–4.

69. Lemm D, Muegge LO, Hoeffken K, et al. Remission with Imatinib mesylate treatment in a patient with

initially unresectable dermatofibrosarcoma protuberans—a case report. Oral Maxillofac Surg 2008;
12(4):209–13.

70. Mattox AK, Mehta AI, Grossi PM, et al. Response of
malignant scalp dermatofibrosarcoma to presurgical targeted growth factor inhibition. J Neurosurg
2010;112(5):965–77.

71. Sciot R, Debiec-Rychter M. GIST under imatinib
therapy. Semin Diagn Pathol 2006;23(2):84–90.

72. Thomison J, McCarter M, McClain D, et al.
Hyalinized collagen in a dermatofibrosarcoma

protuberans after treatment with imatinib mesylate.
J Cutan Pathol 2008;35(11):1003–6.

73. Maki RG, Awan RA, Dixon RH, et al. Differential
sensitivity to imatinib of 2 patients with metastatic
sarcoma arising from dermatofibrosarcoma protuberans. Int J Cancer 2002;100(6):623–6.

74. Haycox CL, Odland PB, Olbricht SM, et al. Immunohistochemical characterization of dermatofibrosarcoma protuberans with practical applications for
diagnosis and treatment. J Am Acad Dermatol
1997;37(3 Pt 1):438–44.

Management of Unusual Cutaneous Malignancies: Atypical Fibroxanthoma, Malignant Fibrous Histiocytoma, Sebaceous Carcinoma, Extramammary Paget Disease

W. Elliot Love, DO[a],*, Adam R. Schmitt, BA[b], Jeremy S. Bordeaux, MD, MPH[c]

KEYWORDS
- Atypical fibroxanthoma • Malignant fibrous histiocytoma
- Sebaceous carcinoma • Extramammary Paget disease
- Skin cancer

ATYPICAL FIBROXANTHOMA
History

Cutaneous sarcomas are primary skin neoplasms of nonepithelial cell origin. They are locally aggressive and have a varying capacity to metastasize. Atypical fibroxanthoma (AFX) is a cutaneous sarcoma of mesenchymal origin that has been referred to in the past by various names including pseudosarcoma and superficial malignant fibrous histiocytoma. It was first identified as a disease sui generis in the early 1960s by Helwig, who later described one of the largest series to date.[1,2] It was once believed to be a benign local reactive proliferation until it was later evident that these tumors possess the capability to metastasize.[3,4]

Treatment of these sarcomas has included cryotherapy, radiation, wide local excision (WLE), and Mohs micrographic surgery (MMS).[5,6]

Epidemiology

AFX arises most commonly in elderly white men with an overall male/female ratio approaching 7:1.[7] The true male/female ratio may extend beyond this as most reports in the literature are on men. The prevalence seems to be bimodal with the highest frequency of tumors occurring in the seventh decade. These occur primarily on the ears, nose, and cheeks. A second smaller subset of patients, whose median age is within the fourth decade, develop AFX more commonly

---

Disclosures: The authors have nothing to disclose.
[a] Department of Dermatology, MetroHealth Medical Center, Case Western Reserve University School of Medicine, 29125 Chagrin Boulevard, Suite 110, Pepper Pike, OH 44122, USA
[b] Department of Dermatology, Case Western Reserve University School of Medicine, 10900 Euclid Avenue, Suite T308, Cleveland, OH 44106, USA
[c] Department of Dermatology, Case Western Reserve University School of Medicine, University Hospitals Case Medical Center, 3909 Orange Place, Suite 4200, Orange Village, OH 44122, USA
* Corresponding author.
E-mail address: wlove@metrohealth.org

Dermatol Clin 29 (2011) 201–216
doi:10.1016/j.det.2011.02.007
0733-8635/11/$ – see front matter © 2011 Published by Elsevier Inc.

on the trunk and extremities.[3,8] The true per capita incidence of AFX has not been meticulously defined given it is relatively uncommon and there is no registry available for these tumors.

Cause and Pathogenesis

AFX may represent a reparative or benign reactive process in previously damaged skin. Ultraviolet (UV) and ionizing radiation are both suspected factors for the development of AFX. Evidence supporting this includes their common occurrence on actinically damaged skin, as portrayed histologically by its background of elastosis. These patients also usually have a history of other malignancies instigated by UV radiation such as basal or squamous cell carcinoma. UV induction has been substantiated by the fact that some AFX have shown P53 gene mutations, specifically on dipyrimidine sites, and the production of cyclobutane pyrimidine dimers.[9,10] Furthermore, AFX has been reported in patients with xeroderma pigmentosum who have an inability to repair UV-induced pyrimidine dimers.[11]

Although generally not a biologically aggressive tumor, when not adequately treated AFX recurs locally in up to 20% of cases; local recurrence portends a significantly higher risk for metastasis.[3,12–15] Time to recurrence may be extremely variable from within 2 months to 13 years, with the average time to recurrence being approximately 27.5 months.[3,7] Although the exact rate of metastases is unknown, it is estimated to occur in 1% of cases. If metastasis does occur, it is within approximately 20 months of the original diagnosis.[16] Factors that lend to higher metastatic potential and a poor prognosis include tumor extension into deep subcutaneous tissue, size, history of ionizing radiation, lymphovascular involvement, and immunocompromised state.[12] Although local and distant metastases rarely occur, it seems that if metastases do occur they are to regional nodal beds.[3,4,16–27]

Tumor depth plays an important roll in the diagnosis of AFX; at times with deeper tumors into fascial planes it is difficult to make a distinction between AFX and superficial malignant fibrous histiocytoma (MFH). This is an important differentiation because the diagnosis of MFH is much more ominous carrying a higher risk of metastasis and poorer prognosis.[20] Because tumor depth in AFX is correlated with metastases, and because of the difficult distinction from superficial MFH, it is prudent to perform sentinel lymph node biopsy on patients with tumors that extend to deep subcutaneous levels. Sentinel lymph node biopsy may also be recommended for recurrent tumors,

however locating the true sentinel node of the original tumor may be an arduous task because of disruption of the drainage patterns as a result of the primary procedure.

Clinical Features

The characteristic presentation of an AFX is that of a single firm painless friable nodule typically less than 2 cm in diameter (**Fig. 1**). Ulceration may be present and bleeding may occur with minimal trauma. The most common locations are head and neck, but in younger patients they may be more common on the trunk and extremities.[3]

Differential diagnosis includes, but is not restricted to, spindle cell squamous cell carcinoma, basal cell carcinoma, leiomyosarcoma, dermatofibrosarcoma protuberans, spindle cell or amelanotic melanoma, as well as the superficial portion of an underlying MFH.

Dermatoscopy may be a useful clinical tool when evaluating these tumors. Superficial white areas or a white veil may be seen. Areas containing polymorphous vascular structures, including dotted, globular, linear, tortuous, and arborizing patterns, can also be appreciated.[28] Although not substantially specific, dermatoscopy may be added to the diagnostic armamentarium for these rare tumors.

Diagnosis

Histologic examination of AFX reveals a proliferation of pleomorphic atypical spindle and polygonal cells in a haphazard arrangement within a fibrous

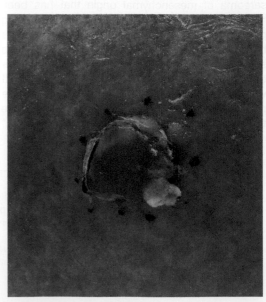

Fig. 1. Atypical fibroxanthoma.

stroma; both of these cell types contain a high nuclear/cytoplasmic ratio, striking nucleoli, and coarse chromatin patterns. A high proportion of atypical mitotic activity is present (**Fig. 2**). Abundant multinucleated giant cells are typical. Although rare, perineural invasion may be present.[29] These features may be indistinguishable from those seen in MFH, which is why many consider AFX to be a variant of this deeper tumor.

Although not typically articulated, AFX has been subcategorized as being histiocyte predominant, spindle cell predominant with a smooth muscle-like pattern, spindle cell predominant with a storiform-like pattern, spindle cell predominant with course nuclear membranes resembling squamous cell carcinoma, and xanthogranulomatous. Other cellular variants have been described and include myxoid, pigmented, clear cell, those containing osteoclast-like giant cells, and granular cell types.[30–37] Monomorphic spindle cells in a fascicular array with eosinophilic cytoplasm and high mitotic rate are seen in the spindle cell nonpleomorphic type; there is a lack of pleomorphism and this variant of AFX is frequently misdiagnosed.[38]

Immunohistochemistry may be helpful in diagnosing AFX; vimentin, CD68, smooth muscle actin, α1-antitrypsin, α1-chemotrypsin, and factor XIIIa are often positive. Other stains that may highlight AFX include CD74, CD117, CD10, CD99, CD163, LN-2, and procollagen-1. CD10 may also be a useful immunohistochemical stain for Mohs sections.[39] In the setting of a difficult to classify tumor, vigilance should be used when interpreting these stains because they do not possess a high degree of specificity.[27,40–47] Cytokeratin, S-100 and HMB-45, desmin and calponin, and CD34 are characteristically negative and are helpful in differentiating spindle cell squamous cell carcinoma, desmoplastic melanoma, leiomyosarcoma, and dermatofibrosarcoma protuberans, respectively.[13]

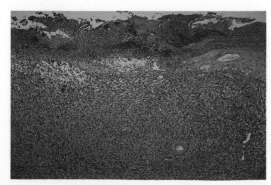

Fig. 2. Atypical fibroxanthoma (original magnification 10×).

Treatment

As previously stated, AFX has been treated with cryotherapy, radiation, WLE, and MMS. Although reported to be efficacious in a small series, because of the risk of recurrence and metastatic potential with AFX, cryotherapy is discouraged.[5] Irradiation is also not recommended because of the potential to further increase the aggressive behavior of the tumor.

WLE has long been the standard modality to treat AFX. Although recurrence rates ranging between 0% and 20% have been reported using WLE, there are sparse data describing the exact surgical margins taken for these tumors. True recurrence rate with WLE is likely around 10%.[3,7,14,15,48] Excisions should extend to the fascial plane because of the potential depth of invasion and associated malignant potential if present. Although no definite surgical margins have been established, margins of at least 1 to 2 cm are recommended to acquire the highest potential clearance.[49,50]

MMS offers the advantage of complete marginal examination as well as sparing of normal surrounding tissue. One hundred percent marginal assessment is extremely valuable because of the risk of metastasis with local recurrence. In addition, the subclinical spread of AFX may typically be greater than 1 cm, which is the margin that is usually taken during WLE.[8,31,51] The mean number of Mohs levels needed to clear AFX is approximately 2.[8,51,52] MMS has been shown to provide superior clearance rates over WLE for AFX.[7] Because of the rarity of this tumor, the number and recurrence rate of AFX treated with MMS has varied in the few studies in which it has been evaluated; studies containing 5-year follow-up rates are also sparse. On average, the available follow-up for AFX treated with MMS is approximately 30.7 months; the average recurrence rate is 3%.[7,8,51,53] Because local recurrence is so highly correlated with metastasis and overall survival, and because fewer recurrences are seen with MMS compared with WLE, MMS should be used to treat AFX when possible.

MFH
History

MFH was first described in 1961 by Kauffman and Stout; previously, it had been referred to by such names as fibroxanthoma, malignant fibrous xanthoma, malignant giant tumor of soft parts, and pleomorphic fibrosarcoma.[54,55] MFH is best regarded as a soft tissue sarcoma and is now referred to by many as pleomorphic sarcoma.

The questions surrounding its origin and its many subtypes have made the diagnosis of MFH as its own entity controversial. Although MFHs arise in subcutaneous tissue, they arise more commonly in soft tissues, such as skeletal muscle. It is among the most common soft tissue sarcomas in late adulthood.[56,57] It is much more aggressive than AFX, with higher recurrence and higher metastatic rates. MFHs are treated surgically with either WLE or MMS.

Epidemiology

Although MFHs occur at a rate of approximately 1.5 per million, they are the third most common cutaneous soft tissue sarcoma after Kaposi sarcoma and dermatofibrosarcoma protuberans. MFHs typically appear between the sixth and eighth decade of life, although childhood tumors have been reported.[58] They are more common in whites and there is a slight male predominance (nearly 3:1). The head and neck are the most common locations for subcuticular MFHs followed closely by the extremities; tumors on upper extremities occur almost twice as often as those on the thighs or legs. Distal tumors have higher 5-year survival than proximal tumors.[56,59,60]

Cause and Pathogenesis

Although originally believed to have a histiocytic origin, evidence suggests that MFHs develop from mesenchymal progenitor cells.[61,62] The exact cause of MFH remains elusive; reports of MFH occurring at surgical sites, burn scars, areas of chronic inflammation, or internal fractures have led to the hypothesis that MFH is a reactive process occurring at sites of trauma.[63–69] Ionizing radiation may also play a role in the development of this malignancy.

It is difficult to ascertain precise rates of recurrence and metastasis for subcutaneous MFH because most reports contain data that combine both subcutaneous and soft tissue MFH. Regardless of location, the tumor is biologically aggressive; recurrence and metastatic rates for both subcutaneous and deep MFHs are taken into account.

Up to 71% of MFHs have recurred after surgical treatment and the time to recurrence is usually within 2 years of treatment. A significant number of patients may develop either recurrence or metastases after 2 years, highlighting the necessity for close follow-up of these patients.[57,60] Deep MFHs have a much higher risk for metastasis than their subcuticular counterpart. Metastasis has occurred in up to 44% of MFHs, but is reported to be as low as 17% of cases in subcuticular tumors. The most common location for metastasis is the lung, followed by regional nodal beds.[57,59,70] Survival is based on tumor size with overall 5-year survival approximately 50%.[57,59] Tumor size and high histologic grade seem to have the greatest effect on metastasis and survival. Despite the histologic grade, tumors less than 5 cm have approximately a 79% survival rate, whereas tumors between 5 and 10 cm and tumors greater than 10 cm have survival rates of 63% and 41%, respectively.[59]

Because of the high metastatic potential of MFH, sentinel lymph node biopsy is recommended for all diagnosed cases. In addition, imaging is not only necessary to rule out metastatic disease at the time of diagnosis but also assists surgeons in planning the initial surgical margins.

Clinical Features

MFHs have a propensity to occur beneath the fascia, and subcutaneous or dermal tumors are less common. It most commonly presents as a deep painless enlarging mass with a rapid rate of growth (Fig. 3). Superficial MFHs extend only down to fascia, whereas deep MFHs go below fascia to muscle and bone; most present as deep tumors.[60] Although previously believed to occur most commonly on the extremities, the head and neck may be the most common location; it is vital to differentiate tumors occurring on the face from AFX. The retroperitoneum is also a common site of occurrence and presents with abdominal symptoms, and this presentation has the worst prognosis. MFHs spread considerably along fascial planes and between muscle fibers, causing difficulty in assessing the full extent of the tumor. The differential diagnosis includes, but is not restricted to, pleomorphic liposarcoma, rhabdomyosarcoma, AFX (when superficial), dermatofibrosarcoma protuberans, epithelioid sarcoma, and fibrosarcoma.

Fig. 3. Malignant fibrous histiocytoma (original magnification 10×).

Diagnosis

The diagnosis of MFH is difficult, and is frequently a diagnosis of exclusion because it shares many histologic similarities with an assortment of poorly differentiated tumors. Five subtypes have been described: storiform-pleomorphic (most common, **Fig. 4**), myxoid, giant cell, inflammatory, and angiomatoid. MFH looks similar to AFX, with the pleomorphic subtype at times being cellularly indistinguishable. This type contains plump pleomorphic spindle cells, numerous atypical mitoses, foam and giant cells, and marked pleomorphism (see **Fig. 3**). Angioinvasion is common.[71] Location plays an important role in the diagnosis of pleomorphic MFH, as superficial tumors typically represent AFX.

Immunohistochemistry may aid in the diagnosis of MFH. Similar to AFX, MFHs stain positive for CD68, smooth muscle actin, and vimentin. α1-antitrypsin and α1-chemotrypsin staining typically displays a varying degree of positivity. The angiomatoid subtype may stain positive for factor VIII–related antigen and *Ulex europaeus*.[72] S-100, HMB-45, CD34, cytokeratin, and desmin are negative.[73] Having such similar histologic and immunologic characteristics as AFX, other immunostains may be useful in differentiating the two. LN-2(CD74) was shown to be expressed to a higher degree in MFH than AFX.[44] As stated earlier, procollagen-1, CD99, CD117, and CD10 tend to show greater affinity for AFX. Molecular studies for mutations in the p53 gene have shown that AFXs have higher immunoreactivity for cyclobutane pyrimidine dimers; mutations in both K-*ras* and H-*ras* genes have been seen in MFH but not AFX.[74,75] Furthermore, AFX shows a diploid distribution on flow cytometry, whereas MFH displays aneuploidy, although aneuploidy may be more of an indicator of malignant potential rather than an indicator of a specific tumor.[76] These molecular findings may not only help to differentiate between AFX and MFH they may also shed light on the pathogenesis of these poorly understood tumors.

Treatment

The standard treatment of MFH is surgical resection, either with WLE, MMS, or amputation in extreme cases. As previously stated, before surgical planning, imaging is necessary to assist in determination of the surgical margins; magnetic resonance imaging (MRI) is more sensitive than computed tomography (CT) for soft tissue detail.

Clearance rates with WLE have been disappointing, with reported recurrence rates of 17% to 71%.[57,59,60,70,77] This can be attributed to the highly infiltrative growth pattern displayed by MFH, with tumor radiating many centimeters from the clinically apparent mass. As many as half of excised tumors may have positive margins that require at least 1 reexcision to achieve negative pathologic margins.[70] Definite parameters have not been set with regard to the surgical margin, but at least a 2-cm margin should be taken from the lateral extent of the tumor unless otherwise directed by MRI/CT. Excisions should be carried to and include the fascia for subcutaneous MFH, and for deeper soft tissue MFH excisions may need to involve bone for tumor clearance.

As previously stated, MFHs that occur in the subcutis have a propensity for growth well beyond the tumor mass, making margin control paramount with resection of the tumor. It would make sense then that MMS would be to the patient's advantage in initial clearance of this tumor. MMS has been used sparsely for the treatment of MFH, but it has been shown to be extremely promising as a therapeutic modality. Of 28 cases of MFH reported to have been treated with MMS, there were only 5 recurrences, yielding a clearance rate of 82%.[31,53,78] Follow-up for these tumors was short, averaging about 2.4 years. MMS allows for immediate evaluation of the entire surgical margin and is not only superior to traditional WLE with regard to clearance of subcuticular MFH it also offers tissue conservation for improved cosmesis. For MFH involving deeper structures, it is unlikely that a Mohs surgeon would perform the primary resection. However, when available a Mohs surgeon would be useful to evaluate the tissue specimen using Mohs histologic techniques to ensure that the entire surgical margin is evaluated. This may provide a higher immediate cure rate and fewer potential surgeries and subsequent

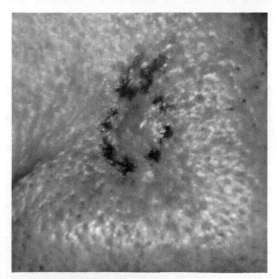

Fig. 4. Sebaceous carcinoma.

exposure to general anesthesia for the patient. Chemotherapy and surgery may also improve long-term survival.[79,80]

SEBACEOUS CARCINOMA
History

Carcinoma of the meibomian gland was first reported in the literature in the late nineteenth century, though sebaceous carcinoma was not classified as a unique type of cutaneous cancer until the early twentieth century.[81–84] Advancements in understanding of the natural history and clinical presentation of sebaceous carcinoma, particularly carcinomas appearing in the eyelid, were then described in several case series throughout the middle twentieth century.[84,85] In recent decades, studies have attempted to further elucidate the epidemiologic and pathologic characteristics of the disease.[83–90] In addition, research has explored the effectiveness of various treatment options.[91–98]

Epidemiology

Sebaceous carcinoma is a rare cutaneous tumor arising from the sebaceous glands. Between 1973 and 2004, 1349 cases were identified and reported to the National Cancer Institute's Surveillance, Epidemiology, and End Results (SEER) database.[86] Sebaceous carcinoma accounts for 0.2% to 5.5% of the cutaneous malignancies occurring on the eyelid.[83,99–101] The SEER study also indicates a yearly incidence of 2.3 cases per million in whites, 1.07 per million in Asian/Pacific Islanders, and 0.48 per million in blacks.[86] Most patients with sebaceous carcinoma are more than 50 years of age (most commonly between ages 60 and 80 years) and most are white.[86,87,90,91,96,102] Furthermore, women have often been labeled as high risk for developing sebaceous carcinoma,[84,90,91,102] but more recent population-wide studies have shown a lack of association between gender and development of the disease.[84,86,87]

Cause and Pathogenesis

The cause of most sebaceous carcinomas is unknown.[88] Most cases arise de novo, and not from a preexisting sebaceous condition,[85] although some cases have been associated with immunosuppression or previous radiation to the tumor site.[85,88,90,102,103] Significant associations with Muir-Torre syndrome have been identified.[88,89,104–106] Because sebaceous carcinomas occur most commonly around the eye,[86–88,90–92,96,102] the tumors types are traditionally divided into 2 categories: ocular and extraocular.[107]

Clinical Features

Most cases of sebaceous carcinoma appear on the head or neck, with up to 75% of cases occurring on the eyelid.[86–88,90–92,105,107] Ocular sebaceous carcinomas typically present as a small, slowly growing, single papule or nodule on the eyelid.[88,107] These papules closely resemble chalazia and tend to occur on the upper eyelid, as more meibomian glands and glands of Zeis are located on the upper lid.[96] The eyelid may also swell diffusely, resembling inflammatory processes such as blepharitis or cicatricial pemphigoid.[108] In addition, the eyelid tissue may be distorted, thus preventing the eyelids from closing. If there is advanced pagetoid spread, the carcinoma may present with eyelash loss, lid eversion or undulation, ocular distortion, and erosion and ulceration.

Extraocular sebaceous carcinoma usually appears as a firm yellow-hued papule (see **Fig. 4**); ulceration may be present. Although other sites may be involved, extraocular tumors are most commonly seen on the head and neck.[103,107] Ocular sebaceous carcinomas share many clinical features with other eyelid lesions, often leading to a delay in proper diagnosis.[87,107,108] Most commonly, sebaceous carcinoma is mistaken for chalazion and blepharoconjunctivitis.[83,90,102] Sebaceous carcinoma may also resemble 3 more common malignancies of the eyelid: basal or squamous cell carcinoma and malignant melanoma.[88,108] Differential diagnosis of sebaceous carcinoma also includes the following: keratoconjunctivitis, unilateral conjunctivitis, cutaneous horn, ocular pemphigoid, leukoplakia, conjunctival carcinoma in situ, granulomatous inflammation, central retinal artery occlusion and proptosis, lacrimal gland tumors, exophthalmos, pyogenic granulomas, metastatic tumors, Merkel cell carcinoma, sarcoidosis, meibomitis, clear-cell eccrine hidradenoma, and benign adnexal tumors.[83,88,102]

As mentioned previously, sebaceous carcinoma is associated with Muir-Torre syndrome and is considered a marker for this disease.[89,102–104,106,107] Sebaceous adenomas and epitheliomas related to this syndrome also tend to appear on the face and may occur as single or multiple papules. They are skin-colored, yellowish, or reddish-brown, and are occasionally ulcerated papules. These tumors may resemble sebaceous hyperplasia.[107] Keratoacanthoma, squamous cell carcinoma, and multiple follicular cysts may also occur as part of this syndrome.

Both ocular and extraocular sebaceous carcinomas have been known to metastasize to regional lymph nodes; preauricular and parotid nodes are the most common sites of metastasis.[85,102,106] Less frequently, they may also metastasize to distant sites such as the liver, lungs, brain, and bones.[85,100] In addition, sebaceous carcinoma is associated with secondary malignancies commonly seen with Muir-Torre syndrome, such as colorectal and genitourinary tumors.[101,103,104]

Diagnosis

Because it mimics a variety of other cutaneous malignancies, identification of sebaceous carcinoma can be problematic. Diagnosis of the disease is often delayed by its clinical and histologic ambiguity, leading to improper treatment as well as increased morbidity and mortality.[83,94,102] Therefore, particular attention should be paid to suspicious chalazia and inflammations that fail to respond to appropriate treatment.[84,103] Biopsies of potential sebaceous carcinomas, coupled with vigilant histologic examination, are crucial components to proper diagnosis.

In addition to its ambiguous clinical presentation, sebaceous carcinoma also mimics a myriad of malignancies histologically.[83,85,102,103,108] Sebaceous carcinomas are centered in the dermis and consist of aggregations of neoplastic cells.[88,107] The tumors may be classified as well, moderately, or poorly differentiated, and most often present as irregular, lobular sebaceous growths.[102,107] The nuclei are commonly pleomorphic, and the cells typically exhibit increased mitotic activity, basaloid features, and hyperchromatic nuclei.[102,103,107] The undifferentiated, neoplastic cells usually present with foamy cytoplasm because of an abundance of small lipid globules (**Fig. 5**).[102,108] Vacuolization of the cytoplasm of moderately differentiated or well-differentiated cells may indicate sebaceous

carcinoma,[108] and sebaceous carcinoma tumors often have areas of central necrosis, similar to the pattern of comedocarcinoma.[90,107] The classic identifier of sebaceous carcinoma, however, is intra-epithelial spread beyond the main site of the tumor into the conjunctival epithelium and the epidermis of the eyelid.[85,90,102,103,108] This pagetoid growth pattern may appear similar to Bowenoid actinic keratosis in the eyelid and carcinoma in situ in the conjunctiva.[108] Moreover, vacuolated sebaceous carcinoma cells show abundant lipid content if stained with Oil Red O and Sudan IV stains.[101,108]

Extraocular and periocular tumors are histologically similar, presenting with large atypical basaloid cells and border infiltration.[103] However, extraocular sebaceous carcinomas exhibit pagetoid intraepithelial spread less often than ocular tumors.

Although histopathologic analysis is usually sufficient to identify cases of sebaceous carcinoma, immunohistochemical analysis may be necessary in highly equivocal cases to make a diagnosis.[101–103] Sebaceous carcinoma stains positive for epithelial membrane antigen (EMA) and androgen receptors, but not for carcinoembryonic antigen (CEA) or S100.[101,102] It is also possible to perform immunostaining for the mismatch repair genes MLH1 and MSH2 on hematoxylin and eosin sections to assess for Muir-Torre syndrome.

Assessment for Muir-Torre syndrome is an important part of the workup for sebaceous carcinoma. Muir-Torre syndrome is an autosomal dominant genodermatosis defined by the presence of at least 1 sebaceous neoplasm of the skin and 1 or more low-grade visceral malignancy.[89,101] About 30% of sebaceous neoplasms associated with Muir-Torre syndrome are sebaceous carcinomas, and the most frequent primary malignancies are colorectal (51%) and genitourinary cancers (25%). Identification of the disease is necessary because patients with Muir-Torre syndrome are at risk for multiple visceral cancers; roughly half of all patients with Muir-Torre syndrome have 2 or more. Therefore, in addition to a baseline chest radiograph, complete metabolic panel, and complete blood count, screening for visceral cancers associated with Muir-Torre syndrome include a rectal examination, full colonoscopy, and barium enema. Because of the autosomal dominant inheritance of the disease, screening should also include a thorough personal and family history of Muir-Torre syndrome or malignancies that indicate Muir-Torre syndrome as well as genetic counseling.

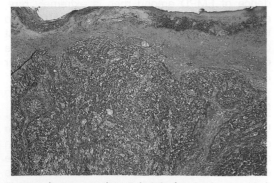

Fig. 5. Sebaceous carcinoma (original magnification 10×).

Treatment

The risk of local recurrence of sebaceous carcinoma varies by treatment modality. Local tumor recurrence has been reported in 6% to 36% of patients within 5 years of surgical treatment.[96,100] Metastasis may occur in 8 to 30% of cases; regional lymph nodes are the most common site of metastatic spread.[85,100] Mortality varies by extent of the disease and treatment used, ranging from 6% to 40%.[85,86,94,99,100]

Several features indicate a poor prognosis; these factors include lesion size greater than 10 mm, delay in diagnosis of more than 6 months, simultaneous upper and lower eyelid involvement, multicentric origin, vascular, lymphatic, orbital, or pagetoid invasion, poor differentiation, and a highly infiltrative pattern.[85,91,94]

The definitive treatment of sebaceous carcinoma is surgical excision,[102,107] although exenteration may be necessary in cases of orbital involvement.[91] WLE has traditionally been used as the primary surgical modality. If WLE is used, margins should be checked in both permanent and frozen sections.[85,91,92,96,99,101] Conjunctival map biopsies may also be used. Reported recurrence rates with this method range between 32% and 36%.[92,96]

Recent studies have shown that MMS results in lower recurrence and mortality than WLE; MMS also offers superior tissue conservation, which is beneficial in this cosmetically demanding area.[91,96,97,102,109] A significant advantage of MMS is that it offers complete margin surveillance at the time of the procedure.[96] This is of great value because of sebaceous carcinoma's tendency to intraepithelial spread. Because of real-time margin monitoring, the final excision margins of MMS may end up being significantly larger than the clinically visible margins.[96] Because of the high potential for recurrence, some have recommended that in cases of intraepithelial pagetoid spread an additional Mohs layer should be removed as a protective measure against local recurrence.[109] Recurrence rates of sebaceous carcinomas treated with MMS have been reported to be around 12%, with an average follow-up of 3 years.[96,109] Moreover, MMS has yielded better outcomes than WLE in case studies of extraocular sebaceous carcinoma, but treatment of extraocular sites is not as well studied.[110,111] MMS may therefore present a more effective treatment of sebaceous carcinoma than traditional surgical methods.[91,96,102,109]

Radiation therapy, cryotherapy, and chemotherapy have been proposed as alternative treatments when the patient either refuses or cannot tolerate surgery, or when there is orbital involvement and the patient refuses exenteration.[91,95,96,98,107,112] Radiotherapy may be useful if surgery is contraindicated.[91,96,98,99,107]

Although studies indicate that radiation is not as effective as surgical treatments, and should be used as a palliative rather than curative therapy,[96,99] previous case studies may not have used adequate amounts of radiation.[98] Cryotherapy may be a viable alternative to exenteration in cases with conjunctival pagetoid involvement, and has palliative uses.[91,96] Use of topical mitomycin C has been successful in initial tumor control in cases of conjunctival pagetoid invasion without evidence of tumor underlying the epithelium.[91,95]

No matter what treatment modality is used, continued surveillance of both ocular and extraocular sebaceous carcinoma is critical in order to assess the patient for local recurrence and metastases.[91,93,112] Because of the aggressive nature of the disease, as well as its proclivity for epithelial infiltration, local recurrence or organ metastases may be detected several years after treatment.

EXTRAMAMMARY PAGET DISEASE
History

In 1874, Sir James Paget described an eczema-like nipple lesion with an associated underlying breast malignancy, now called mammary Paget disease (MPD).[113,114] The cutaneous erosion was a result of invasion of the nipple and areola by characteristic large cells with pleomorphic nuclei, known as Paget cells. Fifteen years later, Crocker was the first to report extramammary Paget disease (EMPD) when he discussed an occurrence of Paget on the penis and scrotum.[115,116] Perianal EMPD was then described in 1893, and Paget disease of the vulva in 1901.[117,118]

Epidemiology

Extramammary Paget disease is a rare neoplasm of apocrine-rich skin, namely the anogenital and axillary regions.[114,118–123] Affected populations are commonly white women between the ages of 50 and 80 years.[114,117,118,121,122,124,125] The incidence of EMPD among men is extremely rare, although men who do present with EMPD also tend to be white and elderly.[115,124,126] The most common location for EMPD is the vulva, yet the disease accounts for only 1% to 2% of all vulvar malignancies.[114,116,118,121,122]

Cause and Pathogenesis

Unlike mammary Paget disease, in which the cutaneous lesion almost always results from an underlying ductal carcinoma,[114,120–122] the cause of EMPD is not uniform. EMPD is generally divided into 2 types: primary and secondary.[114,121,123,125,127,128] The primary form of EMPD is an adenocarcinoma originating in the epidermis; it has no underlying malignancy. Secondary EMPD, on the other hand, is a pagetoid change in the skin associated with either an underlying adnexal carcinoma or an adjacent internal carcinoma.

Primary EMPD occurs much more often than secondary EMPD, with estimates showing that the primary type constitutes somewhere between 75% and 96% of EMPD cases.[114,122,127,128] This primary intraepithelial neoplasm is believed to originate either from intraepidermal apocrine glands or from pluripotent epidermal stem cells.[120,122,127] Primary EMPD may become invasive and invade the dermis and subcutaneous fat[114,121,125,127]; this occurs in 10% to 20% of all EMPD cases, although dermal invasion may not be detected without rigorous sampling. Invasive EMPD may then metastasize via lymphatic spread.[122]

In contrast, secondary EMPD is associated with an underlying adnexal carcinoma or an internal malignancy.[114,118,121,122,128] Up to 25% of all EMPD cases are a result of an underlying adnexal carcinoma, typically of apocrine origin.[114,125] Less commonly, 10% to 15% of cases are associated with a visceral carcinoma, usually of the rectum, bladder, urethra, cervix, prostate, perianal area, vulvar region, glans penis, or groin.[114,122,123,128] These cases are a result of continuous upward extension of malignant cells to the skin. EMPD associated with an underlying adenocarcinoma often metastasizes to both regional and distal lymph nodes.[117,121]

Clinical Features

Extramammary Paget disease usually presents as multicentric lesions that are clinically similar to mammary Paget disease.[118–120,122] EMPD typically presents as an insidious, pruritic, erythematous scaly eroded plaque with well defined borders.[114,117–123,129,130] This plaque may be macerated with shallow ulcers (**Fig. 6**) or appear as an erythematous scaly plaque with scattered crust.[114,123,131] Although the most common features are pruritus, soreness, and erythema, burning and bleeding may also be present.[114,117,122] Furthermore, EMPD may present with regional lymphadenopathy or an underlying palpable mass.[114,120] EMPD arises from areas of high apocrine gland density. The most commonly affected site is the vulva, followed by the anal, perianal and perineal areas, the urethra, the scrotum, and the penis[114,117,122,129]; cases of isolated EMPD of the penis are exceedingly rare.[115,124] Less frequently, EMPD may be

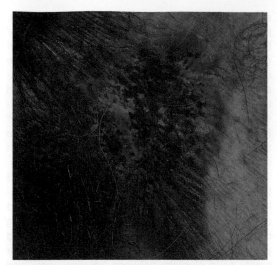

Fig. 6. Extramammary Paget disease.

found in areas with fewer apocrine glands, such as the chest, axillae, abdomen, thigh, eyelids, face, and external auditory canal.[114,122]

Extramammary Paget disease is frequently misdiagnosed, as it resembles a variety of cutaneous conditions. A differential diagnosis of EMPD includes psoriasis, eczema, contact dermatitis, lichen sclerosis, anogenital intraepithelial neoplasia, lichen simplex chronicus, lichen planus, candida intertrigo, tinea corporis, histiocytosis, mycosis funoides, Crohn disease, hidradenitis suppurativa, condylomata accuminata, human papilloma virus–induced intraepithelial neoplasia (when present on the vulvar area or penis), leukoplakia, amelanotic melanoma, basal cell carcinoma, squamous cell carcinoma in situ (SCCIS) (including erythroplasia of Queyrat and Bowen disease), or invasive squamous cell carcinoma.[114,118,119,123]

Diagnosis

Lesions in the areas specified earlier that are unresponsive to topical therapy should be biopsied.[114,115,118,121,123,131,132] Diagnosis of EMPD is delayed by an average of 2 years as treatment of a presumed inflammation or infectious dermatitis is attempted.[116,118,121,122,133] Biopsy should be accompanied by a thorough investigation for both invasive disease and underlying carcinoma[118,121–123]; the results of this investigation affect both the prognosis and treatment considerations. Workup for EMPD should be directed towards detection of associated gastrointestinal or genitourinary malignancies. Appropriate workup may include pelvic ultrasound or MRI, laparoscopy, mammogram, and chest radiograph.[118,122] In cases of perineal/perianal EMPD, suitable tests may include rectal examination, proctoscopy, colonoscopy, sigmoidoscopy, or barium enema.[118,122,123] Moreover, in cases of genital or vulvar EMPD, investigation may include cystoscopy, intravenous pyelogram, hysteroscopy, or pelvic examination. If dermal invasion is present, sentinel node biopsy may be considered to determine if there is nodal involvement.[122] Positron emission tomography scans may also be useful for evaluating invasive EMPD for lymph node involvement and metastases.[122]

Extramammary Paget disease is characterized by the presence of classic Paget cells and is histologically similar to mammary Paget disease.[121–123,130] Paget cells appear as massive round cells with large pleomorphic nuclei and prominent nucleoli. These cells are found either singly or in clusters between keratinocytes, and may extend down into adnexal structures (Fig. 7).[114,117,120,122,123] Paget cells may appear at any level of the epidermis and are distinguished from surrounding epithelial cells by a clear halo; they do not possess intracellular bridges.[114,120,122] The malignant cells arise from abnormal differentiation of basal layer cells.[117,121] Unlike lesions obtained from mammary Paget disease, the finely granular cytoplasm of EMPD Paget cells contains abundant amounts of mucopolysaccharide, indicating a difference in origin (epithelial vs internal ductal adenocarcinoma) between the 2 diseases.[114,120,122,128] Because of their high mucopolysaccharide content, EMPD cells show positive staining for periodic acid–Schiff, mucicarmine, Alcian blue at pH 2.5, and colloidal iron.[114,117,120,122,128]

Even after histologic analysis, immunohistochemistry may be necessary to diagnose EMPD. For instance, SCCIS, melanoma in situ (MIS), MPD, and EMPD can mimic each other throughout the histologic process. Both mammary and EMPD stain positive for CAM 5.2 and cytokeratin 7 and 8 (CK 7, 8), but stain negative for S100 and HMB-45.[114,122,134] SCCIS, on the other hand, stains negative for CAM 5.2 and cytokeratins. Unlike MPD and EMPD, MIS stains positive for S100 and HMB-45. In addition, Paget cells show positive staining for CEA, EMA, mucin core protein, and gross cystic disease fluid protein-15 (GCDFP-15), although GCDFP-15 is often negative in cases of secondary EMPD with an associated malignancy.[114,122]

Prognosis

The prognosis for primary EMPD is good when confined to the epidermis.[121,122,124,127] Because of its high rate of metastasis, the presence of invasive EMPD worsens the prognosis significantly, especially if lymphovascular invasion has already occurred.[122,124,127] The disease is often fatal with regional nodal metastases and lymphovascular invasion.[121,122] The prognosis for EMPD secondary to an underlying adenocarcinoma is poorer than for patients with intraepithelial EMPD.[116,120,127] In cases of secondary EMPD, the prognosis is dependent on the associated carcinoma.[122,127] Prognosis is also poor for patients with a coexisting cancer.[116]

Regardless of the treatment modality, EMPD has a significant proclivity for local recurrence.[120–122,125,133] This property is likely a result of the multifocal origin of EMPD, and because Paget cells may extend beyond grossly visible margins and commonly into adnexal structures.[120,122] Some estimates place the overall local recurrence rate at approximately 33%, with a range of 12% to 60%.[121,124] Thus, treated lesions should be monitored carefully for local recurrence and repeat treatments may be required.[121,122]

Treatment

Surgery is the primary choice for treatment of EMPD.[114,119,121,122,135,136] WLE is used traditionally and local recurrence rates are reported at approximately 44% (range 22%–60%, depending on surgery site).[118,122,132,133] The high recurrence rate is a result of the proclivity of EMPD to spread irregularly beyond gross margins, as well as the multifocal nature of the disease.[117,121–123,133] EMPD remains in situ in 65% to 74% of cases after WLE.[115,123] Intraoperative staining with CK 7, in

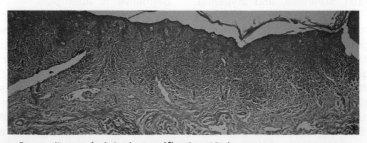

Fig. 7. Extramammary Paget disease (original magnification 10×).

addition to preoperative multiple scouting biopsies, may lead to lower recurrence rates.[115,122,123]

In the event of underlying intraepithelial Paget disease or carcinoma, more radical and extensive surgery may be required.[117,121,125,127] For example, vulvar EMPD secondary to an underlying malignancy should be treated with radical vulvectomy and bilateral inguinal lymph node dissection, as is the standard treatment of any other invasive tumor in the vulvar region.[117,121,125] Furthermore, if Paget cells are found in the dermis, regional lymph nodes are palpable, or there is evidence of lymph node involvement at biopsy, then lymph node dissection should be considered.[123,136]

MMS compares favorably with WLE for treating EMPD. Recurrence rates of EMPD treated with MMS are lower than when treated with WLE.[122,132,133,137] Higher recurrence rates have been reported in patients with vulval and perianal EMPD treated with WLE (43% and 50%, respectively) compared with patients treated with MMS (27% and 28%, respectively).[133] Another study comparing WLE with MMS for a variety of disease sites found recurrence rates of 22% and 8%, respectively.[132] Generally, the recurrence rate for primary EMPD after MMS is 16%, compared with 44% average recurrence rate for WLE.[122,137] Up to 97% of Mohs micrographic surgeries for EMPD require margins 5 cm beyond the gross tumor margin in order to clear residual tumor.[122,137] More radical surgeries may yield better recurrence rates than both MMS and WLE. For instance, 1 study showed that patients with primary vulvar EMPD treated with vulvectomy had a 15% recurrence rate, whereas patients treated with MMS and WLE had recurrence rates of 27% and 43%, respectively.[133] However, significant morbidity is associated with radical surgery, and MMS allows maximal tissue sparing of critical structures often involved in EMPD.[122,138] As with WLE, preoperative scouting biopsies may help in defining disease margins, and CK 7 is useful for intraoperative staining.[114,132]

Alternative treatment modalities exist for patients who are poor candidates for surgery, or for those who are concerned about the extent of surgery that may be necessary for curative treatment. One such option is radiation therapy.[114,119,136] Radiotherapy has been used in cases of local recurrence, as an adjunct to surgery, and as a curative treatment,[122,126] although it should not be considered a curative option in cases of underlying adenocarcinoma. Radiotherapy should be considered in select cases in which lesions are considered inoperable or if a poor functional result is anticipated with surgery.[126,139] In addition, patients with invasive EMPD or underlying adenocarcinoma may benefit from systemic chemotherapy.[122,136,139] Chemotherapeutic regimens for treating EMPD have included 5-fluorouracil (5-FU), cisplatin, mitomycin C, epirubicin, vincristine, docetaxel, etoposide, or adriamycin, or low dose 5-FU combined with cisplatin. Furthermore, topical applications of chemomodulators and immunomodulators, specifically 5-FU and imiquimod, have been reported as potential treatments.[114,119,135] 5-FU may aid in treating EMPD by relieving symptoms, outlining disease margins, cytoreduction before surgery, and postoperative detection of early disease recurrence.[118] Reports indicate that imiquimod 5% cream is useful in cases of primary EMPD, including reports of complete clinical and histologic remission.[135] Other treatments, such as photodynamic therapy and laser ablation, are still under investigation and are likely contraindicated in the event of invasive disease or underlying carcinoma.[114,117,119,122] Nonsurgical treatment modalities should only be considered with patients who are poor surgical candidates, are at risk of significant functional morbidity because of disease location, or have recurrent disease after surgery.

Whatever treatment modality is used, long-term follow-up is required to identify any subsequent recurrence or malignancy.[114,118,124,138] As mentioned previously, EMPD has a high local recurrence rate, and recurrence has been seen in patients up to 15 years after treatment.

SUMMARY

Atypical fibroxanthoma, MFH, sebaceous carcinoma, and EMPD are rare cutaneous tumors. If not recognized and diagnosed in a timely fashion, patient morbidity and mortality may be adversely affected. If atypical fibroxanthoma, MFH, or sebaceous carcinomas do metastasize, the most common location is to regional lymph nodes. Extramammary Paget disease may be associated with an underlying adenocarcinoma; this too may metastasize to either regional or distal lymph nodes. Surgical excision is the treatment of choice for these tumors. Cure rates for MMS have been shown to be as favorable or better than WLE for these tumors. MMS is a favorable treatment option if available.

REFERENCES

1. Levan NE, Hirsch P, Kwong MQ. Pseudosarcomatous dermatofibroma. Arch Dermatol 1963;88: 908–12.
2. Helwig EB. Atypical fibroxanthoma. Tex Med 1963; 59:664–7.

3. Fretzin DF, Helwig EB. Atypical fibroxanthoma of the skin. A clinicopathologic study of 140 cases. Cancer 1973;31:1541–52.

4. Jacobs DS, Edwards WD, Ye RC. Metastatic atypical fibroxanthoma of skin. Cancer 1975;35:457–63.

5. Jacoby WD Jr. Cryosurgical treatment of recurrent atypical fibroxanthoma of the skin. Preliminary report. Cutis 1978;22:599–601.

6. Starink TH, Hausman R, Van Delden L, et al. Atypical fibroxanthoma of the skin. Presentation of 5 cases and a review of the literature. Br J Dermatol 1977;97:167–77.

7. Davis JL, Randle HW, Zalla MJ, et al. A comparison of Mohs micrographic surgery and wide excision for the treatment of atypical fibroxanthoma. Dermatol Surg 1997;23:105–10.

8. Limmer BL, Clark DP. Cutaneous micrographic surgery for atypical fibroxanthoma. Dermatol Surg 1997;23:553–7 [discussion: 557–8].

9. Dei Tos AP, Maestro R, Doglioni C, et al. Ultraviolet-induced p53 mutations in atypical fibroxanthoma. Am J Pathol 1994;145:11–7.

10. Hollstein M, Sidransky D, Vogelstein B, et al. p53 mutations in human cancers. Science 1991;253:49–53.

11. Dilek FH, Akpolat N, Metin A, et al. Atypical fibroxanthoma of the skin and the lower lip in xeroderma pigmentosum. Br J Dermatol 2000;143:618–20.

12. Helwig EB, May D. Atypical fibroxanthoma of the skin with metastasis. Cancer 1986;57:368–76.

13. Farley R, Ratner D. Diagnosis and management of atypical fibroxanthoma. Skinmed 2006;5:83–6.

14. Zalla MJ, Randle HW, Brodland DG, et al. Mohs surgery vs wide excision for atypical fibroxanthoma: follow-up. Dermatol Surg 1997;23:1223–4.

15. Kroe DJ, Pitcock JA. Atypical fibroxanthoma of the skin. Report of ten cases. Am J Clin Pathol 1969;51:487–92.

16. New D, Bahrami S, Malone J, et al. Atypical fibroxanthoma with regional lymph node metastasis: report of a case and review of the literature. Arch Dermatol 2010;146:1399–404.

17. Grosso M, Lentini M, Carrozza G, et al. Metastatic atypical fibroxanthoma of skin. Pathol Res Pract 1987;182:443–7.

18. Rizzardi C, Angiero F, Melato M. Atypical fibroxanthoma and malignant fibrous histiocytoma of the skin. Anticancer Res 2003;23:1847–51.

19. Kemp JD, Stenn KS, Arons M, et al. Metastasizing atypical fibroxanthoma. Coexistence with chronic lymphocytic leukemia. Arch Dermatol 1978;114:1533–5.

20. Cooper JZ, Newman SR, Scott GA, et al. Metastasizing atypical fibroxanthoma (cutaneous malignant histiocytoma): report of five cases. Dermatol Surg 2005;31:221–5 [discussion: 225].

21. Sahn RE, Lang PG. Sentinel lymph node biopsy for high-risk nonmelanoma skin cancers. Dermatol Surg 2007;33:786–92 [discussion: 792–3].

22. Kargi E, Güngör E, Verdi M, et al. Atypical fibroxanthoma and metastasis to the lung. Plast Reconstr Surg 2003;111:1760–2.

23. Giuffrida TJ, Kligora CJ, Goldstein GD. Localized cutaneous metastases from an atypical fibroxanthoma. Dermatol Surg 2004;30:1561–4.

24. Dahl I. Atypical fibroxanthoma of the skin. A clinico-pathological study of 57 cases. Acta Pathol Microbiol Scand A 1976;84:183–97.

25. Glavin FL, Cornwell ML. Atypical fibroxanthoma of the skin metastatic to a lung. Report of a case, features by conventional and electron microscopy, and a review of relevant literature. Am J Dermatopathol 1985;7:57–63.

26. Sankar NM, Pang KS, Thiruchelvam T, et al. Metastasis from atypical fibroxanthoma of skin. Med J Aust 1998;168:418–9.

27. Lum DJ, King AR. Peritoneal metastases from an atypical fibroxanthoma. Am J Surg Pathol 2006;30:1041–6.

28. Bugatti L, Filosa G. Dermatoscopic features of cutaneous atypical fibroxanthoma: three cases. Clin Exp Dermatol 2009;34:e898–900.

29. Dettrick A, Strutton G. Atypical fibroxanthoma with perineural or intraneural invasion: report of two cases. J Cutan Pathol 2006;33:318–22.

30. Patton A, Page R, Googe PB, et al. Myxoid atypical fibroxanthoma: a previously undescribed variant. J Cutan Pathol 2009;36:1177–84.

31. Dzubow LM. Mohs surgery report: spindle cell fibrohistiocytic tumors: classification and pathophysiology. J Dermatol Surg Oncol 1988;14:490–5.

32. Murali R, Palfreeman S. Clear cell atypical fibroxanthoma-report of a case with review of the literature. J Cutan Pathol 2006;33:343–8.

33. Orosz Z. Atypical fibroxanthoma with granular cells. Histopathology 1998;33:88–9.

34. Wright NA, Thomas CG, Calame A, et al. Granular cell atypical fibroxanthoma: case report and review of the literature. J Cutan Pathol 2010;37:380–5.

35. Diaz-Cascajo C, Weyers W, Borghi S. Pigmented atypical fibroxanthoma: a tumor that may be easily mistaken for malignant melanoma. Am J Dermatopathol 2003;25:1–5.

36. Ferrara N, Baldi G, Di Marino MP, et al. Atypical fibroxanthoma with osteoclast-like multinucleated giant cells. In Vivo 2000;14:105–7.

37. Rudisaile SN, Hurt MA, Santa Cruz DJ. Granular cell atypical fibroxanthoma. J Cutan Pathol 2005;32:314–7.

38. Luzar B, Calonje E. Cutaneous fibrohistiocytic tumours-an update. Histopathology 2010;56:148–65.

39. Thosani MK, Marghoob A, Chen CS. Current progress of immunostains in Mohs micrographic surgery: a review. Dermatol Surg 2008;34:1621–36.

40. Ma CK, Zarbo RJ, Gown AM. Immunohistochemical characterization of atypical fibroxanthoma and dermatofibrosarcoma protuberans. Am J Clin Pathol 1992;97:478–83.

41. Mirza B, Weedon D. Atypical fibroxanthoma: a clinicopathological study of 89 cases. Australas J Dermatol 2005;46:235–8.

42. Mathew RA, Schlauder SM, Calder KB, et al. CD117 immunoreactivity in atypical fibroxanthoma. Am J Dermatopathol 2008;30:34–6.

43. Jensen K, Wilkinson B, Wines N, et al. Procollagen 1 expression in atypical fibroxanthoma and other tumors. J Cutan Pathol 2004;31:57–61.

44. Lazova R, Moynes R, May D, et al. LN-2 (CD74). A marker to distinguish atypical fibroxanthoma from malignant fibrous histiocytoma. Cancer 1997;79: 2115–24.

45. Luzar B, Calonje E. Morphological and immunohistochemical characteristics of atypical fibroxanthoma with a special emphasis on potential diagnostic pitfalls: a review. J Cutan Pathol 2010; 37:301–9.

46. Monteagudo C, Calduch L, Navarro S, et al. CD99 immunoreactivity in atypical fibroxanthoma: a common feature of diagnostic value. Am J Clin Pathol 2002;117:126–31.

47. Kanner WA, Brill LB 2nd, Patterson JW, et al. CD10, p63 and CD99 expression in the differential diagnosis of atypical fibroxanthoma, spindle cell squamous cell carcinoma and desmoplastic melanoma. J Cutan Pathol 2010;37:744–50.

48. Silvis NG, Swanson PE, Manivel JC, et al. Spindle-cell and pleomorphic neoplasms of the skin. A clinicopathologic and immunohistochemical study of 30 cases, with emphasis on "atypical fibroxanthomas". Am J Dermatopathol 1988;10:9–19.

49. Stadler FJ, Scott GA, Brown MD. Malignant fibrous tumors. Semin Cutan Med Surg 1998;17:141–52.

50. Wollina U, Schönlebe J, Koch A, et al. Atypical fibroxanthoma: a series of 25 cases. J Eur Acad Dermatol Venereol 2010;24:943–6.

51. Seavolt M, McCall M. Atypical fibroxanthoma: review of the literature and summary of 13 patients treated with mohs micrographic surgery. Dermatol Surg 2006;32:435–41 [discussion: 439–41].

52. Leibovitch I, Huilgol SC, Richards S, et al. Scalp tumors treated with Mohs micrographic surgery: clinical features and surgical outcome. Dermatol Surg 2006;32:1369–74.

53. Huether MJ, Zitelli JA, Brodland DG. Mohs micrographic surgery for the treatment of spindle cell tumors of the skin. J Am Acad Dermatol 2001;44: 656–9.

54. Kauffman SL, Stout AP. Histiocytic tumors (fibrous xanthoma and histiocytoma) in children. Cancer 1961;14:469–82.

55. O'Brien JE, Stout AP. Malignant fibrous xanthomas. Cancer 1964;17:1445–55.

56. Rouhani P, Fletcher CD, Devesa SS, et al. Cutaneous soft tissue sarcoma incidence patterns in the U.S: an analysis of 12,114 cases. Cancer 2008;113:616–27.

57. Weiss SW, Enzinger FM. Malignant fibrous histiocytoma: an analysis of 200 cases. Cancer 1978;41: 2250–66.

58. Corpron CA, Black CT, Raney RB, et al. Malignant fibrous histiocytoma in children. J Pediatr Surg 1996;31:1080–3.

59. Pezzi CM, Rawlings MS Jr, Esgro JJ, et al. Prognostic factors in 227 patients with malignant fibrous histiocytoma. Cancer 1992;69:2098–103.

60. Kearney MM, Soule EH, Ivins JC. Malifnant fibrous histiocytoma: a retrospective study of 167 cases. Cancer 1980;45:167–78.

61. Nascimento AF, Raut CP. Diagnosis and management of pleomorphic sarcomas (so-called "MFH") in adults. J Surg Oncol 2008;97:330–9.

62. Gazziola C, Cordani N, Wasserman B, et al. Malignant fibrous histiocytoma: a proposed cellular origin and identification of its characterizing gene transcripts. Int J Oncol 2003;23:343–51.

63. Foti C, Giannelli G, Berloco A, et al. Malignant fibrous histiocytoma arising on chronic osteomyelitis. J Eur Acad Dermatol Venereol 2002;16:390–2.

64. Iglesias ME, Vázquez Doval FJ, Idoate F, et al. Malignant fibrous histiocytoma at the site of total knee replacement. J Dermatol Surg Oncol 1994; 20:848–9.

65. Spirtos G, Qadri A, Phillips AK. Malignant fibrous histiocytoma (MFH) arising within a cholecystectomy incision: a cause-and-effect relationship is possible between previous surgery and the development of a malignant fibrous histiocytoma within the operative site. J Surg Oncol 1988;38:267–70.

66. Farber JN, Koh HK. Malignant fibrous histiocytoma arising from discoid lupus erythematosus. Arch Dermatol 1988;124:114–6.

67. Yamamura T, Aozasa K, Honda T, et al. Malignant fibrous histiocytoma developing in a burn scar. Br J Dermatol 1984;110:725–30.

68. Berth-Jones J, Graham-Brown RA, Fletcher A, et al. Malignant fibrous histiocytoma: a new complication of chronic venous ulceration. BMJ 1989;298:230–1.

69. Inoshita T, Youngberg GA. Malignant fibrous histiocytoma arising in previous surgical sites. Report of two cases. Cancer 1984;53:176–83.

70. Fanburg-Smith JC, Spiro IJ, Katapuram SV, et al. Infiltrative subcutaneous malignant fibrous histiocytoma: a comparative study with deep malignant

fibrous histiocytoma and an observation of biologic behavior. Ann Diagn Pathol 1999;3:1–10.

71. Headington JT, Niederhuber JE, Repola DA. Primary malignant fibrous histiocytoma of skin. J Cutan Pathol 1978;5:329–38.

72. Pettinato G, Manivel JC, De Rosa G, et al. Angiomatoid malignant fibrous histiocytoma: cytologic, immunohistochemical, ultrastructural, and flow cytometric study of 20 cases. Mod Pathol 1990;3: 479–87.

73. Marcet S. Atypical fibroxanthoma/malignant fibrous histiocytoma. Dermatol Ther 2008;21:424–7.

74. Sakamoto A, Oda Y, Itakura E, et al. Immunoexpression of ultraviolet photoproducts and p53 mutation analysis in atypical fibroxanthoma and superficial malignant fibrous histiocytoma. Mod Pathol 2001;14:581–8.

75. Sakamoto A, Oda Y, Itakura E, et al. H-, K-, and N-ras gene mutation in atypical fibroxanthoma and malignant fibrous histiocytoma. Hum Pathol 2001;32:1225–31.

76. Worrell JT, Ansari MQ, Ansari SJ, et al. Atypical fibroxanthoma: DNA ploidy analysis of 14 cases with possible histogenetic implications. J Cutan Pathol 1993;20:211–5.

77. Hashimoto H, Enjoji M. Recurrent malignant fibrous histiocytoma. A histologic analysis of 50 cases. Am J Surg Pathol 1981;5:753–60.

78. Brown MD, Swanson NA. Treatment of malignant fibrous histiocytoma and atypical fibrous xanthomas with micrographic surgery. J Dermatol Surg Oncol 1989;15:1287–92.

79. Glenn J, Kinsella T, Glatstein E, et al. A randomized, prospective trial of adjuvant chemotherapy in adults with soft tissue sarcomas of the head and neck, breast, and trunk. Cancer 1985;55:1206–14.

80. Gherlinzoni F, Bacci G, Picci P, et al. A randomized trial for the treatment of high-grade soft-tissue sarcomas of the extremities: preliminary observations. J Clin Oncol 1986;4:552–8.

81. Beach A, Severance AO. Sebaceous gland carcinoma. Ann Surg 1942;115:258–66.

82. Collins DC. Carcinoma originating in sebaceous cysts. Can Med Assoc J 1936;35:370–2.

83. Kass LG, Hornblass A. Sebaceous carcinoma of the ocular adnexa. Surv Ophthalmol 1989;33:477–90.

84. Zürcher M, Hintschich CR, Garner A, et al. Sebaceous carcinoma of the eyelid: a clinicopathological study. Br J Ophthalmol 1998;82:1049–55.

85. Shields JA, Demirci H, Marr BP, et al. Sebaceous carcinoma of the ocular region: a review. Surv Ophthalmol 2005;50:103–22.

86. Dasgupta T, Wilson LD, Yu JB. A retrospective review of 1349 cases of sebaceous carcinoma. Cancer 2009;115:158–65.

87. Dores GM, Curtis RE, Toro JR, et al. Incidence of cutaneous carcinoma and risk of associated neoplasms: insight into Muir-Torre syndrome. Cancer 2008;113:3372–81.

88. Nelson BR, Hamlet KR, Gillard M, et al. Sebaceous carcinoma. J Am Acad Dermatol 1995;33:1–15.

89. Schwartz RA, Torre DP. The Muir-Torre syndrome: a 25-year retrospect. J Am Acad Dermatol 1995; 33:90–104.

90. Shields JA, Demirci H, Marr BP, et al. Sebaceous carcinoma of the eyelids: personal experience with 60 cases. Ophthalmology 2004;111:2151–7.

91. Callahan EF, Appert DL, Roenigk RK, et al. Sebaceous carcinoma of the eyelid: a review of 14 cases. Dermatol Surg 2004;30:1164–8.

92. Dim-Jamora KC, Perone JB. Management of cutaneous tumors with mohs micrographic surgery. Semin Plast Surg 2008;22:247–56.

93. Duman DG, Ceyhan BB, Celikel T, et al. Extraorbital sebaceous carcinoma with rapidly developing visceral metastases. Dermatol Surg 2003; 29:987–9.

94. Rao NA, Hidayat AA, McLean IW, et al. Sebaceous carcinomas of the ocular adnexa: a clinicopathologic study of 104 cases, with five-year follow-up data. Hum Pathol 1982;13:113–22.

95. Shields CL, Naseripour M, Shields JA, et al. Topical mitomycin-C for pagetoid invasion of the conjunctiva by eyelid sebaceous gland carcinoma. Ophthalmology 2002;109:2129–33.

96. Spencer JM, Nossa R, Tse DT, et al. Sebaceous carcinoma of the eyelid treated with Mohs micrographic surgery. J Am Acad Dermatol 2001;44: 1004–9.

97. Thomas CJ, Wood GC, Marks VJ. Mohs micrographic surgery in the treatment of rare aggressive cutaneous tumors: the Geisinger experience. Dermatol Surg 2007;33:333–9.

98. Yen MT, Tse DT, Wu X, et al. Radiation therapy for local control of eyelid sebaceous cell carcinoma: report of two cases and review of the literature. Ophthal Plast Reconstr Surg 2000;16:211–5.

99. Cook BE Jr, Bartley GB. Treatment options and future prospects for the management of eyelid malignancies: an evidence-based update. Ophthalmology 2001;108:2088–98.

100. Lan MC, Lan MY, Lin CZ, et al. Sebaceous carcinoma of the eyelid with neck metastasis. Otolaryngol Head Neck Surg 2007;136:670–1.

101. Martinelli PT, Cohen PR, Schulze KE, et al. Sebaceous carcinoma. In: Nouri K, editor. Skin cancer. New York: McGraw-Hill; 2008. p. 240–50.

102. Buitrago W, Joseph AK. Sebaceous carcinoma: the great masquerader: emerging concepts in diagnosis and treatment. Dermatol Ther 2008; 21:459–66.

103. Lazar AJ, Lyle S, Calonie E. Sebaceous neoplasia and Torre-Muir syndrome. Curr Diagn Pathol 2007;13:301–19.

104. Higgins HJ, Voutsalath M, Holland JM. Muir-Torre syndrome: a case report. J Clin Aesthet Dermatol 2009;2:30–2.

105. Hybarger CP. Cutaneous malignant neoplasms. In: Lalwani AK, editor. Current diagnosis & treatment in otolaryngology–head & neck surgery. 1st edition. New York: McGraw-Hill; 2004. p. 221–38.

106. Wick MR, Goellner JR, Wolfe JT III, et al. Adnexal carcinomas of the skin: II. extraocular sebaceous carcinomas. Cancer 1985;56:1163–72.

107. Taylor RS, Perone JB, Kaddu S, et al. Appendage tumors and hamartomas of the skin. In: Wolff K, Goldsmith LA, Katz SI, et al, editors. Fitzpatrick's dermatology in general medicine, vol. 1. 7th edition. New York: McGraw-Hill; 2008. p. 1068–87.

108. Folberg R. The eye. In: Kumar V, Abbas AK, Fausto N, editors. Pathologic basis of disease. 7th edition. Philadelphia: Elsevier Saunders; 2005. p. 1424–5.

109. Snow SN, Larson PO, Lucarelli MJ, et al. Sebaceous carcinoma of the eyelids treated by mohs micrographic surgery: report of nine cases with review of the literature. Dermatol Surg 2002;28:623–31.

110. Berlin AL, Amin SP, Goldberg DJ. Extraocular sebaceous carcinoma treated with Mohs micrographic surgery: report of a case and review of literature. Dermatol Surg 2008;34:254–7.

111. Reina RS, Parry E. Aggressive extraocular sebaceous carcinoma in a 52-year-old man. Dermatol Surg 2006;32:1283–6.

112. Husain A, Blumenschein G, Esmaeli B. Treatment and outcomes for metastatic sebaceous cell carcinoma of the eyelid. Int J Dermatol 2008;47:276–9.

113. Calhoun KE, Giuliano AE. Breast cancer. In: Berek JS, editor. Berek & Novak's gynecology. 14th edition. Philadelphia: Lippincott Williams & Wilkins; 2007. p. 1605–31.

114. Tannous Z. Paget's disease. In: Nouri K, editor. Skin cancer. New York: McGraw-Hill; 2008. p. 371–4.

115. Yang WJ, Kim DS, Im YJ, et al. Extramammary Paget's disease of penis and scrotum. Urology 2005; 65:972–5.

116. Parker LP, Parker JR, Bodurka-Bevers D, et al. Paget's disease of the vulva: pathology, pattern of involvement, and prognosis. Gynecol Oncol 2000; 77:183–9.

117. Addis IB, Hatch KD, Berek JS. Intraepithelial disease of the cervix, vagina, and vulva. In: Berek JS, editor. Berek & Novak's gynecology. 14th edition. Philadelphia: Lippincott Williams & Wilkins; 2007. p. 561–600.

118. Shepherd V, Davidson EJ, Davies-Humphreys J. Extramammary Paget's disease. BJOG 2005;112: 273–9.

119. Bunker CB. Diseases and disorders of the male genitalia. In: Wolff K, Goldsmith LA, Katz SI, et al, Fitzpatrick's dermatology in general medicine, vol. 1. 7th edition. New York: McGraw-Hill; 2008. p. 654–75.

120. Crum CP. The female genital tract. In: Kumar V, Abbas AK, Fausto N, editors. Pathologic basis of disease. 7th edition. Philadelphia: Elsevier Saunders; 2005. p. 1068–9.

121. Landay M, Satmary WA, Memarzadeh S, et al. Premalignant & malignant disorders of the vulva & vagina. In: DeCherney AH, Goodwin TM, Nathan L, et al, editors. Current diagnosis & treatment obstetrics & gynecology. 10th edition. New York: McGraw-Hill; 2007. p. 819–32.

122. Neuhaus IM, Grekin RC. Mammary and extramammary Paget disease. In: Wolff K, Goldsmith LA, Katz SI, et al, editors, Fitzpatrick's dermatology in general medicine, vol. 1. 7th edition. New York: McGraw-Hill; 2008. p. 1094–8.

123. Wolff K, Johnson RA. Skin signs of systemic cancers. In: Fitzpatrick's color atlas & synopsis of clinical dermatology. 6th edition. New York: McGraw-Hill; 2009. p. 486–503.

124. Ekwueme KC, Zakhour HD, Parr NJ. Extramammary Paget's disease of the penis: a case report and review of the literature. J Med Case Reports 2009;3:4.

125. Fanning J, Lambert HC, Hale TM, et al. Paget's disease of the vulva: prevalence of associated vulvar adenocarcinoma, invasive Paget's disease, and recurrence after surgical excision. Am J Obstet Gynecol 1999;180:24–7.

126. Guerrieri M, Back MF. Extramammary Paget's disease: role of radiation therapy. Australas Radiol 2002;46:204–8.

127. Lloyd J, Flanagan AM. Mammary and extramammary Paget's disease. J Clin Pathol 2000;53:742–9.

128. Sitakalin C, Ackerman AB. Mammary and extramammary Paget's disease. Am J Dermatopathol 1985;7:335–40.

129. Berger TG. Dermatologic disorders. In: McPhee SJ, Papadakis MA, Tierney LM Jr, editors. Current medical diagnosis & treatment. 47th edition. New York: McGraw-Hill; 2008. p. 85–140.

130. Cole P, Heller L, Bullocks J, et al. The skin and subcutaneous tissue. In: Brunicardi FC, Andersen DK, Billiar TR, et al, editors. Schwartz's principles of surgery. 9th edition. New York: McGraw-Hill; 2010. p. 405–21.

131. Adams Hillard PJ. Benign diseases of the female reproductive tract. In: Berek JS, editor. Berek & Novak's gynecology. 14th edition. Philadelphia: Lippincott Williams & Wilkins; 2007. p. 431–504.

132. O'Connor WJ, Lim KK, Zalla MJ, et al. Comparison of Mohs micrographic surgery and wide excision for extramammary Paget's disease. Dermatol Surg 2003;29:723–7.

133. Zollo JD, Zeitouni NC. The Roswell Park Cancer Institute experience with extramammary Paget's disease. Br J Dermatol 2000;142:59–65.

134. Lau J, Kohler S. Keratin profile of intraepidermal cells in Paget's disease, extramammary disease,

and pagetoid squamous cell carcinoma in situ. J Cutan Pathol 2003;30:449–54.

135. Cohen PR, Schulze KE, Tschen JA, et al. Treatment of extramammary Paget disease with topical imiquimod cream: case report and literature review. South Med J 2006;99:396–402.

136. Tsutsumida A, Yamamoto Y, Minakawa H, et al. Indications for lymph node dissection in the treatment of extramammary Paget's disease. Dermatol Surg 2003;29:21–4.

137. Hendi A, Brodland DG, Zitelli J. Extramammary Paget's disease: surgical treatment with Mohs micrographic surgery. J Am Acad Dermatol 2004; 51:767–73.

138. Coldiron BM, Goldsmith BA, Robinson JK. Surgical treatment of extramammary Paget's disease: a report of six cases and a reexamination of Mohs micrographic surgery compared with conventional surgical excision. Cancer 1991;67: 933–8.

139. Luk NM, Yu KH, Yeung WK, et al. Extramammary Paget's disease: outcome of radiotherapy with curative intent. Clin Exp Dermatol 2003;28: 360–3.

Flaps and Grafts Reconstruction

Alexandra Y. Zhang, MD, Jon G. Meine, MD*

KEYWORDS

• Flaps • Grafts • Reconstruction

Reconstruction of Mohs surgical defects is a challenging venture. A thorough understanding of skin physiology and anatomy (cosmetic subunits, relaxed skin tension lines, underlying neurovascular structures at risk, potential functional compromise, character of adjacent skin, and so forth), careful wound analysis, and meticulous operative techniques is key to a successful reconstruction.

One of the cardinal principles in reconstructive surgery is function before form (ie, contour), and form before cosmesis. Preservation of the function is of utmost importance. Regardless of how beautiful a scar is, it is worthless if a patient's ability to breathe or vision is impaired, for example. Change of contour (depressions or elevations) is more difficult to hide than a suboptimal scar. A reconstructive ladder is also often used in considering options for reconstruction with the order of from the least invasive to the most invasive. Healing by secondary intention is at the bottom of the ladder, followed by primary closure, graft, flap, and free flap (**Fig. 1**). When there are multiple cosmetic subunits involved in a defect, combination closures with flap and/or graft and/or secondary intention should be considered to achieve an optimal reconstruction. This article discusses in detail the use of local skin flaps and graft reconstruction.

PREOPERATIVE PLANNING

Preoperative consultation establishes an open communication between surgeon, patient, and family members. It provides a patient with a better understanding of the procedure by discussing the limitations and advantages of different reconstruction options. It also provides the opportunity for a surgeon to understand a patient's aesthetic expectations and to evaluate a patient's overall comorbidities, risk factors (**Box 1**), and character and extent of the defect (**Box 2**). In general, the simplest closure (healing by secondary intention or primary closure) is often the best option; it makes the fewest number of incisions and produces the least rearrangement of the tissue. Yet, when a defect is under high tension or with functional compromise, a flap is a good choice for redirecting tension lines, minimizing distortion of the tissue, and keeping the contours intact.

FLAP RECONSTRUCTION

A skin flap is defined as a construct of skin and subcutaneous tissue containing a direct vascular supply that is transferred to a primary surgical site adjacent to or near the flap.

Physiology of Skin Flaps

Adequate vascular supply to the flap and neovascularization between the flap and the recipient wound bed are critical factors to the survival of a flap. A wide interconnecting network of dermal and subdermal plexuses fed by septocutaneous and musculocutaneous arteries provides ample vascular supply to the skin.

Random pattern skin flaps and axial skin flaps are the primary flaps used in facial reconstruction. Random pattern skin flaps are supplied by musculocutaneous arteries close to the base of the flap that empty into the dermal plexus. Therefore, a good perfusion pressure from the supplying vascular network is important to prevent flap necrosis. Variable length-to-width ratios (2–4:1) have been suggested when designing random

The authors have no conflicts of interest to disclose.
Department of Dermatology, Cleveland Clinic Foundation, 9500 Euclid Avenue, A61, Cleveland, OH 44195, USA
* Corresponding author.
E-mail address: meinej@ccf.org

derm.theclinics.com

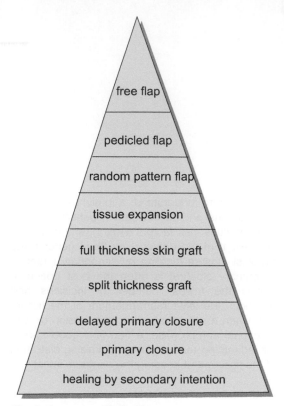

Fig. 1. Reconstructive ladder.

Box 2
Defect analysis

What type of cancer type does the patient have? Are the margins clear? What is the chance for recurrence?

What is the location and size of the defect?

What is the depth of the defect (partial thickness, full thickness, fat, fascia, muscle, cartilage, or bone; Any key structures exposed)?

What and how many cosmetic units and/or subunits are involved?

In which direction do the regional relaxed skin tension lines run?

How are the adjacent cosmetic boundaries associated with the defect?

Are free margins involved—nose, eyelids, and lips?

Is there compromise of function (ie, collapse of nasal valve, named nerve damage, and so forth)?

What are the quality, texture, laxity, and mobility of adjacent skin?

Box 1
Preparation of the patient

What are the patient's age, occupation, and other daily activities?

Did the patient have previous radiation to the surgical site?

What is the patient's aesthetic expectation?

Is the patient willing to go through and tolerate a multistaged repair?

Is the patient compliant in wound care? What is his/her living situation (family support system)?

What comorbidities may cause delayed wound healing (hypertension, heart disease, diabetes, organ transplant, immunosuppression, bleeding disorders, and smoking)?

Does the patient have a pacemaker/defibrillator?

Does the patient need prophylactic antibiotics?

Is the patient taking anticoagulants (aspirin, warfarin, clopidogrel, nonsteroidal anti-inflammatory drugs, vitamin E, fish oil, or herbal supplements)?

pattern skin flaps, depending on variable blood supplies at different wound defect locations. A wider skin flap, however, does not necessarily guarantee better survival.[1]

The axial pattern flap (arterial flap) contains a specific named artery. Because of its dependable blood supply from the specific artery, it allows for the reconstruction of a more complex defect at a relative distant location, using the axial pattern flap. For example, the paramedian forehead flap, based on the supratrochlear artery, is often used in repairing large nasal defects. Axial pattern flaps are multistage flaps that are usually divided in 3 weeks after flap transfer once enough collateral vascular supply is established at the distal portion of the flap from the wound bed.[2]

Flap Classification and Design

Flaps are classified in many ways based on:

- Location—local, regional, or distant
- Blood supply—random pattern or axial
- Configuration—bilobe or rhombic
- Method of transfer—pivotal, advancement, or hinge.

Flap design by method of transfer is the most common means of discussing the use of cutaneous facial flaps.

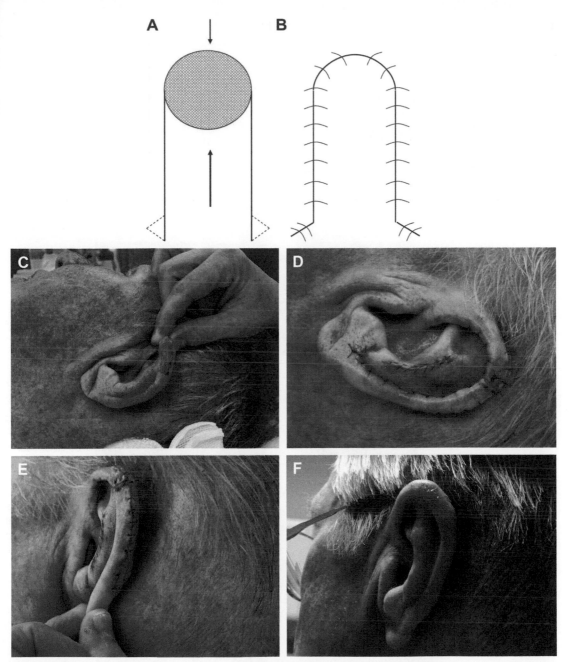

Fig. 2. (*A*) Diagram showing the planning of a unipedicle advancement flap. Incisions are made along the lateral borders of a defect. (*B*) A U-shaped flap is created and advanced into the defect. (*C*) A defect on the right helical rim after Mohs micrographic surgery. (*D, E*) The defect is repaired with the advancement flap. (*F*) One year postoperative. (*G–L*) T-plasty (O to T) is used for reconstruction of a circular wound. (*G, H*) Diagram showing planning for O to T. Incision is made at the inferior border of a circular wound. Two flaps are advanced toward to each other into the defect. Standing cone deformity formed superiorly is excised (*dotted lines*) and becomes part of the vertical branch of the T. The final suture line of the wound closure is in a T configuration. (*I*) Defect on the left lower lip after Mohs micrographic surgery. (*J*) The defect is repaired with a T-plasty. (*K*) Results at 6-week follow-up. (*L–N*) A defect on lateral forehead above the eyebrow after Mohs micrographic surgery (*L*) is repaired with a T-plasty (*M*). Well-healed wound at 6-week follow-up (*N*) without elevation of the eyebrow.

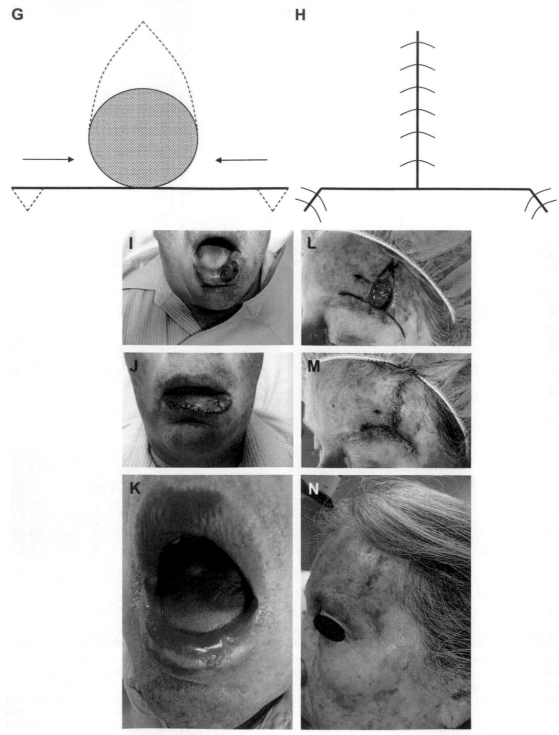

Fig. 2. (*continued*)

Advancement flaps

In advancement flaps, incisions are made so that the tissue is transferred by sliding toward the defect. They are usually constructed in a linear configuration. Unipedicle, bipedicle, and V-Y flaps are the principle types of advancement flaps.

1. Unipedicle advancement flaps

In unipedicle advancement flaps, parallel incisions (often along the relaxed skin tension lines) are made to allow the flap and its pedicle to slide toward the defect. Undermining of the flap, around the pedicle and the defect, is important to reduce the tension and facilitates tissue movement. Because the length of advancement (defect width plus flap incision) is longer than the length of flap, it usually results in standing cone deformities. There are two main ways to eliminate the standing cones. Burow triangles can be excised along the longer sides to remove the standing cones. Alternatively, the rule of halves may be used when placing sutures to redistribute the extra length along the borders of the wound (defect plus the wound incision) evenly to eliminate the standing cones. Variations of unipedicle advancement flaps, such as U-plasty, H-plasty, and T-plasty (O to T or A to T), work particularly well in reconstructing certain locations: helical rim, chin, eyebrows, eyelids, medial cheek, and forehead (Fig. 2).

2. Bipedicle advancement flaps

The bipedicle advancement flap is designed near the primary defect and allows for advancement into the primary defect at an angle often perpendicular to the flap axis. A secondary defect is created that can be repaired either by primary closure or a graft. Bipedicle advancement flaps are often used in reconstruction of large defects on the scalp and forehead and in realigning full-thickness defects on the nasal ala or hemitip with a vertical dimension less than 1 cm.[3,4] These flaps are rarely used in dermatologic surgery and little has been published about them in the literature.

3. V-Y advancement flaps

In a V-Y advancement flap, V-shaped incisions are made, which result in a triangular donor flap that can be pushed forward to cover the primary defect with minimal tension. This leaves

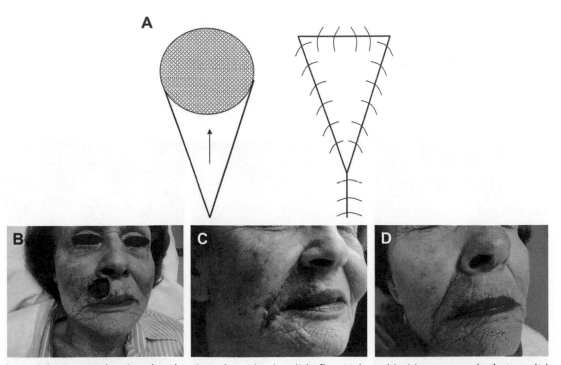

Fig. 3. (A) Diagram showing the planning of an island pedicle flap. V-shaped incisions are made that result in a triangular-shaped donor flap that is based on a subcutaneous tissue stalk. The flap is stretched into the defect. The primary and secondary wounds are closed and the suture line is in a Y configuration. (B) A large defect on the right upper cutaneous lip after Mohs micrographic surgery. Island pedicle flap designed for reconstruction. (C) The defect is repaired with an island pedicle flap. Sutures are removed at 1 week postoperative. (D) Six weeks postoperative.

a secondary defect that is closed primarily as a straight line. It results in Y-shaped suture lines once both primary and secondary defects are closed. The V-Y flaps are especially helpful in releasing a contracted scar by lengthening the scar. The island pedicle flap is technically a type of unipedicle advancement flap. The donor flap is stretched into the primary defect, however, based on a pedicle that consists of underlying subcutaneous tissue (**Fig. 3**).

Pivotal flaps

1. Rotation flaps

Rotation flaps are curvilinear in configuration and are rotated into the defect moving about a pivotal point. In general, the flap is designed so that the ratio of the length of the incision to the width of the defect is 4:1. A standing cone often develops at the base of the flap that can be removed. Sometimes a back-cut at the base of the flap is needed to lengthen the flap, which shifts the pivotal point of the flap. This also changes the

location of the standing cone and tension vectors for wound closure. Rotation flaps work well in closing defects on the scalp, temple, and lateral forehead region as well as large defects on the lower lateral cheek (**Fig. 4**). The dorsal nasal flap is a variation of a rotation flap that is useful in closing certain defects on the nasal dorsum, tip, and sidewall.[5,6]

2. Transposition flaps

Transposition flaps are linear in configuration and move in a pivotal fashion. In these flaps, noncontiguous tissue is transposed across the intervening area of unaffected skin into the primary defect. The donor flap may or may not immediately border the primary defect. The ability to recruit the donor flap from a relatively remote site offers great flexibility in selecting donor sites based on skin laxity, elasticity, color and texture match, and scar camouflage. One rule to keep in mind when designing a transposition flap is that the size of standing cone at the base increases and the effective length of the flap decreases as the arc of

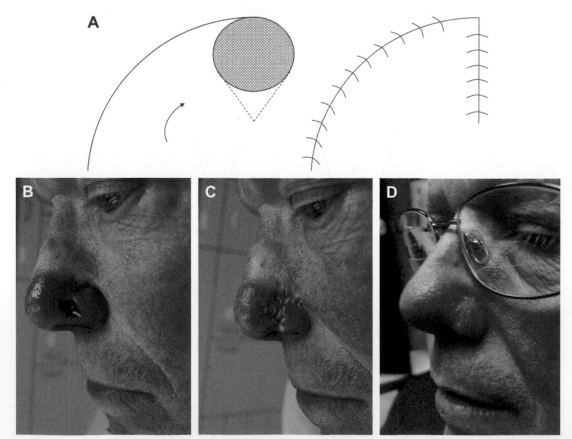

Fig. 4. (*A*) Diagram showing the planning of a rotation flap. A standing cone deformity can be excised (*dotted lines*). (*B*) Defect on the nasal ala after Mohs micrographic surgery. (*C*) Rotation flap is used for reconstruction; flap in place. (*D*) Six weeks postoperative.

pivotal movement increases. Therefore, a longer design of the flap is needed if flap is transposed at a greater pivotal angle from its original position.[7] Rhombic (**Fig. 5**) and bilobe flaps (**Fig. 6**) are two types of commonly used transposition flaps.

3. Interpolation flaps

Interpolation flaps are staged flaps. In the first stage, the flap is harvested and a pedicle is created. The pedicle then crosses over or under the intervening area of unaffected skin when the flap is transposed into the primary defect. In 2 to 3 weeks, once neovascularization is established, the pedicle is divided and the flap is then detached, which finalizes the reconstruction. Interpolation flaps can be either axial pattern flaps (eg, paramedian forehead flap) (**Fig. 7**) or random pattern flaps (eg, melolabial interpolation flap) (**Fig. 8**). Interpolation flaps work particularly well in reconstructing large, deep defects that involve greater than 50% of the cosmetic subunit and/or defects with infrastructure loss.

GRAFT RECONSTRUCTION

Skin grafting involves transplanting skin and sometimes underlying tissue from its donor site to a distant site. As a skin graft is harvested, its vascular supply is also separated; this needs to be re-established at the recipient site in order for the graft to survive.

There are three physiologic stages that the graft endures before it is fully sustained by the recipient wound bed. The first stage, imbibition, occurs within the first 24 hours after emplacement of the graft to the recipient site. The graft is attached to the recipient wound bed with the help of fibrin. The graft becomes edematous by absorbing nutrients and exudates from the wound through capillary action.[8] Inosculation occurs within 48 to 72 hours of grafting. In this stage, dermal plexuses begin to anastomose with the wound bed.[9] This process bestows on the graft a red and occasionally somewhat cyanotic appearance. The third stage is neovascularization, during which complete vascular circulation is re-established 4 to 7 days after grafting.

Graft Classification

Skin grafts are classified into three categories: full-thickness, split-thickness, and composite skin grafts.

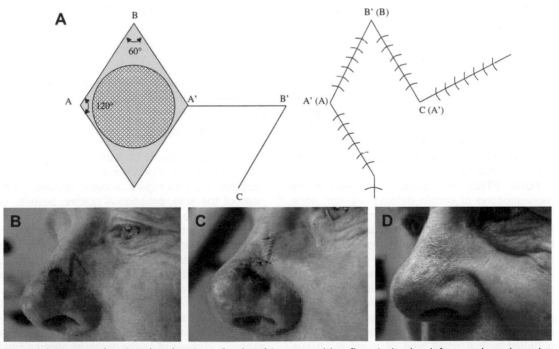

Fig. 5. (*A*) Diagram showing the planning of a rhombic transposition flap. A circular defect can be enlarged to rhombus in shape. The 4 sides of the rhombus are equal in length with 2 opposing 60° and 120° angles. The extension of the short diagonal (A′C) should be equal to the length of each side of the rhombus (A′B). (*B*) Defect superior to the nasal ala after Mohs micrographic surgery. (*C*) A rhombic transposition flap is used for reconstruction. Flap in place. (*D*) Six weeks postoperative.

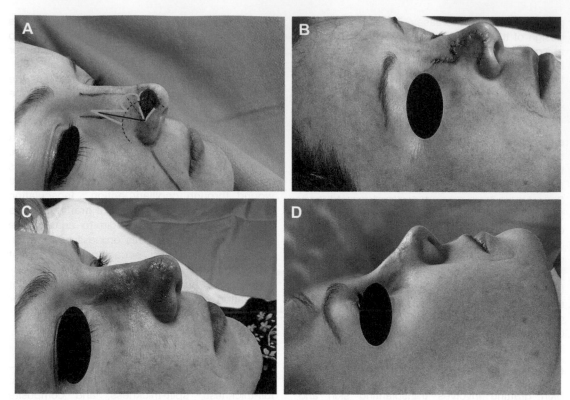

Fig. 6. Bilobe transposition flap (Zitelli modification). (*A*) Defect on the nasal ala after Mohs micrographic surgery. The flap is designed laterally based. The standing cone deformity is placed at the alar crease. The total transposition is approximately 90° (between the blue running lines) and the angles between the 2 lobes of flaps are 45°. The planned incisions are indicated by the green lines. (*B*) Flap in place. (*C*) One week postoperative. (*D*) Six weeks postoperative.

Full-thickness skin graft

Full-thickness skin grafts (FTSGs) contain the full thickness of epidermis, dermis, and dermal adnexal structures, which minimize wound contraction.[10] They offer acceptable cosmesis in the right setting by providing good depth, texture, and color matches for defects after skin cancer removal. FTSGs are particularly useful in the reconstruction of certain defects (eg, ear, nose, and eyelids), where there is minimal surrounding laxity, and when other options, such as healing by secondary intention, primary closure, and local flaps, are not suitable.

It is important to evaluate the vascularity of the recipient wound bed before harvesting an FTSG to ensure the survival of the graft. An FTSG should not be placed over a large area of avascular tissue, such as exposed tendon, cartilage, or bone. In a defect with a small area of avascular tissue, however, delayed grafting may be considered to allow the recipient bed to granulate and revascularize. Alternatively, a hinge flap, using adjacent fat that is lifted and turned over to cover exposed underlying cartilage or bone, can be used in conjunction with FTSG to allow immediate repair of the defect.

1. Donor site selection

The principle criteria for donor site selection are based on whether it provides a good match to the recipient site with regard to color, texture, thickness of the skin, sebaceous quality, severity of actinic damage, and presence or absence of hair. Depending on the size and location of the defect, common donor sites available for FTSGs include the preauricular cheek, postauricular sulcus, glabella, conchal bowl, nasolabial fold, upper eyelid, lateral neck, and supraclavicular area. Another donor source for FTSG comes from the excision of a Burow triangle (a standing cone deformity), which is known as a Burow graft. For example, in cases of a large defect involving almost the entire nasal tip, an FTSG harvested from preauricular cheek provides an excellent cosmetic result without going through a large staged repair with a paramedian forehead flap (**Fig. 9**).

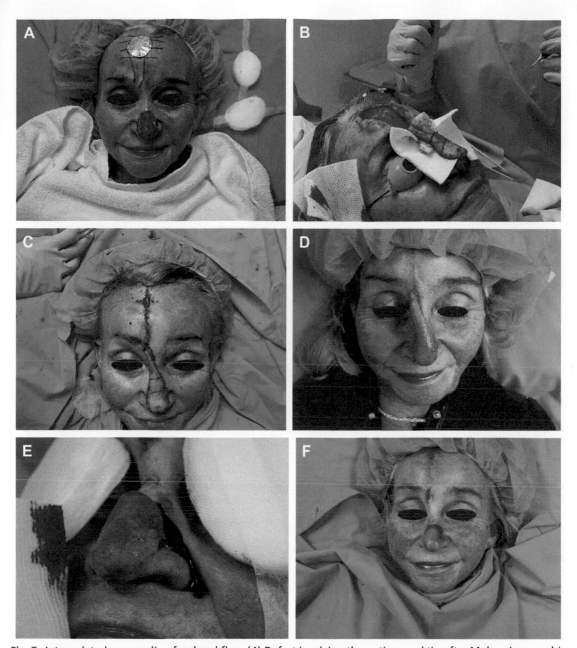

Fig. 7. Interpolated paramedian forehead flap. (*A*) Defect involving the entire nasal tip after Mohs micrographic surgery. A template of the defect is created. (*B*) The flap is lifted. (*C*) Flap in place. The secondary defect on the forehead is closed. (*D*) Three weeks post paramedian forehead flap transfer. (*E*) The pedicle is separated. (*F*) Flap sutured in place after division; donor site wound is also repaired. (*G–I*) Long-term follow-up result.

2. Technique

A template of the defect is made by using gauze, cardboard labels, or foil from suture packaging. The template is then transposed to the donor site. The graft excised from the donor site should be slightly larger than the template, because FTSGs contract approximately 10% to 15% after excision.[11] Donor tissue is often excised in elliptical configuration to facilitate the primary closure of the donor site defect. It is important to defat the graft using curved iris scissors before placement of the graft to the recipient bed to allow for better revascularization. Keeping the FTSG in iced sterile saline prolongs the viability of the graft up to 24 hours. Once a graft is transferred to the defect in the correct orientation, a few tacking sutures can be placed to secure the graft. The

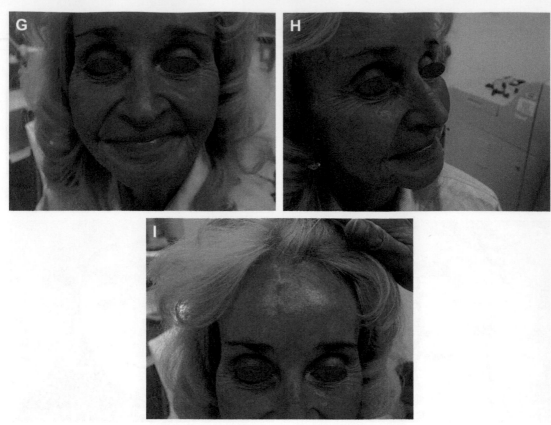

Fig. 7. (*continued*)

graft can be trimmed as needed to make an exact fit to the recipient wound bed. Simple interrupted sutures are placed from the graft to the borders of the recipient site with precise wound edge approximation. A bolster that contains cotton balls, petrolatum-based ointment, and Xeroform gauze may be tied over the graft to enhance the direct contact between the graft and the recipient site and to keep the graft moist (**Fig. 10**). The bolster may be removed in 5 to 7 days.

Split-thickness skin graft

Split-thickness skin grafts (STSGs) consist of the epidermis and a part of the underlying dermis. Depending on the amount of dermis included, the STSGs are subdivided into thin (0.13–0.31 mm), medium (0.31–0.47 mm), and thick (0.47–0.78 mm) grafts. STSGs are indicated in repairing large surgical defects and defects at high risk of tumor recurrence. Unlike FTSGs, STSGs contain less tissue that demands a robust vascular supply; thus, they have better chance of survival in recipient beds with suboptimal vascularity. The main disadvantages of STSGs include significant graft contraction and suboptimal color, texture, and

thickness match, resulting in a more prominent tire-patch appearance.

1. Donor site selection

After harvesting an STSG, the donor site usually heals by secondary intention and appears hypopigmented. Thus, unexposed areas that can be hidden under clothing, such as the medial or lateral upper thigh, medial or lateral upper arm, abdomen, and buttocks, are popular donor sites for STSGs. Donor sites that offer large flat surfaces also facilitate the harvesting of STSGs.

2. Techniques

Either the freehand or an electric dermatome can be used to harvest STSGs. Examples of freehand dermatomes include double-blade razor blades, scalpel blades, and Weck knives. They are useful in harvesting small STSGs. Electric dermatomes, such as the Davol dermatome (with fixed graft width and thickness), the Brown and Padgett dermatomes (with adjustable graft width and thickness), and the Zimmer dermatome (with uniform predetermined graft width and thickness), are used in harvesting large STSGs.

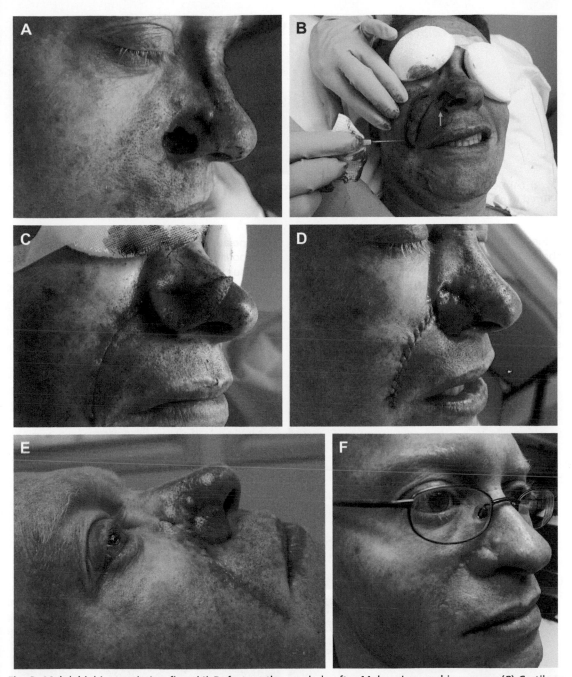

Fig. 8. Melolabial interpolation flap. (*A*) Defect on the nasal ala after Mohs micrographic surgery. (*B*) Cartilage graft (*arrow*) harvested from the antihelix is placed into the defect providing structural support. (*C*) Donor flap harvested from melolabial fold is lifted. Donor site wound closed with sutures. (*D*) Flap in place. (*E*) The pedicle is divided at 3 weeks post flap transfer. Flap in place. Superior donor site wound is closed with sutures. (*F*) Five months postoperative.

Once the dermatome is ready, the donor site is sterilized, anesthetized, and then lubricated with sterile saline or mineral oil.

The dermatome is held at a 30° to 45° angle to the skin on the donor site with a consistent pressure applied as the dermatome slides across the donor skin. A gentle countertraction can be applied to pull the skin away from the donor site to build a smooth surface. Once the graft is harvested, it should be kept in sterile iced saline.

The STSG can be meshed by using a graft-meshing machine or by making slits using a scalpel

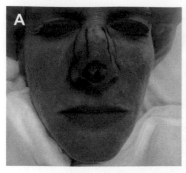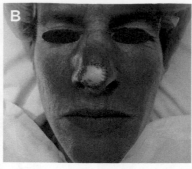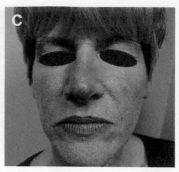

Fig. 9. (*A*) Defect on nasal tip after Mohs micrographic surgery. (*B*) FTSG harvested from preauricular cheek is sutured in place. (*C*) Six weeks postoperative.

if the graft needs to be expanded. The STSG should be trimmed and then secured to the recipient bed by sutures with good wound edge approximation. Like FTSGs, basting sutures can be placed in the center of the STSGs, and a bolster can also be used to maximize the direct contact between the graft and the recipient bed to enhance graft survival.

Composite Graft

Composite grafts are composed of multiple layers of tissue, such as skin and fat, skin and perichondrium, or skin and cartilage, among which, composite grafts, consisting of skin and cartilage, are most commonly used in dermatologic surgery. Composite grafts are useful in reconstruction of full-thickness defects with loss of structural

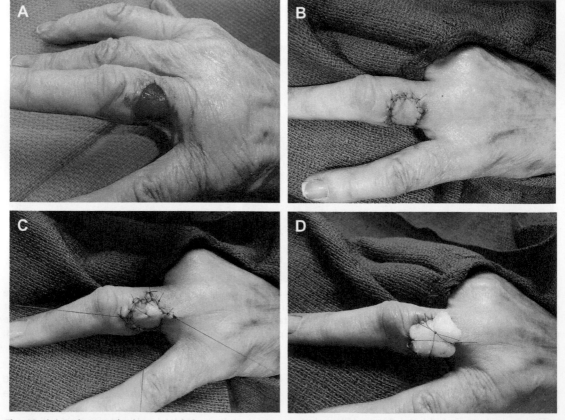

Fig. 10. (*A*) Defect on the base of left fourth finger after Mohs micrographic surgery. (*B*) FTSG harvested from left dorsal wrist sutured in place. (*C*) A basting suture is placed in the center of the graft. (*D*) A bolster dressing is placed over the graft.

support, such as nasal ala rim defects and nasal tip defects with cartilage loss. Because of their high demand of rapid vascular supply, the composite grafts should be kept small in size (usually <1 cm).

The ear is a common donor site for composite grafts used in repairing nasal defects. Both the crus of the helix and the helical rim serve as good donor sites for nasal ala defects with cartilage loss. The conchal bowl is used as a donor site in repairing more substantial defects, such as deep nasal ala defects. The donor site can be closed in most situations by primary closure if the graft is taken from the helical crus. Wedge resection may be used in repairing the helical rim donor defect. The conchal bowl donor defect usually heals by secondary intention.

A template of the defect can be created (described previously). Before harvesting, the graft may be designed to have a cartilage wing on each end extending beyond the cutaneous portion. The cartilage wings can be inserted into the pockets created at the recipient site and then aligned and secured by sutures.

Complications

Hematoma/seroma

A hematoma or seroma blocks the blood and nutrient supply to the graft, thereby compromising the graft's survival. Meticulous hemostasis and an adequate pressure dressing are the keys to preventing hematoma or seroma formation underneath the graft. Other risk factors contributing to the development of a hematoma include strenuous activity, hypertension, trauma to the graft site, consumption of anticoagulants, and other factors. As described previously, basting sutures and a tie-over bolster are helpful in minimizing the dead space between the graft and recipient bed, thereby decreasing the risk of hematoma/seroma formation.

Graft necrosis

Partial or full necrosis of the graft may occur, presenting as a black eschar due to inadequate blood supply. It is recommended to leave the necrotic graft intact and keep it moist with a petrolatum-based dressing, so that the necrotic graft serves as a natural dressing for the viable tissue underneath until it falls off on its own.

Wound infection

Wound infection can occur after graft placement, especially in patients who are immunocompromised, diabetic, or undergoing a prolonged operation. Incision and drainage of abscesses, performing wound cultures to identify the causative organisms followed by appropriate oral antibiotics, and vigilant wound care are mainstays in the treatment of wound infections.

Graft contraction

Graft contraction can result in substantial functional and cosmetic problems. One study demonstrated a mean contraction of 38% by 16 weeks after placement of FTSGs. Graft contracture is more significant in grafts that are placed on the nose and periorbital region than those placed on scalp and temple.[12] In general, graft contraction is more significant in STSGs when compared with FTSG. Surgical revision may be warranted if the graft contraction results in significant functional impairment.

Pigment alteration

Color and texture mismatch may occur after grafting. This can be improved with certain revision procedures, such as superficial dermabrasion or ablative laser resurfacing, using an erbium:YAG or carbon dioxide laser at 6 weeks to 6 months after graft placement. These procedures, along with gentle massage and/or intralesional injection of corticosteroids, also help to soften firm and elevated scars. In addition, vascular lasers can be used in reducing the visible and clinically apparent surface neovascularization at the graft site.

POSTOPERATIVE CARE

The principle goals of wound care after flap and graft reconstruction are to prevent postoperative bleeding and wound infection and to protect the flap or graft from environmental insults, therefore ensuring flap or graft survival. An initial pressure dressing is often applied over the flap or graft for 24 to 48 hours after reconstruction, because hematomas are most likely to occur during the first 48 hours postoperatively. Intraoperative sterile technique is essential in preventing postoperative wound infection. In certain practices, intraincisional antibiotic injection has been routinely used in preventing postoperative wound infections with excellent results. One study demonstrated the efficacy of preoperative intraincisional clindamycin injection as antibiotic prophylaxis treatment in dermatologic surgery.[13] Before discharge, patients should be educated about postoperative wound care, the wound healing process, and potential complications. Written wound care instructions are especially helpful to serve as a reminder and guide for patients and their caretakers in wound care management after reconstructive surgery.

REFERENCES

1. Daniel R, Kerrigan C. The anatomy and hemodynamics of the cutaneous circulation and their influence on skin flap design. In: Grabb W, Myers M, editors. Skin flaps. Boston: Little, Brown & Co; 1975. p. 111–31.
2. Converse JM, Wood-Smith D. Experiences with the forehead island flap with a subcutaneous pedicle. Plast Reconstr Surg 1963;31:521–7.
3. Flint ID, Siegle RJ. The bipedicle flap revisited. J Dermatol Surg Oncol 1994;20(6):394–400.
4. Stoner JG, Swanson NA. Use of the bipedicled scalp flap for forehead reconstruction. J Dermatol Surg Oncol 1984;10(3):213–5.
5. Rieger RA. A local flap for repair of the nasal tip. Plast Reconstr Surg 1967;40(2):147–9.
6. Rigg BM. The dorsal nasal flap. Plast Reconstr Surg 1973;52(4):361–4.
7. Gorney M. Tissue dynamics and surgical geometry. In: Kernahan D, Vistnes L, editors. Biological aspects of reconstructive surgery. Boston: Little, Brown & Co; 1977.
8. Converse JM, Uhlschmid GK, Ballantyne DL Jr. "Plasmatic circulation" in skin grafts. The phase of serum imbibition. Plast Reconstr Surg 1969;43(5):495–9.
9. Converse JM, Smahel J, Ballantyne DL, et al. Inosculation of vessels of skin graft and host bed: a fortuitous encounter. Br J Plast Surg 1975;28(4):274–82.
10. Walden JL, Garcia H, Hawkins H, et al. Both dermal matrix and epidermis contribute to an inhibition of wound contraction. Ann Plast Surg 2000;45(2):162–6.
11. Hill TG. Reconstruction of nasal defects using full-thickness skin grafts: a personal reappraisal. J Dermatol Surg Oncol 1983;9(12):995–1001.
12. Stephenson AJ, Griffiths RW, La Hausse-Brown TP. Patterns of contraction in human full thickness skin grafts. Br J Plast Surg 2000;53(5):397–402.
13. Huether MJ, Griego RD, Brodland DG, et al. Clindamycin for intraincisional antibiotic prophylaxis in dermatologic surgery. Arch Dermatol 2002;138(9):1145–8.

Management of Skin Cancer in Solid-organ Transplant Recipients: A Multidisciplinary Approach

Judah N. Greenberg, MD[a], Fiona O. Zwald, MD, MRCPI[b,c],*

KEYWORDS

- Multidisciplinary clinic • Skin cancer
- Solid-organ transplant • Immunosuppression

There are presently more than 170,000 solid-organ transplant recipients (SOTR) living in the United States alone, compared with 120,000 SOTR 10 years ago.[1] This increase is attributable to an increase in the number of transplants performed and to improved posttransplant survival as a result of refinement of surgical techniques and medical management of the SOTR. As transplant medicine continues to advance, posttransplant survival may be expected to improve further and the numbers to increase accordingly. These trends are of particular interest to the dermatologist because SOTR are known to be at markedly increased risk for cutaneous malignancies. More than 50% of SOTR are ultimately diagnosed with at least 1 skin cancer.[2] Skin cancers remain the most commonly diagnosed neoplasms among SOTR, comprising nearly 40% of all posttransplant malignancies.[3] In addition to the increased incidence of these tumors in the SOTR population, the tumors tend to behave more aggressively than those in nontransplant hosts.

The significant burden of morbidity and mortality conferred by these aggressive skin cancers demands a systematic response by dermatologists caring for the SOTR population. In the past, these patients were typically not brought to the attention of dermatologists until after they were discovered to have cutaneous malignances, obviating the possibility of implementing effective preventive strategies. This suboptimal approach to a population already known to be at higher risk for skin cancer has been characterized as reactive rather than proactive.[4] In recent years, an alternative approach has been developed at several centers: the organization of a dedicated dermatology subspecialty clinic within a multidisciplinary clinical environment in the transplant center.[5] Such a multidisciplinary clinic may integrate transplant surgeons, dermatologists (including dermatopathologists and Mohs micrographic surgeons), nephrologists, hepatologists, medical and radiation oncologists, and representatives of other relevant subspecialties. This multidisciplinary environment facilitates collaboration and close communication between the wide array of specialties responsible for the various facets of the care of a complex patient population. In addition, it serves to simplify the expeditious scheduling of follow-up with the necessary specialists, such that the

Disclosures: the authors have nothing to disclose.

[a] Department of Medicine, Emory University School of Medicine, 1724 Briarvista Way North East, Atlanta, GA 30329, USA

[b] Mohs Micrographic Surgery, Transplant Dermatology, Department of Dermatology, Emory University School of Medicine, A Building, 1365 Clifton Road North East, Suite 1400, Atlanta, GA 30322, USA

[c] Division of Transplantation, Department of Surgery, Emory University School of Medicine, A Building, 1365 Clifton Road North East, Suite 1400, Atlanta, GA 30322, USA

* Corresponding author.

E-mail address: taranadine@aol.com

Dermatol Clin 29 (2011) 231–241

doi:10.1016/j.det.2011.02.004

0733-8635/11/$ – see front matter © 2011 Published by Elsevier Inc.

dermatologist may routinely see the SOTR in the pretransplant phase to undertake baseline risk assessment and initiation of appropriate interventions. Fundamentally, the role of the dermatologist in this multidisciplinary approach follows the paradigm of prevention (via education, chemoprophylaxis, and revision of immunosuppression), surveillance for the purpose of early detection, and treatment of cutaneous malignancies.

EPIDEMIOLOGY

Most the cutaneous malignancies diagnosed in SOTR are nonmelanoma skin cancers (NMSC), with squamous cell carcinomas (SCC) and basal cell carcinomas (BCC) accounting for 90% to 95% of the total in multiple reported cohorts.[6–9] The mean interval between transplantation and diagnosis of NMSC varies with patient age at transplantation: 8 years for patients transplanted around 40 years of age, but approximately 3 years for those transplanted after 60 years of age.[6,10] Although the incidence of both tumor types is markedly increased in SOTR, the rate of SCC is disproportionately higher (Table 1). Although the incidence of BCC is increased tenfold to 16-fold, SCC occurs at a frequency of between 65 and 250 times that of the general population.[8,11,12] This results in the inversion of the SCC/BCC ratio of 1:4 in the general population to a ratio of at least 4:1 in SOTR.[2,13] This reversal becomes even more pronounced with decreasing latitude (ie, in sunnier climates) and length of time after transplant.[10,14]

In an Australian cohort, the cumulative incidence of NMSC has been reported to be 45% by ~10 years after transplantation, and 70% by 20 years after transplantation.[15] In a UK cohort, the mean annual risk of developing NMSC was found to be 3.27% for SOTR less than 5 years after transplantation, 5.86% for SOTR 5 to 10 years after transplantation, and 11.1% for those more than 10 years after transplantation.[16] The considerable acceleration of SCC incidence in SOTR is such

that the diagnosis of a first SCC has been shown to be predictive of multiple subsequent NMSC within 5 years.[17] In addition to the increased incidence of SCC, the tumors display a more aggressive phenotype in SOTR than in the general population, with more rapid growth, local recurrence in 13.4% of SOTR, and a metastatic rate of approximately 8%.[8,18]

The risk of other types of skin cancer is also increased in the SOTR population (see Table 1). The incidence of melanoma seems to be increased 2.2-fold to 8-fold in SOTR.[8,19,20] The largest study to date of melanoma in SOTR found that risk of melanoma increased with increasing age in male patients, but not in female patients.[19] The incidence of Kaposi sarcoma has been shown to be increased 84-fold in SOTR.[11] SOTR may be at increased risk for other rare skin cancers, including Merkel cell carcinoma, atypical fibroxanthoma, angiosarcoma, verrucous carcinoma, leiomyosarcoma, and cutaneous T-cell and B-cell lymphomas, but evidence is scant and anecdotal at present owing to the rarity of these tumors.[21–23]

RISK FACTORS

The determinants of skin cancer development in SOTR are well defined (Box 1). As in the general population, the most significant risk factor in SOTR is exposure to ultraviolet radiation (UVR).[24] Fair skin (Fitzpatrick skin types I, II, or III) also predisposes SOTR to cutaneous malignancies.[25] Increased age is correlated with the development of skin cancer, probably because of greater total UVR exposure in older patients.[26]

Several additional risk factors are unique to the SOTR population. The most important of these is the immunosuppression that accompanies organ

Table 1 Population-based standardized incidence ratios of skin cancers in organ transplant recipients	
Skin Cancer	Fold Increase in Incidence
Squamous cell carcinoma	65–250
Basal cell carcinoma	10–16
Melanoma	2.2–8
Kaposi sarcoma	84

Box 1 Risk factors for the development of skin cancer after solid-organ transplantation
Exposure to UVR
Fitzpatrick skin types I, II, or III
Increased age at transplantation
Duration, degree, and type of immunosuppression
Type of organ transplant: heart/lung > kidney > liver
Previous organ transplant
Personal history of actinic keratosis (AK), NMSC, or melanoma
Human papillomavirus (HPV) infection

transplantation. Pharmacologic suppression of the immune system increases the risk of developing malignancies, particularly those of the skin.[27] Moreover, it has been shown that their incidence is proportional to the dosage, duration, and even the type of immunosuppression.[7,28,29] Among SOTR, heart transplant recipients seem to be at the highest risk for developing skin cancers after transplantation (2–3 times that of kidney transplant recipients), because of the greater intensity of immunosuppression demanded by the cardiac allograft.[8,10,30] Kidney transplant recipients tend to develop more individual tumors in the course of time, possibly as a result of their younger average age at transplantation and consequent longer ultimate duration of immunosuppression.[17] Liver transplant recipients seem to be at the lowest relative risk for skin cancers.[31,32] Repeat or multiple transplantation seems to further increase skin cancer risk, likely as a result of the greater cumulative burden of immunosuppression.

Although human papillomavirus (HPV) is a known oncovirus (implicated in the carcinogenesis of ano-genital malignancies), its role in the pathogenesis of NMSC has been uncertain.[2] However, recent data seem to confirm that HPV does contribute to the development of SCC (especially in the immuno-compromised host), although the precise mechanism remains a matter of debate.[33–35] Several genetic polymorphisms, including those in gluta-thione S-transferase, interleukin 10, the folate pathway, and vitamin D receptor genes, may also contribute to skin cancer development in kidney transplant recipients in particular, although it remains to be elucidated whether this applies to SOTR in general.[36,37] Another important risk factor among SOTR is pretransplant personal history of AK, NMSC, or melanoma, which significantly increases the risk of subsequent skin cancer development in the posttransplant period.[24,38]

Such factors as sex of the recipient, type of donor (live vs cadaveric), and duration of pretransplant dialysis (in kidney transplant recipients) do not seem to increase the risk of cutaneous malignancies in SOTR.[25,39]

PRETRANSPLANT CONSIDERATIONS

In addition to management of the posttransplant patient, the dermatologist may serve a significant advisory role in the pretransplant phase. As noted earlier, a personal history of skin cancer (or prema-lignant skin lesions) is known to be an independent risk factor for development of further skin cancers after transplantation. There has therefore been some discussion in the recent literature as to whether a previous diagnosis of high-risk skin

cancer should, a priori, be considered a relative contraindication to organ transplantation.[40]

A guiding principle of the organ transplantation process is the judicious allocation of a scarce resource to those likely to derive the most benefit. Accordingly, as with other malignancies, patients with active metastatic skin cancer would not qualify as transplant candidates. However, the question remains whether patients with a history of intermediate-risk to high-risk tumors should be transplanted, given that the aggressiveness and metastatic potential of their malignancy may even be increased in the posttransplant setting. Little evidence yet exists to guide transplant physi-cians in answering this question. Therefore, a multidisciplinary approach is warranted. The decision must be based on careful examination of the historical and pathologic data of the cuta-neous malignancy in the potential transplant candidate, in consultation with appropriate specialists, including dermatopathologists and dermatologic surgeons. Otley and colleagues[40] proposed suggested waiting intervals for reevalu-ation before transplantation after various cuta-neous malignancies. These proposals have been cited with approval by other investigators,[41] and may form the basis of a standard approach to pre-transplant evaluation of such patients in the multi-disciplinary setting.

PREVENTIVE EDUCATION

Because the most important element of skin cancer prevention in SOTR is minimization of exposure to UVR, education regarding sun protection and avoidance is the cornerstone of any effective prevention program. However, numerous studies have shown both knowledge of the importance of photoprotection and compliance with photoprotec-tive measures to be consistently inadequate among SOTR.[42–44] Before the advent of multidisciplinary transplant clinics, Seukeran and colleagues[45] proposed that these deficiencies may be attribut-able, at least in part, to insufficient input by derma-tologists in the process of preventive education.

It is thus incumbent on the dermatologist to provide rigorous, repetitive, and persuasive instruction to patients regarding the necessity of photoprotection and the most efficacious means thereof. Several studies have shown that the multi-disciplinary approach is particularly well suited to the accomplishment of this goal. Ismail and colleagues[46] reported that, among patients attending their specialist organ transplant recipient dermatology clinic, 98% recalled receiving photo-protection advice and 95% reported regular sunscreen use, compared with 77% and 67%, respectively, of patients who did not attend. Clowers-Webb and colleagues[47] described significantly more compliant sun-protective behavior among SOTR in a multidisciplinary setting who received intensive versus standard preventive education. Ulrich and colleagues[48] found that, regardless of general photoprotection education, provision of free sunscreen and specific training regarding its correct application resulted in significantly more photoprotection compliance (measured as sunscreen use 5.6 d/wk, compared with 0.3 d/wk in the control group), with a concomitant decline in NMSC incidence. The dermatologist in the multidisciplinary setting should frequently and repeatedly encourage all SOTR to apply sunscreen (of sufficient sun protection factor) every day, not just when sun exposure is expected, and counsel avoidance of sun exposure between 10:00 AM and 2:00 PM, abstention from exposure to artificial sources of UVR (ie, tanning beds), and dressing in sun-impermeable clothes including long-sleeved shirts, long pants, and broad-brimmed hats. Patients practicing optimal photoprotection may be at risk for vitamin D deficiency, because of reduction of vitamin D production in non–sun-exposed skin.[49] Therefore, the American Academy of Dermatology recommends oral supplementation of these patients with a total daily dose of 1000 IU of vitamin D to prevent deficiency while minimizing skin cancer risk.

REVISION OF IMMUNOSUPPRESSION

Although pharmacologic suppression of the host immune system is indispensable to graft survival in SOTR, an unintended consequence of chronic immunosuppression is acceleration of the development of cutaneous malignancies. Immunosuppressant medications promote tumorigenesis by 2 mechanisms. First, the agents may be directly carcinogenic.[50] Second, the immunosuppressive milieu impairs endogenous detection and destruction of cells harboring mutations, which may progress to malignancy if left unchecked.[51] Reducing the degree of immunosuppression may be a viable adjuvant strategy for retarding tumor development in select cases.[52] Conceptually, the usefulness of such an approach is contingent on weighing the benefit conferred by reducing skin cancer incidence against the risk of precipitating graft rejection.

To date, only 1 randomized controlled trial (RCT) has evaluated reduction of immunosuppression. Dantal and colleagues[53] found that reduction of immunosuppression did not result in significant impairment of graft survival (compared with a standard-dose control group), whereas it did decrease the incidence of new skin cancers during the duration of follow-up. Based on observational data, reduction of immunosuppression may also serve to mitigate the aggressiveness, as well as the multiplicity, of high-risk or metastatic NMSC.[54] Although no guidelines yet exist regarding reduction of immunosuppression, the International Transplant Skin Cancer Collaborative (ITSCC) and Skin Care in Organ Transplant Patients Europe (SCOPE) have published an expert consensus survey of transplant dermatologists recommending this strategy for secondary prevention in high-risk cases of NMSC and melanoma.[55] A follow-up study surveyed non-dermatologist transplant physicians and found them to be even more amenable to aggressive reduction of immunosuppression in similar clinical circumstances.[56] Both these studies emphasize that decisions regarding reduction of immunosuppression should be undertaken via a multidisciplinary approach with appropriate input from both dermatologists and transplant physicians.

Another method of revising immunosuppression in SOTR entails altering the type of immunosuppressant regimen itself. In the past, this was commonly accomplished by maintaining SOTR on fewer total immunosuppressant agents, which seems to be efficacious in reducing the incidence of skin cancers.[8,57] In recent years, evidence has begun to accumulate that mammalian target of rapamycin (mTOR) inhibitors, such as sirolimus and everolimus, may confer a decreased risk of skin cancer relative to traditional calcineurin inhibitors.[58,59] Moreover, data suggest that mTOR inhibitors may exert a protective effect on the development of skin cancers via their incidental antineoplastic activity.[60,61] Several RCT are ongoing to prospectively evaluate the effect of mTOR inhibitors (compared with calcineurin inhibitors) on skin cancer risk in SOTR, which will help to elucidate the future role of these promising agents.[62–65] Studies in the transplant literature have already shown the safety and efficacy of mTOR inhibitors in graft function and survival.[66] The mTOR inhibitors have their own side effects (including hyperlipidemia, myelosuppression, impaired wound healing, proteinuria, and pneumonitis) and there is insufficient evidence to recommend their use as first-line agents in de novo SOTR.[67] Any decision regarding conversion of immunosuppression must be made on a case-by-case basis involving close consultation between the dermatologist and the primary transplant team.

CHEMOPROPHYLAXIS

The tendency of skin cancers to arise from premalignant keratotic lesions on sun-damaged skin in

SOTR suggests field cancerization.[24,39] The concept of field cancerization denotes a process whereby an area subject to an ongoing carcinogenic insult may accumulate repeated mutations until 1 focus of that area undergoes malignant transformation and clonal expansion, forming a clinically apparent tumor. Although the malignant neoplasm may arise from a single offending cell, a concentric field of surrounding tissue still harbors an analogous complement of mutations and consequent malignant potential, which standard excisional or ablative techniques for skin cancer fail to eliminate. Thus, modalities for the suppression of these reservoirs of malignant precursors are indicated in SOTR at high risk for future cancer development.[68]

Retinoid derivatives have been shown to be the most efficacious agents available for this purpose. The usefulness of systemic retinoids for suppression of SCC development has been widely investigated, although study designs vary. Two RCT have shown a significant decrease in the incidence of both AK and SCC with administration of oral acitretin.[69,70] A third RCT noted a reduction in AK but did not show a significant decrease in the incidence of SCC.[71] Two other studies also found a decrease in the incidence of both AK and SCC with acitretin, although both were small and lacked formal control groups.[72,73] A retrospective longitudinal study published recently confirmed the long-term efficacy of acitretin for suppression of SCC.[74] Accordingly, the available evidence supports the adjuvant use of retinoid chemoprophylaxis in select SOTR at high risk for developing multiple, recurrent, and aggressive NMSC.[75] Indications for the initiation of systemic retinoid therapy are presented in **Box 2**.

Poor tolerability adversely affects compliance with systemic retinoids. Patients commonly complain of mucocutaneous xerosis and arthralgias/myalgias, frequently leading to self-discontinuation of the drug. Because these effects are generally dose dependent, acitretin should be started at a low dose (10 mg/d) and increased incrementally at 2-week to 4-week intervals to target dose of 20 to 25 mg/d, enabling patients to acclimate gradually to any adverse effects.[76] Laboratory abnormalities such as increased transaminases and hyperlipidemia are also common, requiring regular monitoring. In the interest of minimizing systemic side effects, topical retinoid formulations have also been studied, but with inconsistent results.[77,78]

Notable among all the retinoid studies mentioned earlier is the consistent observation of a rebound effect: relapse of SCC on discontinuation of the drug. Thus, barring severe adverse

Box 2
Indications for systemic retinoid chemoprophylaxis in SOTR
Development of multiple SCC per year (5–10/y)
Development of multiple SCC in high-risk locations (eg, head and neck)
SOTR with SCC and a history of lymphoma/leukemia
Single SCC with high metastatic risk
Metastatic SCC
Explosive SCC development
Eruptive keratoacanthomas

effects necessitating discontinuation, maintenance of retinoid chemoprophylaxis should be lifelong. To promote compliance, patients should be counseled extensively regarding expectation and manageability of side effects, and the importance of continuing retinoid therapy once initiated. Patients should be encouraged to discuss their concerns with their transplant dermatologist so that strategies for mitigating intolerable side effects (such as dose reduction) may be implemented without sacrificing chemosuppression.

SURVEILLANCE

Once appropriate preventive measures have been undertaken, SOTR must be followed closely for the development of cutaneous malignancies. To that end, the multidisciplinary clinical environment offers a distinct advantage, enabling efficient scheduling of appointments and the opportunity for standardization of follow-up intervals in conjunction with those of the primary transplant team. All SOTR should undergo an initial dermatologic history and physical including total body skin examination before transplantation, to establish a baseline for future comparison and to define initial follow-up intervals (**Box 3**). At each subsequent visit, patients should be evaluated and treated for any new lesions, and follow-up intervals adjusted accordingly. In addition, SOTR should be counseled to be vigilant for new or changing skin lesions, and self-examination of the skin should be taught and encouraged on a monthly basis. SOTR with a history of high-risk SCC or melanoma should also be taught lymph node self-examination. Such systematic surveillance facilitates the early detection and rapid treatment of skin cancers and premalignant lesions as they develop.

Box 3 Follow-up intervals for dermatologic examination of SOTR	
Patient History	Follow-up Interval (mo)
No skin cancer or actinic keratoses	12
Actinic keratoses	3–6
One nonmelanoma skin cancer	3–6
Multiple nonmelanoma skin cancers	3
High-risk SCC or melanoma	3
Metastatic SCC or melanoma	1–3

TREATMENT
Actinic Keratosis

Consistent with the concept of field cancerization, actinic keratosis (AK) represents a nonobligate precursor lesion to SCC and should be managed aggressively. Standard destructive techniques for AK include cryotherapy and electrodessication with curettage (ED&C). Other modalities target not only discrete dysplastic lesions but also the surrounding field of potentially premalignant tissue. Application of topical 5-fluorouracil (5-FU) has proved efficacious for this purpose.[79] More recently, the topical immunomodulator imiquimod has also been shown to be effective in the treatment of these premalignant skin lesions. Early concerns regarding the use of such an immunomodulator in SOTR have been dispelled, because imiquimod seems to have no effect on systemic immunity and has been shown to be safe in SOTR, with efficacy comparable with that in nontransplant hosts.[80,81] These topical agents may be implemented in cyclic rotation to maximize the beneficial effect of each. Combination of 5-FU and imiquimod may result in faster response rates and fewer adverse effects.[82]

A novel, field-directed modality for the suppression of premalignant skin lesions is photodynamic therapy (PDT). PDT involves the topical application of a photosensitizer compound (aminolevulinate [ALA] or methyl-aminolevulinate [MAL]) to a desired area of the skin, followed by irradiation with visible light to selectively destroy cells in the sensitized target area. Two early studies by Dragieva and colleagues[83,84] were encouraging regarding the efficacy of PDT in treating AK in SOTR. Several subsequent studies have reached concordant conclusions.[85,86] Perrett and colleagues[87] found PDT to be superior to 5-FU in efficacy, tolerability, and cosmesis. However, de Graaf and colleagues[88] reported that 1 or 2 PDT treatments failed to prevent

the development of SCC, casting doubt on its usefulness as a prophylactic modality. More recently, Willey and colleagues[89] treated SOTR with cyclic PDT at regular intervals for 2 years, and observed a reduction in SCC incidence of 79% after 12 months, and 95% after 24 months. Presently, an RCT is recruiting participants to compare ALA-PDT against sham PDT (with application of a topical placebo vehicle) regarding reduction in AK and NMSC incidence.[90] Additional prospective investigation is warranted to determine the efficacy and clinical usefulness of PDT to suppress NMSC development in the long-term.

Squamous Cell Carcinoma

According to ITSCC guidelines, SCC should be stratified by clinicopathologic criteria into low-risk and high-risk categories for purposes of treatment.[91] Characteristics defining high-risk SCC are reviewed in **Box 4**. Low-risk SCC should optimally be treated with Mohs micrographic surgery or traditional surgical excision, although ED&C may be used in the case of multiple low-risk lesions not amenable to excision.[92] High-risk SCC demands early and aggressive surgical intervention. Mohs micrographic surgery is the treatment of choice, but excision with postoperative margin assessment (with margins of at least 6–10 mm beyond surrounding erythema and resection into

Box 4 Clinical and pathologic characteristics of high-risk SCC

Size:
    >0.6 cm, face (excluding cheeks and forehead)
    >1 cm, cheeks, forehead, neck, and scalp
    >2 cm, trunk and extremities

Multiple SCC
Recurrence
Ulceration
Presence of satellite lesions
High-risk location: central face, lips, over parotid glands, ear, temple, scalp, digits, and genitalia

Histology:
    Poor differentiation
    Deep extension of tumor into subcutaneous fat
    Perineural, perivascular, or intravascular invasion

subcutaneous fat) is acceptable if Mohs surgery is not available. Mohs surgery may not adequately achieve complete tumor clearance in the setting of in-transit metastasis, deep-tissue (eg, bone or parotid gland) invasion, or perineural extension, especially along major nerve branches of the head and neck. In such cases, the optimal treatment strategy involves a multidisciplinary approach, including preoperative radiologic imaging and collaboration with craniofacial or head and neck surgeons.[93] Several other multidisciplinary modalities may have an adjunctive role in the treatment of high-risk SCC. Small observational studies have suggested the usefulness of sentinel lymph node (SLN) biopsy for the detection of subclinical nodal metastasis.[94–96] Further prospective investigation is needed to define the role of SLN biopsy in high-risk SCC in the SOTR population.

Adjuvant radiation therapy (XRT) may be indicated in the setting of SCC with postoperative margins positive for residual tumor, perineural invasion, or nodal metastasis. XRT may also be considered as a primary treatment modality for inoperable SCC, although it is generally less efficacious than radical excision.[97] The role of systemic chemotherapy in the management of high-risk SCC remains ill-defined in the SOTR population. Platinum-based regimens have yielded inconsistent outcomes and high rates of adverse effects, which may include toxicity to the transplanted organ. Capecitabine, an oral prodrug of 5-FU, has shown promise in recent small studies for the treatment and prevention of recurrence of advanced cutaneous SCC.[98–100] Epidermal growth factor receptor (EGFR) inhibitors are another emerging chemotherapeutic option for high-risk SCC that overexpress EGFR promoting cellular proliferation, angiogenesis, and metastasis.[101] Cetuximab, a chimeric (human/mouse) monoclonal antibody that competitively inhibits EGFR, has shown benefit in several case reports.[102,103] Presently, an ongoing clinical trial is investigating cetuximab for the treatment of cutaneous SCC.[104] The small-molecule EGFR inhibitor erlotinib and the fully human anti-EGFR monoclonal antibody panitumumab may also prove beneficial in high-risk SCC.[105] The adverse effects and toxicities of these agents remain to be characterized in SOTR,[106] but they represent promising additions to the multidisciplinary armamentarium for the treatment of high-risk SCC.

Melanoma

Treatment of melanoma in SOTR parallels management of the disease in nontransplant hosts. Suspicious-appearing pigmented lesions should be biopsied expeditiously. Definitive therapy for localized tumors entails wide local excision, with margins dictated by Breslow thickness. SLN biopsy is indicated for lesions deeper than 1 mm, and may be considered for thinner lesions showing clinicopathologic risk factors for metastasis, including high mitotic figure counts or ulceration. In the SOTR population, SLN biopsy may help to identify patients who might benefit from revision of immunosuppression or other adjuvant therapy.[41] For metastatic melanoma, limited systemic therapy exists. Prolonged treatment with interferon α, which confers a marginal survival benefit in nontransplant hosts, may not be used in SOTR because of the risk of graft rejection. In SOTR with metastatic or high-risk melanoma, discontinuation of immunosuppression may be warranted and must be addressed with the transplant team. Because advanced melanoma lacks effective treatment options and carries a poor prognosis, careful surveillance and aggressive surgical intervention are essential in the SOTR population.

SUMMARY

Management of skin cancer in patients who have undergone solid-organ transplantation is a challenging clinical problem for both dermatologists and transplant physicians. Long-term immunosuppression results in a higher incidence of skin cancers and more aggressive tumors in the SOTR population. In the interest of developing an optimal management strategy for these patients, multidisciplinary transplant clinics have been established, integrating multiple specialties in a comprehensive care environment. The role of the dermatologist in this clinic encompasses patient education, emphasizing rigorous sun protection, initiation of chemoprophylaxis with systemic retinoids, and early detection and aggressive treatment of cutaneous malignant and premalignant lesions. The dermatologist may also serve as an advisor to the transplant team in the collaborative environment of the transplant clinic, particularly with respect to negotiating revision of immunosuppression in the setting of accelerating or catastrophic cutaneous carcinogenesis. In addition to facilitating cooperation and collaboration between providers from various specialties, the multidisciplinary clinical environment affords the opportunity to educate not just patients but also other providers about the unique dermatologic concerns pertaining to transplant recipients and the importance of effective preventive measures. The refinement of the care of SOTR enabled by the multidisciplinary approach should continue to ameliorate dermatologic morbidity and mortality in this expanding population.

REFERENCES

1. Annual Report of the U.S. Organ procurement and transplantation network and the scientific registry of transplant recipients: transplant data 1998–2007. Rockville (MD): USDHHS/HRSA/HSB/DOT; 2008. Available at: www.ustransplant.org. Accessed February 1, 2011.
2. Euvrard S, Kanitakis J, Claudy A. Skin cancers after organ transplantation. N Engl J Med 2003; 348(17):1681–91.
3. Penn I. Post-transplant malignancy: the role of immunosuppression. Drug Saf 2000;23(2):101–13.
4. Otley CC. Organization of a specialty clinic to optimize the care of organ transplant recipients at risk for skin cancer. Dermatol Surg 2000;26(7):709–12.
5. Christenson LJ, Geusau A, Ferrandiz C, et al. Specialty clinics for the dermatologic care of solid-organ transplant recipients. Dermatol Surg 2004;30(4 Pt 2):598–603.
6. Webb MC, Compton F, Andrews PA, et al. Skin tumours posttransplantation: a retrospective analysis of 28 years' experience at a single centre. Transplant Proc 1997;29(1–2):828–30.
7. Edwards NM, Rajasinghe HA, John R, et al. Cardiac transplantation in over 1000 patients: a single institution experience from Columbia University. Clin Transpl 1999;249–61.
8. Jensen P, Hansen S, Moller B, et al. Skin cancer in kidney and heart transplant recipients and different long-term immunosuppressive therapy regimens. J Am Acad Dermatol 1999;40(2 Pt 1):177–86.
9. Winkelhorst JT, Brokelman WJ, Tiggeler RG, et al. Incidence and clinical course of de-novo malignancies in renal allograft recipients. Eur J Surg Oncol 2001;27(4):409–13.
10. Euvrard S, Kanitakis J, Pouteil-Noble C, et al. Comparative epidemiologic study of premalignant and malignant epithelial cutaneous lesions developing after kidney and heart transplantation. J Am Acad Dermatol 1995;33(2 Pt 1):222–9.
11. Hartevelt MM, Bavinck JN, Kootte AM, et al. Incidence of skin cancer after renal transplantation in The Netherlands. Transplantation 1990;49(3):506–9.
12. Lindelöf B, Sigurgeirsson B, Gäbel H, et al. Incidence of skin cancer in 5356 patients following organ transplantation. Br J Dermatol 2000;143(3): 513–9.
13. Ulrich C, Schmook T, Sachse MM, et al. Comparative epidemiology and pathogenic factors for non-melanoma skin cancer in organ transplant patients. Dermatol Surg 2004;30(4 Pt 2):622–7.
14. Ramsay HM, Fryer AA, Hawley CM, et al. Non-melanoma skin cancer risk in the Queensland renal transplant population. Br J Dermatol 2002;147(5): 950–6.
15. Bouwes Bavinck JN, Hardie DR, Green A, et al. The risk of skin cancer in renal transplant recipients in Queensland, Australia. A follow-up study. Transplantation 1996;61(5):715–21.
16. Ramsay HM, Reece SM, Fryer AA, et al. Seven-year prospective study of nonmelanoma skin cancer incidence in U.K. renal transplant recipients. Transplantation 2007;84(3):437–9.
17. Euvrard S, Kanitakis J, Decullier E, et al. Subsequent skin cancers in kidney and heart transplant recipients after the first squamous cell carcinoma. Transplantation 2006;81(8):1093–100.
18. Martinez JC, Otley CC, Stasko T, et al. Defining the clinical course of metastatic skin cancer in organ transplant recipients: a multicenter collaborative study. Arch Dermatol 2003;139(3):301–6.
19. Hollenbeak CS, Todd MM, Billingsley EM, et al. Increased incidence of melanoma in renal transplantation recipients. Cancer 2005;104(9):1962–7.
20. Le Mire L, Hollowood K, Gray D, et al. Melanomas in renal transplant recipients. Br J Dermatol 2006; 154(3):472–7.
21. Douds AC, Mellotte GJ, Morgan SH. Fatal Merkel-cell tumour (cutaneous neuroendocrine carcinoma) complicating renal transplantation. Nephrol Dial Transplant 1995;10(12):2346–8.
22. Wehrli BM, Janzen DL, Shokeir O, et al. Epithelioid angiosarcoma arising in a surgically constructed arteriovenous fistula: a rare complication of chronic immunosuppression in the setting of renal transplantation. Am J Surg Pathol 1998;22(9):1154–9.
23. Hafner J, Kunzi W, Weinreich T. Malignant fibrous histiocytoma and atypical fibroxanthoma in renal transplant recipients. Dermatology 1999;198(1):29–32.
24. Bavinck JN, De Boer A, Vermeer BJ, et al. Sunlight, keratotic skin lesions and skin cancer in renal transplant recipients. Br J Dermatol 1993;129(3): 242–9.
25. España A, Martínez-González MA, García-Granero M, et al. A prospective study of incident nonmelanoma skin cancer in heart transplant recipients. J Invest Dermatol 2000;115(6):1158–60.
26. Ramsay HM, Fryer AA, Reece S, et al. Clinical risk factors associated with nonmelanoma skin cancer in renal transplant recipients. Am J Kidney Dis 2000;36(1):167–76.
27. Penn I, Starzl TE. Malignant tumors arising de novo in immunosuppressed organ transplant recipients. Transplantation 1972;14(4):407–17.
28. Ducloux D, Carron PL, Rebibou JM, et al. CD4 lymphocytopenia as a risk factor for skin cancers in renal transplant recipients. Transplantation 1998; 65(9):1270–2.
29. Kauffman HM, Cherikh WS, Cheng Y, et al. Maintenance immunosuppression with target-of-rapamycin

inhibitors is associated with a reduced incidence of de novo malignancies. Transplantation 2005;80(7): 883–9.

30. Adamson R, Obispo E, Dychter S, et al. High incidence and clinical course of aggressive skin cancer in heart transplant patients: a single-center study. Transplant Proc 1998;30(4):1124–6.

31. Kelly DM, Emre S, Guy SR, et al. Liver transplant recipients are not at increased risk for nonlymphoid solid organ tumors. Cancer 1998;83(6):1237–43.

32. Jensen AO, Sv Aelig Rke C, Farkas D, et al. Skin cancer risk among solid organ recipients: a nationwide cohort study in Denmark. Acta Derm Venereol 2010;90(5):474–9.

33. Struijk L, Bouwes Bavinck JN, Wanningen P, et al. Presence of human papillomavirus DNA in plucked eyebrow hairs is associated with a history of cutaneous squamous cell carcinoma. J Invest Dermatol 2003;121(6):1531–5.

34. Iftner A, Klug SJ, Garbe C, et al. The prevalence of human papillomavirus genotypes in nonmelanoma skin cancers of nonimmunosuppressed individuals identifies high-risk genital types as possible risk factors. Cancer Res 2003;63(21):7515 9.

35. Karagas MR, Nelson HH, Sehr P, et al. Human papillomavirus infection and incidence of squamous cell and basal cell carcinomas of the skin. J Natl Cancer Inst 2006;98(6):389–95.

36. Laing ME, Kay E, Conlon P, et al. Genetic factors associated with skin cancer in renal transplant patients. Photodermatol Photoimmunol Photomed 2007;23(2–3):62–7.

37. Ramsay HM, Harden PN, Reece S, et al. Polymorphisms in glutathione S-transferases are associated with altered risk of nonmelanoma skin cancer in renal transplant recipients: a preliminary analysis. J Invest Dermatol 2001;117(2):251–5.

38. Penn I. The effect of immunosuppression on pre-existing cancers. Transplantation 1993;55(4):742–7.

39. London NJ, Farmery SM, Will EJ, et al. Risk of neoplasia in renal transplant patients. Lancet 1995;346(8972):403–6.

40. Otley CC, Hirose R, Salasche SJ. Skin cancer as a contraindication to organ transplantation. Am J Transplant 2005;5(9):2079–84.

41. Zwald FO, Christenson LJ, Billingsley EM, et al. Melanoma in solid organ transplant recipients. Am J Transplant 2010;10(5):1297–304.

42. Cowen EW, Billingsley EM. Awareness of skin cancer by kidney transplant patients. J Am Acad Dermatol 1999;40(5 Pt 1):697–701.

43. Robinson JK, Rigel DS. Sun protection attitudes and behaviors of solid-organ transplant recipients. Dermatol Surg 2004;30(4 Pt 2):610–5.

44. Donovan JC, Rosen CF, Shaw JC. Evaluation of sun-protective practices of organ transplant recipients. Am J Transplant 2004;4(11):1852–8.

45. Seukeran DC, Newstead CG, Cunliffe WJ. The compliance of renal transplant recipients with advice about sun protection measures. Br J Dermatol 1998;138(2):301–3.

46. Ismail F, Mitchell L, Casabonne D, et al. Specialist dermatology clinics for organ transplant recipients significantly improve compliance with photoprotection and levels of skin cancer awareness. Br J Dermatol 2006;155(5):916–25.

47. Clowers-Webb HE, Christenson LJ, Phillips PK, et al. Educational outcomes regarding skin cancer in organ transplant recipients: randomized intervention of intensive vs standard education. Arch Dermatol 2006;142(6):712–8.

48. Ulrich C, Jürgensen JS, Degen A, et al. Prevention of non-melanoma skin cancer in organ transplant patients by regular use of a sunscreen: a 24 months, prospective, case-control study. Br J Dermatol 2009;161(Suppl 3):78–84.

49. Reichrath J, Nürnberg B. Solar UV-radiation, vitamin D and skin cancer surveillance in organ transplant recipients (OTRs). Adv Exp Med Biol 2008;624:203–14.

50. Hojo M, Morimoto T, Maluccio M, et al. Cyclosporine induces cancer progression by a cell-autonomous mechanism. Nature 1999;397(6719): 530–4.

51. Servilla KS, Burnham DK, Daynes RA. Ability of cyclosporine to promote the growth of transplanted ultraviolet radiation-induced tumors in mice. Transplantation 1987;44(2):291–5.

52. Otley CC, Maragh SL. Reduction of immunosuppression for transplant-associated skin cancer: rationale and evidence of efficacy. Dermatol Surg 2005;31(2):163–8.

53. Dantal J, Hourmant M, Cantarovich D, et al. Effect of long-term immunosuppression in kidney-graft recipients on cancer incidence: randomised comparison of two cyclosporin regimens. Lancet 1998;351(9103):623–8.

54. Moloney FJ, Kelly PO, Kay EW, et al. Maintenance versus reduction of immunosuppression in renal transplant recipients with aggressive squamous cell carcinoma. Dermatol Surg 2004;30(4 Pt 2): 674–8.

55. Otley CC, Berg D, Ulrich C, et al. Reduction of immunosuppression for transplant-associated skin cancer: expert consensus survey. Br J Dermatol 2006;154(3):395–400.

56. Otley CC, Griffin MD, Charlton MR, et al. Reduction of immunosuppression for transplant-associated skin cancer: thresholds and risks. Br J Dermatol 2007;157(6):1183–8.

57. Glover MT, Deeks JJ, Raftery MJ, et al. Immunosuppression and risk of non-melanoma skin cancer in renal transplant recipients. Lancet 1997; 349(9049):398.

58. Campistol JM, Eris J, Oberbauer R, et al. Sirolimus therapy after early cyclosporine withdrawal reduces the risk for cancer in adult renal transplantation. J Am Soc Nephrol 2006;17(2):581–9.

59. Mathew T, Kreis H, Friend P. Two-year incidence of malignancy in sirolimus-treated renal transplant recipients: results from five multicenter studies. Clin Transplant 2004;18(4):446–9.

60. Koehl GE, Andrassy J, Guba M, et al. Rapamycin protects allografts from rejection while simultaneously attacking tumors in immunosuppressed mice. Transplantation 2004;77(9):1319–26.

61. Amornphimoltham P, Leelahavanichkul K, Molinolo A, et al. Inhibition of mammalian target of rapamycin by rapamycin causes the regression of carcinogen-induced skin tumor lesions. Clin Cancer Res 2008; 14(24):8094–101.

62. TUMORAPA 1: efficacy of rapamycin in secondary prevention of skin cancers in kidney transplant recipients. Multicentric randomized, open-label study of rapamycin vs calcineurin inhibitors. ClinicalTrials.gov identifier: NCT00133887. Available at: http://clinicaltrials.gov/ct2/show/NCT00133887. Accessed September 7, 2010.

63. RESCUE: recurrent cutaneous squamous cell carcinoma under rapamune-a randomized, prospective, open-label, multi-center study comparing the efficacy and safety of conversion to sirolimus in stable renal or liver transplant recipients with a cutaneous squamous cell carcinoma. Netherlands Trial Register identifier: NTR388. Available at: http://apps.who.int/trialsearch/Trial.aspx?TrialID=NTR388. Accessed September 7, 2010.

64. PROSKIN: prevention of skin cancer in high risk patients after conversion to a sirolimus-based immunosuppressive protocol. ClinicalTrials.gov identifier: NCT00866684. Available at: http://clinicaltrials.gov/ct2/show/NCT00866684. Accessed September 7, 2010.

65. Study evaluating sirolimus in non-melanoma skin cancer in kidney transplant recipients: a randomized, open-label study to compare the rate of new non-melanoma skin cancer in maintenance renal allograft recipients converted to a sirolimus-based regimen versus continuation of a calcineurin inhibitor-based regimen. ClinicalTrials.gov identifier: NCT00129961. Available at: http://clinicaltrials.gov/ct2/show/NCT00129961. Accessed September 6, 2010.

66. Schena FP, Pascoe MD, Alberu J, et al. Conversion from calcineurin inhibitors to sirolimus maintenance therapy in renal allograft recipients: 24-month efficacy and safety results from the CONVERT trial. Transplantation 2009;87(2):233–42.

67. Rostaing L, Kamar N. mTOR inhibitor/proliferation signal inhibitors: entering or leaving the field? J Nephrol 2010;23(2):133–42.

68. De Graaf YG, Euvrard S, Bouwes Bavinck JN. Systemic and topical retinoids in the management of skin cancer in organ transplant recipients. Dermatol Surg 2004;30(4 Pt 2):656–61.

69. Bavinck JN, Tieben LM, Van der Woude FJ, et al. Prevention of skin cancer and reduction of keratotic skin lesions during acitretin therapy in renal transplant recipients: a double-blind, placebo-controlled study. J Clin Oncol 1995;13(8):1933–8.

70. George R, Weightman W, Russ GR, et al. Acitretin for chemoprevention of non-melanoma skin cancers in renal transplant recipients. Australas J Dermatol 2002;43(4):269–73.

71. de Sévaux RG, Smit JV, de Jong EM, et al. Acitretin treatment of premalignant and malignant skin disorders in renal transplant recipients: clinical effects of a randomized trial comparing two doses of acitretin. J Am Acad Dermatol 2003;49(3):407–12.

72. McKenna DB, Murphy GM. Skin cancer chemoprophylaxis in renal transplant recipients: 5 years of experience using low-dose acitretin. Br J Dermatol 1999;140(4):656–60.

73. McNamara IR, Muir J, Galbraith AJ. Acitretin for prophylaxis of cutaneous malignancies after cardiac transplantation. J Heart Lung Transplant 2002;21(11):1201–5.

74. Harwood CA, Leedham-Green M, Leigh IM, et al. Low-dose retinoids in the prevention of cutaneous squamous cell carcinomas in organ transplant recipients: a 16-year retrospective study. Arch Dermatol 2005;141(4):456–64.

75. Kovach BT, Sams HH, Stasko T. Systemic strategies for chemoprevention of skin cancers in transplant recipients. Clin Transplant 2005;19(6):726–34.

76. Otley CC, Stasko T, Tope WD, et al. Chemoprevention of nonmelanoma skin cancer with systemic retinoids: practical dosing and management of adverse effects. Dermatol Surg 2006;32(4):562–8.

77. Euvrard S, Verschoore M, Touraine JL, et al. Topical retinoids for warts and keratoses in transplant recipients. Lancet 1992;340(8810):48–9.

78. Smit JV, Cox S, Blokx WA, et al. Actinic keratoses in renal transplant recipients do not improve with calcipotriol cream and all-trans retinoic acid cream as monotherapies or in combination during a 6-week treatment period. Br J Dermatol 2002; 147(4):816–8.

79. Weiss J, Menter A, Hevia O, et al. Effective treatment of actinic keratosis with 0.5% fluorouracil cream for 1, 2, or 4 weeks. Cutis 2002;70(Suppl 2):22–9.

80. Brown VL, Atkins CL, Ghali L, et al. Safety and efficacy of 5% imiquimod cream for the treatment of skin dysplasia in high-risk renal transplant recipients: randomized, double-blind, placebo-controlled trial. Arch Dermatol 2005;141(8):985–93.

81. Ulrich C, Bichel J, Euvrard S, et al. Topical immunomodulation under systemic immunosuppression: results

of a multicentre, randomized, placebo-controlled safety and efficacy study of imiquimod 5% cream for the treatment of actinic keratoses in kidney, heart, and liver transplant patients. Br J Dermatol 2007; 157(Suppl 2):25–31.

82. Price NM. The treatment of actinic keratoses with a combination of 5-fluorouracil and imiquimod creams. J Drugs Dermatol 2007;6(8):778–81.

83. Dragieva G, Hafner J, Dummer R, et al. Topical photodynamic therapy in the treatment of actinic keratoses and Bowen's disease in transplant recipients. Transplantation 2004;77(1):115–21.

84. Dragieva G, Prinz BM, Hafner J, et al. A randomized controlled clinical trial of topical photodynamic therapy with methyl aminolaevulinate in the treatment of actinic keratoses in transplant recipients. Br J Dermatol 2004;151(1):196–200.

85. Wulf HC, Pavel S, Stender I, et al. Topical photodynamic therapy for prevention of new skin lesions in renal transplant recipients. Acta Derm Venereol 2006;86(1):25–8.

86. Piaserico S, Belloni Fortina A, Rigotti P, et al. Topical photodynamic therapy of actinic keratosis in renal transplant recipients. Transplant Proc 2007;39(6):1847–50.

87. Perrett CM, McGregor JM, Warwick J, et al. Treatment of post-transplant premalignant skin disease: a randomized intrapatient comparative study of 5-fluorouracil cream and topical photodynamic therapy. Br J Dermatol 2007;156(2):320–8.

88. de Graaf YG, Kennedy C, Wolterbeek R, et al. Photodynamic therapy does not prevent cutaneous squamous-cell carcinoma in organ-transplant recipients: results of a randomized-controlled trial. J Invest Dermatol 2006;126(3):569–74.

89. Willey A, Mehta S, Lee PK. Reduction in the incidence of squamous cell carcinoma in solid organ transplant recipients treated with cyclic photodynamic therapy. Dermatol Surg 2010;36(5): 652–8.

90. ALA-PDT versus vehicle PDT for treatment of AK and reduction of new NMSC in solid organ transplant recipients-a randomized, evaluator-blinded, parallel group comparison of PDT with Levulan topical solution + blue light vs Levulan topical solution vehicle + blue light for the treatment of AK and reduction of new NMSC in organ transplant recipients. Clinicaltrials.gov identifier: NCT00865878. Available at: http://clinicaltrials.gov/ct2/show/NCT00865878. Accessed September 7, 2010.

91. Stasko T, Brown MD, Carucci JA, et al. Guidelines for the management of squamous cell carcinoma in organ transplant recipients. Dermatol Surg 2004;30(4 Pt 2):642–50.

92. de Graaf YG, Basdew VR, van Zwan-Kralt N, et al. The occurrence of residual or recurrent squamous cell carcinomas in organ transplant recipients after

curettage and electrodesiccation. Br J Dermatol 2006;154(3):493–7.

93. Jennings L, Schmults CD. Management of high-risk cutaneous squamous cell carcinoma. J Clin Aesthet Dermatol 2010;3(4):39–48.

94. Altinyollar H, Berberoglu U, Celen O. Lymphatic mapping and sentinel lymph node biopsy in squamous cell carcinoma of the lower lip. Eur J Surg Oncol 2002;28(1):72–4.

95. de Hullu JA, Hollema H, Piers DA, et al. Sentinel lymph node procedure is highly accurate in squamous cell carcinoma of the vulva. J Clin Oncol 2000;18(15):2811–6.

96. Wagner JD, Evdokimow DZ, Weisberger E, et al. Sentinel node biopsy for high-risk nonmelanoma cutaneous malignancy. Arch Dermatol 2004;140(1):75–9.

97. Kwan W, Wilson D, Moravan V. Radiotherapy for locally advanced basal cell and squamous cell carcinomas of the skin. Int J Radiat Oncol Biol Phys 2004;60(2):406–11.

98. Wollina U, Hansel G, Koch A, et al. Oral capecitabine plus subcutaneous interferon alpha in advanced squamous cell carcinoma of the skin. J Cancer Res Clin Oncol 2005;131(5):300–4.

99. Endrizzi BT, Lee PK. Management of carcinoma of the skin in solid organ transplant recipients with oral capecitabine. Dermatol Surg 2009;35(10):1567–72.

100. Jirakulaporn T, Mathew J, Lindgren BR, et al. Efficacy of capecitabine in secondary prevention of skin cancer in solid organ-transplanted recipients (OTR). J Clin Oncol 2009;27(15S):1519.

101. Shimizu T, Izumi H, Oga A, et al. Epidermal growth factor receptor overexpression and genetic aberrations in metastatic squamous-cell carcinoma of the skin. Dermatology 2001;202(3):203–6.

102. Bauman JE, Eaton KD, Martins RG. Treatment of recurrent squamous cell carcinoma of the skin with cetuximab. Arch Dermatol 2007;143(7):889–92.

103. Suen JK, Bressler L, Shord SS, et al. Cutaneous squamous cell carcinoma responding serially to single-agent cetuximab. Anticancer Drugs 2007;18(7):827–9.

104. Study of Cetuximab in Squamous Cell Carcinoma of the Skin Expressing EGFR (CTXSCC)-Phase II Study of cetuximab as monotherapy and first line treatment in patients with locally advanced or metastatic squamous cell carcinoma of the skin expressing EGFR. Clinicaltrials.gov identifier: NCT00240682. Available at: http://clinicaltrials.gov/ct2/show/NCT00240682. Accessed September 7, 2010.

105. Read WL. Squamous carcinoma of the skin responding to erlotinib: three cases. J Clin Oncol 2007;25(18S):16519.

106. Leard LE, Cho BK, Jones KD, et al. Fatal diffuse alveolar damage in two lung transplant patients treated with cetuximab. J Heart Lung Transplant 2007;26(12):1340–4.

Imaging in Cutaneous Oncology: Radiology for Dermies

Allison T. Vidimos, RPh, MD[a],*, Todd W. Stultz, DDS, MD[b]

KEYWORDS

- Nonmelanoma skin cancer • Preoperative imaging • MRI
- CT • Ultrasound • PET • PET-CT

Diagnostic imaging has a supporting role in the evaluation and management of cutaneous neoplasms. As in radiology, the appearance of a lesion is a major factor in the process of reaching a diagnosis. When evaluating an aggressive skin tumor, cross-sectional imaging augments physical examination to refine the assessment of local spread, assist in determining regional nodal and distant metastatic involvement, and provide whole-body staging for cutaneous malignancies, such as melanoma, utilizing positron emission tomography-computed tomography (PET-CT).[1]

The following issues should be kept in mind by the clinician when considering imaging for the evaluation of a suspected aggressive cutaneous neoplasm. First, the clinician must clearly communicate the pathologic diagnosis or suspected pathology and anticipated biologic behavior to the radiologist if a biopsy has not been performed. Secondly, the clinician should include specific references to particular concerns based upon the examination and patients' symptoms: perineural invasion, depth of tumor, contiguous involvement of adjacent structures, and potential for local or distant metastases. Finally, the clinician should consult with the radiologist concerning the most appropriate and cost-effective examination to answer the clinical questions.

From the radiologist's perspective, imaging has several general goals:

1. Display anatomy desired
2. Provide adequate detail
3. Differentiate normal from abnormal structures
4. Minimize risk to patients.

Within the broader field of surgical oncology, imaging also plays a role intraoperatively. For example, intraoperative magnetic resonance imaging (MRI) or ultrasound is employed during resection of some brain tumors; intraoperative cone beam CT, MRI, or ultrasound are employed during cryotherapy for solid neoplasms; and catheter angiography is utilized during solid-tumor embolization. Sentinel lymph node identification with vital dye and nuclear pharmaceuticals guides sampling intraoperatively.[2] The accessibility of cutaneous neoplasms visually and the systematic mapping obtained during Mohs surgery likely in part account for the lesser role of intraoperative imaging for surgical management of the primary tumor. In the field of dermatologic oncology, imaging can certainly play a role in preoperative planning, discussion of potential morbidity with patients, preoperative staging, and post-therapeutic follow-up.

The authors have nothing to disclose.
[a] Section of Dermatologic Surgery and Cutaneous Oncology, Department of Dermatology, Cleveland Clinic Foundation, 9500 Euclid Avenue, Cleveland, OH 44195, USA
[b] Section of Neuroradiology, Imaging Institute, Cleveland Clinic Foundation, 9500 Euclid Avenue, Cleveland, OH 44195, USA
* Corresponding author.
E-mail address: vidimoa@ccf.org

Dermatol Clin 29 (2011) 243–260
doi:10.1016/j.det.2011.01.009
0733-8635/11/$ – see front matter © 2011 Elsevier Inc. All rights reserved.

IMAGING MODALITIES
Plain Film

Most exhaustive dermatologic texts contain plain-film images of multiple odontogenic keratocysts, bifid ribs, and calcified falx cerebri seen in patients with nevoid basal cell carcinoma syndrome, sub-ungual osteomas, or, unfortunately, enlargement of skull base foramina in patients with an aggressive cutaneous tumor. Medical imaging has advanced substantially since these images found their way into medical textbooks. The visual appearance and tactile characteristics of a cutaneous neoplasm often suggests the diagnosis prior to biopsy and sophisticated cross-sectional imaging serves to map out the extent of the abnormality or assist in staging if this is necessary prior to definitive intervention. As an example, evaluation of perineural tumor by plain film requires sufficient tumor spread and nerve expansion to cause smooth remodeling of bony foramina or gross erosion of adjacent bone caused by tumor infiltration. CT scanning improves sensitivity for bone changes, but still requires substantial soft-tissue abnormality to create visible secondary bone remodeling. Contrast-enhanced MRI provides greater soft-tissue resolution, and allows earlier detection of tumor infiltration along nerves or tissue planes prior to bulky nerve expansion or bone remodeling. Plain films are an interesting historical footnote but currently play no significant role in the workup of aggressive cutaneous malignancies, except perhaps with screening chest radiographs for metastatic disease.

Computed Tomography

Modern CT scanners employ a circular rotating x-ray tube head and detector array in combination with a continuously movable patient gantry to permit rapid scanning of a contiguous anatomic segment. Native collimation for multidetector CT scanners typically ranges from 0.5 mm to 1.0 mm and allows reconstruction of images with near isotropic resolution. This capability means that the smallest individual volumes (voxels) that make up the 3-dimensional data set are either only slightly rectangular or cubic at this 0.5-mm to 1.0-mm resolution allowing patient anatomy to be reviewed with reasonable fidelity in multiple planes. Image acquisition with modern equipment is quite rapid. For example, image acquisition time for the entire cervical, thoracic, and lumbar spine on a currently available 64-row scanner at 0.75-mm collimation is less than 30 seconds. The term *spiral* or more appropriately *helical* CT is applied to imaging performed in this manner. Tissue differences are displayed as a function of x-ray beam attenuation related to the predominant atomic number of the tissue or foreign material imaged. The relative attenuation of the x-ray beam is responsible for the areas of relative brightness or darkness on the image. Hounsfield units (HU) represent an arbitrarily defined scale of attenuation, with air at a value of -1000, fat at a value of -100, water at a value of 0, muscle at a value of approximately 40 to 50, acute blood at a value of approximately 70, and calcium and metal ranging from 200 to greater than 1000.[3,4] Intrinsic differences between tissues often provide substantial resolution. For example, extraocular muscles and globes are clearly visualized against the lower density of the retrobulbar fat and inflammatory processes, which cause edema, and infiltration within subcutaneous fat is often visible without the addition of intravenous contrast.

Contrast is utilized to highlight normal and abnormal structures. For example, in the neck, contrast causes a typical enhancement pattern within major salivary glands, lymph nodes, and vascular structures, rendering this anatomy in greater detail than possible with an unenhanced scan. The thyroid also enhances after contrast, but has significant density caused by intrinsic iodine content and is usually easily visualized on an unenhanced scan.

Iodine linked to an organic molecule is utilized to provide contrast enhancement for CT. As described previously, x-ray beam attenuation is related to the atomic number of the material in the field of view. A typical dose of intravenous contrast (100 mL Ultravist 300) for a neck CT will cause attenuation reaching a value of approximately 180 to 200 HU within the vasculature, and will accumulate in tissues with impaired vascular barrier related to tumor, direct extravasation, or inflammation.

Commonly used iodinated contrast materials are iso-osmolar or slightly greater than typical whole blood osmolarity. High osmolar contrast agents are no longer widely utilized, and are associated with a higher incidence of nausea and vomiting. True allergy is uncommon, but mild reactions, including itching and hives, can be controlled or substantially blunted by the use of a combined oral premedication regimen, including prednisone and diphenhydramine. More serious reactions, including hypertension and airway compromise, should prompt strong consideration for withholding contrast. Renal insufficiency is primarily a concern with regards to precipitating acute renal injury in patients with borderline renal function.[5] At one time, gadolinium-enhanced MRI was considered a viable alternative to the use of iodinated contrast in patients with borderline renal function. Subsequent experience with nephrogenic systemic fibrosis has obviously changed this approach.[6] Consultation with a radiologist at your institution regarding optimal imaging for a given situation and protocols for managing contrast-related issues is advised.

The main advantages of computed tomography include speed, intermediate cost, easy accessibility at most institutions, and, in particular, fine bone detail permitting assessment for subtle sclerotic change or superficial bony erosion. Skull-base foraminal enlargement can be identified, but in the setting of suspected perineural spread indicates gross bulky disease. Benign entities, such as schwannoma or neurofibroma, may also enlarge bony foramina. In either case, MRI is superior to assess the skull-base foraminal contents or intracranial spread of disease. As previously mentioned, intrinsic attenuation differences between tissues with or without the addition of contrast provide some soft tissue resolution. Gross tumor extent, extracapsular nodal spread, central nodal necrosis, and broad survey for gross enlargement along draining lymph node groups can also be determined with contrast-enhanced CT.[7]

CT has come under scrutiny as concerns over radiation exposure have risen.[8] Many practices are now including the dose-length product, an estimate of radiation absorption for the body part and technical parameters in CT reports. Eventually, a total ionizing radiation exposure profile may be maintained as a part of a patient's electronic medical record.

Ultrasound

Diagnostic ultrasound involves the use of a hand-held transducer containing a piezoelectric crystal array, which generates sound waves within a narrow frequency spectrum. These sound waves travel through tissue and reflect back towards the transducer from areas of tissue interface. Mathematical reconstruction of this data creates a 2-dimensional, with some devices a 3-dimensional, image that can be viewed at any angle because of the free movement of the transducer held by the operator. Imaging is in real time and can include measurements of vascularity/quantitative blood flow because of the Doppler effect created by the moving blood through the vasculature included in the field of view. For the assessment of small or superficial lesions, a semisolid gel disk larger than the width of the transducer and approximately 1.0 to 1.5 cm in thickness (standoff pad) in conjunction with acoustically conductive gel is used to move the face of the transducer away from the surface of the skin.

The lack of ionizing radiation; real-time image reconstruction; small size of the transducer; and suitability for use with ancillary equipment, such as needle guides and cryogenic probes, makes ultrasound a key modality for intraprocedural imaging and, in particular, image-guided procedures. High-frequency, high-resolution ultrasound before Mohs surgery for basal cell carcinoma (BCC) and squamous cell carcinoma (SCC) has been studied and found to be suboptimal for identification of subtle areas of tumor extension, such as foci of dermal invasion for micronodular BCC and infiltrative SCC.[9,10] Ultrasound is also useful for assessment of regional lymph node groups and is significantly more sensitive than CT alone to evaluate suspicious nodes and guide minimally invasive needle sampling.[11,12] Experimental techniques, such as sonoelastography, show promise in identifying differentiating benign versus metastatic lymph nodes, but the offline processing is too time consuming to be useful in a busy clinical environment.[13] Imaging depth limitations and the small size of the transducers make ultrasound less useful for wide survey examinations. Whole-body staging is primarily accomplished with PET or hybrid PET-CT scanners.

Nuclear Medicine

PET imaging utilizes 18-fluorodeoxyglucose (PET-FDG) to identify tissues with high metabolic activity. In particular, tumors with high glycolytic activity will accumulate 18-FDG, as the initial glycolytic metabolite becomes trapped within the cell after initial phosphorylation. PET scanning alone provides moderate-resolution cross-sectional information. Software can be employed to coregister PET data sets to a CT scan of the same patient's anatomy, but is most effective in brain imaging because of the rigid outline of the skull and constraint of the intracranial contents. Hybrid PET-CT scanners improve upon this difficulty, with a PET detector ring merged on the same gantry with a multidetector CT scanner. Patients remain immobile during the scan, the 2 data sets are coregistered, and the low-dose CT scan obtained for coregistration also provides attenuation correction data for the PET study. The moderate-resolution metabolic information provided by the PET scan is displayed in an overlay with the higher-resolution CT scan for better anatomic correlation.[14] Early work is underway on hybrid PET-MRI scanners,[15,16] which would reduce the total ionizing radiation to patients and also benefit from the improved soft-tissue resolution obtainable with MRI.

PET staging sensitivity may be reduced for tumor volumes less than 1 cm^3 and tumors with low metabolic activity. PET-FDG can detect metastases in areas of necrosis, scarring, and fibrosis secondary to radiotherapy.[17] However, little data is available regarding staging for cutaneous nonmelanoma skin cancer. Fosko and colleagues[18] reported on PET in 6 BCC greater than 1 cm of the head and neck, and in 3 subjects the PET imaging correlated with the size and extent of the soft-tissue invasion. All 3 of these tumors were of the nodular subtype. Two of the 3 tumors that did not highlight on PET imaging were infiltrative, and 1 was the nodular subtype. PET imaging did not detect perineural spread demonstrated by tissue biopsy. Beer and Weibel[19] reported a recurrent BCC beneath a scar on the back from prior electrodesiccation and curettage that was detected at the time of a PET-CT performed for surveillance of other internal malignancies. Boswell and colleagues[20] reported a subjects with metastatic BCC to the lung that was detected on PET-CT.

There are few reports of PET or PET-CT for evaluation of cutaneous SCC. Conrad and colleagues[21] reported a subject with invasion of SCC into the pterygoid musculature and perineural SCC extending along V3 to the skull base confirmed on PET-CT. Cho and colleagues[22] employed PET-FDG to subjects with stage 11 cutaneous SCC, 9 subjects had high-risk cutaneous SCC. A total of 25% of subjects had lymph node metastases, and 1 subject had lung metastases. All 9 high-risk SCC showed FDG uptake. Incidentally, 1 subject was also diagnosed with stomach cancer. Leach and colleagues[23] reported 4 subjects with cutaneous SCC and 2 with melanoma who presented with cranial neuropathy as a sign of recurrent aggressive skin cancer, all 6 subjects exhibited symptoms associated with trigeminal nerve and 3 with facial nerve involvement. MRI confirmed perineural disease in all 6 subjects, and 1 subject had PET-CT imaging findings that correlated well with the MRI findings. The investigators emphasized the importance of early radiologic evaluation when patients present with signs of cranial neuropathy so that aggressive surgical and adjunctive therapy may be performed.

The clinical utility of PET/CT for head and neck tumors has been documented for initial staging and follow-up in rare head and neck tumors,[24] evaluation of patients with an unknown primary,[25] as well as follow-up for treatment response and surveillance for regional and distant metastases.[26,27] Roh and colleagues[24] reported on 24 subjects with rare head and neck tumors,

10 with melanoma, 9 with sarcoma, 3 with olfactory neuroblastomas, and 2 with BCC. PET/CT and CT/MRI scanning were performed at the initial staging or follow-up, and the diagnostic accuracy of CT and PET-FDG for detecting primary tumors and metastases were compared with histopathology. The PET-FDG and CT/MRI accuracies for detecting primary tumors were 92% and 79% respectively, and 91% and 74% respectively for nodal metastases. The sensitivity and specificity of PET-FDG for detecting distant metastases and second primary tumors were 100% and 87%, respectively. Rudmik and colleagues[25] reported on 20 subjects with cervical metastases from an unknown head and neck primary. PET/CT increased the detection of a primary tumor from 25% with a standard work-up to 55%; there was 1 false negative PET/CT scan.

Kao and colleagues[26] reported 80 subjects who received radiation therapy for head and neck cancer who were followed for a median of 21 months with clinical examination, PET/CT, and correlative imaging. The sensitivity, specificity, and positive and negative predictive values of PET/CT for detecting locoregional recurrence were 92%, 82%, 42%, and 98%, respectively; and distant metastases or second primary tumors were 93%, 96%, 81%, and 98%, respectively. Negative PET/CT results within 6 months after radiation therapy correlated with statistically significant improved 2-year overall survival rates. Gourin and colleagues[27] reported 64 subjects with suspected recurrent head and neck SCC. Distant metastases were detected in 15 of 64 subjects, 13 of which were unsuspected prior to PET-CT. The sensitivity and specificity, and positive and negative predictive value of PET-CT in detecting distant metastases were 86%, 84%, 60%, and 95%, respectively.

MRI

Protons behave as small dipole magnets in the presence of the strong main magnetic field of an MRI scanner. A slightly higher proportion of the protons (hydrogen in organic molecules and water) align parallel to the main magnetic field along the z-axis of patients, which is the slightly lower energy state in comparison with antiparallel alignment, which is a slightly higher energy state. Within the static main magnetic field, these protons wobble or precess about the z-axis in an analogous fashion to a top that slowly wobbles about the vertical axis of gravity. The precession of the protons in the main magnetic field is rapid. At 1.5 T, which is the typical field strength of a clinical MRI scanner, protons precess about the z-axis at

63.7 MHz. This steady-state equilibrium is modified by applying a short-duration radiofrequency pulse, which causes these protons to be deflected from the main magnetic field axis, and also causes the protons to precess in phase with one another rather than the usual random precession. This brief change yields a weak but measurable signal, providing the data that is ultimately reconstructed to form an MR image. Intuitively, one might imagine a rapid realignment of the protons with the main magnetic field and a rapid return to random precession as soon as the radiofrequency (RF) pulse ends. Although this is a simplistic description, these 2 phenomena define T1 and T2 relaxation. The terms T1 or T2 are in essence time constants, which are unique for particular tissues or substances at particular magnet field strengths. Manipulation of the technical parameters of each individual scan yields the image characteristics specific for that particular pulse sequence. As one would expect, patient motion, abrupt changes in the local magnetic environment (for example, the dense bone of the petrous ridge and aeration of the mastoid air cells immediately adjacent to the ventral temporal lobes), and metallic or paramagnetic substances can sharply alter the data obtained and grossly distort the images.

In general, common substances responsible for a high signal on a T1-weighted scan include acute blood, highly proteinaceous material, fat, some valence states of calcium, and paramagnetic gadolinium contrast. A high signal on T2-weighted scans primarily reflect free fluid and tissues with high free water content, including areas of edema, tumors with moderate to high intracellular fluid; cerebrospinal fluid; cysts; vitreous and aqueous humor; and low-velocity intraluminal contents such as encountered in the hepatobiliary, gastrointestinal, and genitourinary tracts. Short tau inversion recovery (STIR) sequence suppresses all substances with short T1 relaxation, such as acute blood, fat, pus, certain valent states of calcium, and so forth. The purpose is to make tissues or collections with high free water content stand out intensely from a background of low signal.

Gadolinium-based contrast agents provide contrast by shortening T1 relaxation by a factor of approximately 680 yielding a high signal on a T1-weighted pulse sequence. Enhancement is increased in the presence of highly vascularized tissues, and in particular tissues with incomplete blood/tissue barrier as encountered in many tumors and in the presence of active inflammation. As previously stated, fat is also high signal on a T1-weighted pulse sequence. Application of an additional pulse sequence can be employed to null the high signal from fat and improve the visualization of normal structures or pathology exhibiting gadolinium enhancement. As an example, this reduces the intensity of fat signal surrounding the various neurovascular bundles exiting through skull base foramina, making these structures more conspicuous when there is abnormal enhancement from tumor infiltration, which is the purpose for postgadolinium fat suppressed T1-weighted scans commonly employed in the head and neck, body, and musculoskeletal MRI.[28] Nemzek and colleagues[29] reported a 95% sensitivity for MRI detection of perineural invasion, but only a 63% sensitivity for mapping the entire extent of perineural tumor.

For many years, gadolinium was thought to be a safe option for patients at risk for exacerbation of renal insufficiency from intravenous administration of iodinated CT contrast. More recently, nephrogenic systemic fibrosis (NSF) has come to attention and has sharply curtailed the use of gadolinium-based contrast agents in patients with renal insufficiency. A full review of NSF is beyond the scope of this discussion; the reader is referred to the recently published overview of NSF by Chen and colleagues.[30] The key differences between the use of CT and MR contrast agents in patients with renal insufficiency revolve around the different mechanisms for possible adverse sequelae. Intravenous iodinated CT contrast administered to patients with marginal renal function can be associated with acute renal injury. The concern for NSF gadolinium-based contrast agents in patients with renal insufficiency is thought to be related to release and accumulation of free gadolinium in tissues. Normal or near normal estimated glomerular filtration rate (eGFR) is associated with significantly reduced risk for this complication. Adoption of restrictive policies regarding gadolinium-based contrast administration, and a switch from gadodiamide to gadobenate dimeglumine has reduced the number of NSF cases at the reporting institutions.[31] Consult with the radiology department at your institution regarding the policies in place regarding administration of gadolinium-based contrast agents to patients with borderline renal function. At the authors' institution, the cutoffs for mandatory postscan dialysis, nephrology consult and hydration, and proceeding with the examination are eGFR less than 15 mL/min, 15 to 30 mL/min, and greater than 30 mL/min, respectively.

Patient Characteristics and Imaging Modality

Radiologic studies may be indicated to assess the extent if the primary tumor, rule out metastatic spread, as well as follow up for local or regional recurrence or distant metastatic disease. The choice of imaging modality will not only be based on the suspected tumor biology and location but also on patient characteristics. Allergy to radio-contrast materials must be taken into account as previously discussed, as must renal function. MRI is contraindicated in patients with pace-makers and automated implanted cardiac defibril-lators, ferromagnetic aneurysm clips, and spine stimulators. Other devices require modifications in scanning protocol. Implanted medication pumps must be turned off prior to scanning, inter-rogated for normal functioning, and turned on after the procedure. Vagal nerve stimulators may be scanned with modification to the typical pulse sequences employed. An exhaustive reference of implanted devices and relative safety at various field strengths is available in print[32] and online at www.mrisafety.com.

CASE PRESENTATIONS AND DISCUSSION
Case 1: Recurrent Perineural BCC

A 53-year-old Caucasian woman with a history of Mohs surgery for a basal cell carcinoma of the right naso-facial sulcus 8 years prior presented with progressive elevation of the right ala and paresthesias of the right cheek (**Fig. 1**). A punch biopsy adjacent to the linear scar revealed infiltra-tive basal cell carcinoma. Preoperative MRI revealed perineural tumor of the infraorbital nerve extending to the infraorbital foramen (**Fig. 2**).

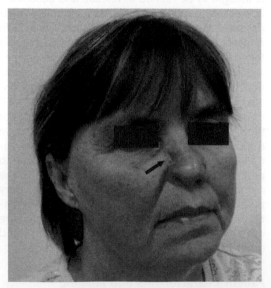

Fig. 1. A 53-year-old Caucasian woman with scar (*arrow*) from prior Mohs surgery at right naso-facial sulcus with right alar retraction.

A multidisciplinary approach with the facial plastic surgeon excising the tumor under general anes-thesia and Mohs mapping of the excised tissue revealed clear peripheral margins, but perineural tumor extension to the infraorbital foramen (**Fig. 3**). An anterior maxillotomy was performed, and V2 was traced posteriorly to the pterygopala-tine fossa and foramen rotundum at skull base. The segment of V2 proximal to the infraorbital foramen was not involved with tumor, confirming the MRI findings. The patient underwent a complex reconstruction by the facial plastic surgeon with a right paramedian forehead flap, septal mucosal flap, auricular and septal cartilage grafts, and cer-vicofacial advancement flap with subsequent revi-sions of the right ala and a vascularized fat graft to the right cheek (**Fig. 4**). She received postopera-tive radiation therapy, 6000 cGy in 30 fractions, and has no evidence of recurrence at 36 months postoperatively (see **Fig. 4**).

The incidence of perineural BCC is 0.1% to 3.0%.[33–35] Risk factors for perineural BCC include sclerosing, infiltrative and morpheaform growth patterns, recurrent BCC, and radiation treated tumors. Preoperative MRI was chosen for this patient in light of the clinical symptoms of perineu-ral involvement of V2 and the recurrent nature of the BCC and the superior ability for MRI to detect the perineural tumor and the extent of soft-tissue invasion. Tumor appeared to extend to, but not beyond the infraorbital foramen. Knowledge of the potential extent of tumor spread centrally prompted the multidisciplinary surgical approach to include the Mohs surgeon, facial plastic surgeon, and skull base surgeon. Aggressive surgical resection of the involved nerve with clear histologic margins and adjunctive radiation therapy allow for the greatest chance of local control and lasting cure.

Case 2: Perineural SCC

A 62-year-old Caucasian man presented with an incompletely excised SCC after 2 wide excisions above the left eyebrow, with perineural invasion noted on the second excision specimen. Physical examination revealed a linear scar over the left eyebrow with paresis of the temporal branch of left facial nerve (noted after second excision, unclear as to whether this nerve deficit was from surgery or tumor involvement of the nerve) (**Fig. 5**). There was no palpable lymphadenopathy. Chest radiograph was normal. Five stages of Mohs surgery were performed, and the tumor extended medially from the left temple, almost exclusively along nerves, to involve the left supraorbital and supratrochlear nerve branches as well as the

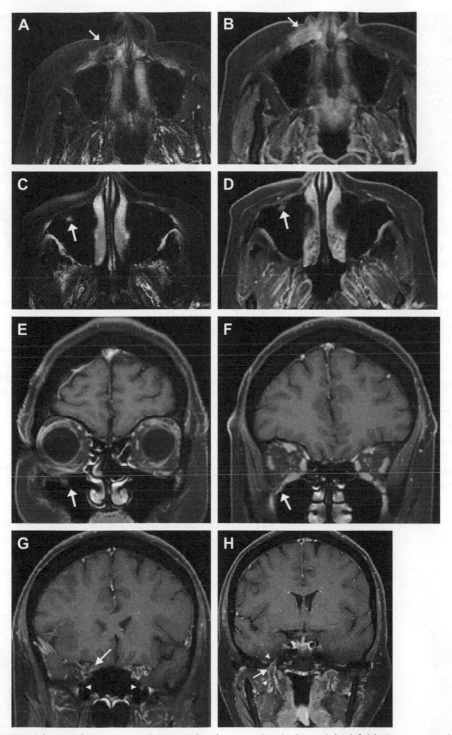

Fig. 2. (*A*) MRI with axial fat suppressed T2-weighted scan at level of nasolabial fold. Tumor mass (*arrow*). (*B*) Axial postgadolinium T1-weighted scan at same level showing enhancing tumor (*arrow*). (*C*) MRI with axial fat suppressed T2-weighted scan. Tumor showing increased signal and expansion superficial aspect of infraorbital nerve (*arrow*). (*D, E*) Axial and coronal postgadolinium T1-weighted scan showing enhancing tumor (*arrow*). (*F*) Coronal postgadolinium T1-weighted scan showing normal caliber infraorbital nerve 2 cm posterior to foramen (*arrow*). (*G, H*) Coronal postgadolinium T1-weighted scans at level of central skull base. (*G*) Normal orbital apex (*arrow*) and foramen rotundum (*arrowheads*). No tumor at posterior aspect of second division of right trigeminal nerve. (*H*) Normal third division of right trigeminal nerve (*arrowheads*), foramen ovale (*arrow*).

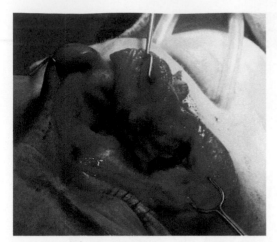

Fig. 3. Thickened infraorbital nerve extending to in-fraorbital foramen.

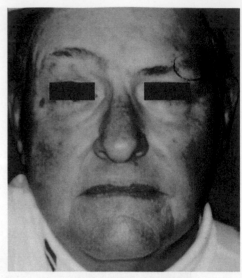

Fig. 5. A 62-year-old Caucasian man with linear scar over left lateral brow at site of incompletely excised perineural SCC.

temporal branch of the left facial nerve, resulting in a 5.5 x 7.0-cm wound (Fig. 6). MRI was performed and revealed no gross tumor surrounding the temporal branch of the facial nerve or the supraorbital nerve at the foramen (Fig. 7). The wound was repaired with a combination of rotation flaps and the patient received postoperative radiation therapy. Three months following completion of radiation therapy, he developed a left-sided Bells palsy and left ear pain. MRI revealed thickening of the left facial nerve at the skull base extending through the stylomastoid foramen and into the vertical portion of the facial nerve canal (Fig. 8). CT of the chest revealed a single bronchial

metastasis, and a bone scan performed for right thigh pain revealed a single bone metastasis. The patient expired 18 months later despite chemotherapy and further radiation therapy to the lung and bone metastases.

The incidence of perineural SCC is reported to be as high as 14%; risk factors include adenosquamous, spindle cell, and poorly differentiated subtypes.[36–38] Only 30% or less of patients with perineural SCC or BCC will experience any neurologic sign or symptom associated with their neoplasm.[36,39] Almost all patients with radiologic evidence of perineural invasion will be clinically symptomatic; the most commonly involved nerves

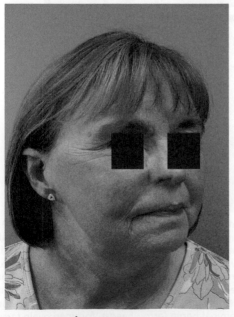

Fig. 4. One year after surgery.

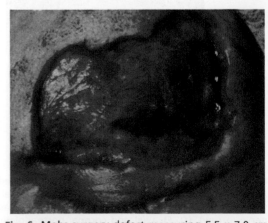

Fig. 6. Mohs surgery defect measuring 5.5 x 7.0 cm. Perineural SCC was noted around the temporal branch of the facial nerve, as well as the supraorbital and supratrochlear nerves, extending to the supraorbital foramen.

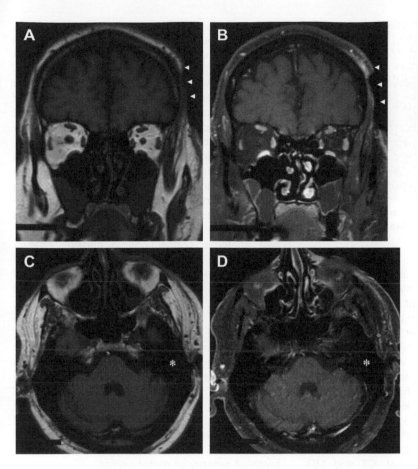

Fig. 7. (*A, B*) MRI with prega-dolinium and postgadolinium coronal T1-weighted scans showing scalp defect and some enhancing scar (*arrow-heads*) at the margin of the resection. No gross tumor. (*C, D*) Pregadolinium and postga-dolinium axial T1-weighted scans showing no tumor associated with the facial nerve in the left temporal bone (*asterisk*).

are the trigeminal and facial nerves.[39] Conversely, patients with clinical signs and symptoms of peri-neural tumor invasion may have negative MRI find-ings and should undergo surgical exploration.[40,41]

The rate of metastases to regional lymph nodes and distant sites is significantly higher with peri-neural head and neck SCC.[35] Ballantyne and colleagues[42] reported a case series of 80 subjects

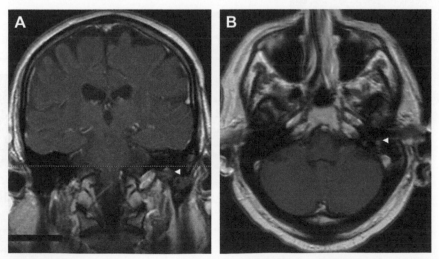

Fig. 8. (*A, B*) MRI with postgadolinium coronal and axial T1-weighted scans. Reference line on coronal scan (*A*) is the axial plane in (*B*). Abnormal enhancement at the entrance to the stylomastoid foramen in the coronal plane and vertical portion of the facial nerve canal in the axial plane (*arrowheads*).

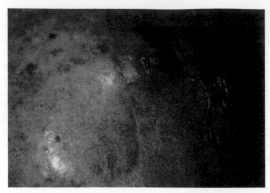

Fig. 9. A 72-year-old Caucasian man with 4-cm fixed erythematous nodule overlying flap scar on left parietal scalp.

with head and neck SCC, 26 of which were primary cutaneous SCC. They noted that early major nerve trunk involvement could occur when invasive SCC developed near a nerve trunk, and that SCC invasion of smaller nerve fibers progressed axially to the central nervous system. Mendenhall and colleagues[39] reported that perineural tumor spread can also extend peripherally.

Case 2 illustrates the need for aggressive initial surgery and radiologic work-up with MRI to detect perineural tumor, and that microscopic perineural tumor escapes detection by current MRI technology, as seen in the MRI performed immediately after Mohs surgery. CT and MRI

have both been effectively used in the past to detect perineural SCC or BCC, prompting more aggressive treatment and resulting in improved outcomes.[43,44] The development of Bell's palsy in patients with facial SCC should prompt an immediate clinical and radiologic work-up and subsequent aggressive surgery with or without adjunctive radiation therapy in order to provide patients with the best possible long-term outcomes.[23] In addition, in this patient the spread of SCC from the temporal branch of the facial nerve to branches of the first division of the trigeminal nerve illustrates the anatomic connections reported in cadaver studies by Li and colleagues.[45] These investigators reported extensive anatomic connections in cadaver studies between the infraorbital nerve to the buccal branch of the facial nerve; the auriculotemporal nerve to the buccal, zygomatic, and temporal branches of the facial nerve; the supraorbital nerve to the zygomatic and temporal branches of the facial nerve; the mental nerve to the marginal mandibular nerve; and the buccinator nerve to the zygomatic, buccal, and marginal mandibular branches of the facial nerve. Clinicians should keep these anatomic connections in mind and perform both sensory and motor examinations on patients with tumors located near major nerve trunks on the face, as well as request radiologic surveillance of potentially involved sensory or motor nerves.

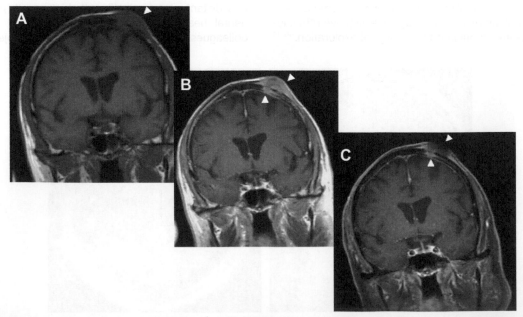

Fig. 10. (A–C) MRI coronal pregadolinium T1 (A), postgadolinium T1 (B), and postgadolinium fat-suppressed T1-weighted images (C). Scalp nodule invades calvarium and erodes through inner table to involve adjacent dura (arrowheads). No gross brain parenchymal involvement.

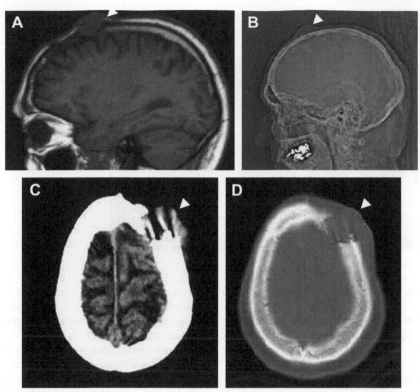

Fig. 11. (*A–D*) Sagittal T1-weighted MRI without gadolinium (*A*), scout view from CT scan (*B*), brain (*C*), and bone (*D*) windows from axial CT scan through tumor (*arrowhead*) showing soft tissue with greatest detail on MRI (*A*), and bone detail on CT (*C, D*). The scout view approximates the limited detail available with a plain-film image (*B*).

Case 3: Recurrent SCC of the Scalp

A 72-year-old Caucasian man presented with a fixed, tender 4-cm erythematous nodule on the left side of the vertex in the center of a surgical scar (**Fig. 9**). This SCC had been widely excised twice and then treated with Mohs surgery and tissue expander-assisted rotation flap repair elsewhere for a SCC at this site 6 months prior. Review of outside operative reports revealed that the outer table had been burred down prior to the flap repair. There was no palpable lymphadenopathy. An MRI was performed, which revealed tumor extending through the skull to involve dura (**Figs. 10** and **11A**). CT of the head was also performed showing tumor erosion through the calvarium and subtle thickening of the meninges suspicious for dural involvement (see **Fig. 11B–D**). CT of the neck was negative. The patient underwent wide excision of skin, bone, and dura by a plastic surgeon and neurosurgeon. Intraoperative frozen sections and paraffin-embedded sections confirmed clear margins in the skin, bone, and dura specimens. The dural defect was repaired with a tensor fascia lata graft. Titanium mesh was secured and cranioplasty was completed with methyl methacrylate. The cutaneous 10 x 8-cm defect was repaired

with a vascularized free flap from the anterolateral aspect of the left thigh. The patient received postoperative radiation therapy to the scalp and draining nodes. Two years later he presented with a left-sided neck mass that was biopsied by fine-needle aspiration and found to be metastatic SCC. He received radiation therapy to the neck

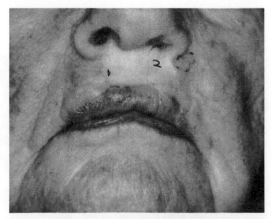

Fig. 12. An 86-year old Caucasian woman with indurated pink papules at periphery of skin graft placed after Mohs surgery for presumed morpheaform BCC 8 years prior.

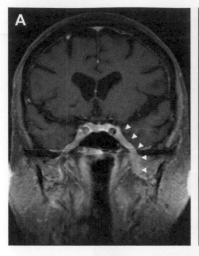
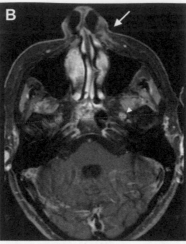

Fig. 13. (A, B) MRI postgadolinium T1-weighted scans showing tumor in left cavernous infiltrating the third division of the trigeminal nerve, and exiting through foramen ovale into the infratemporal fossa. (arrowheads). Infiltrating tumor in L nasolabial fold (arrow).

and was without evidence of disease at 3 months follow-up.

Case 3 illustrates that fine bone detail is more visible with CT, but overall management is best determined by MRI as both gross degree of bone infiltration and assessment of intracranial extension are optimally demonstrated.

Case 4: Recurrent Microcystic Adnexal Carcinoma

An 86-year-old Caucasian woman presented with a 6-month history of diplopia and pain/paresthesias of the left cheek. She had Mohs surgery 8 years prior for 2 recurrent morpheaform BCC of the left side of the upper lip and left alar crease with a full-thickness skin graft and primary linear repair, respectively. The examination revealed indurated papules at the inferior edge of the skin

graft at the vermilion border and at the superior aspect of the graft at the nasolabial crease (Fig. 12). She had decreased sensation to light touch and pin prick in the left V2 distribution. Two punch biopsies revealed microcystic adnexal carcinoma with perineural invasion.

An MRI was ordered to assess for tumor invasion in the cavernous sinus in light of her diplopia and V2 nerve dysfunction. Thickening of the infraorbital nerve was seen extending to the cavernous sinus, with tumor filling the cavernous sinus and traveling distally along V3 (Fig. 13).

Stereotactic gamma knife radiation therapy was administered to the left cavernous resulting in shrinkage of the tumor and resolution of her diplopia and left cheek paresthesias (Fig. 14). In light of her frailty and advanced age, no surgery was pursued. She started palliative radiation therapy to the tumor on her upper lip and cheek;

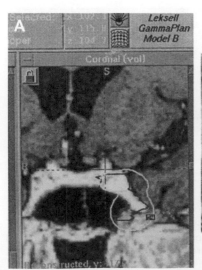
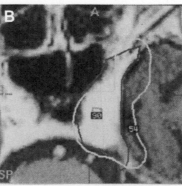

Fig. 14. (A, B) Stereotactic gamma knife treatment outline for palliative radiosurgery to left cavernous sinus. 1500 cGy were delivered in 12 shots.

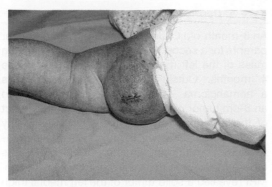

Fig. 15. An 8-month-old girl with 8-cm tumor left medial proximal thigh with central incisional biopsy wound. (*From* Thornton S, Reid J, Papay FA, Vidimos AT. Childhood dermatofibrosarcoma protuberans: role of preoperative imaging. J Amer Acad Dermatol 2005;53:76–83; with permission.)

however, the series of treatments were discontinued because of mucositis. The patient expired 5 years later of unrelated causes.

Microcystic adnexal carcinomas (MAC) have a high incidence of perineural invasion, which is frequently asymptomatic. MACs are frequently initially misdiagnosed, mainly because of inadequate biopsy sampling that fails to show the characteristic histologic findings and depth of tumor infiltration. Case 4 illustrates the utility of MRI in assessing perineural spread to the central nervous system, and also the ability of tumor cells to track axially along V2 to the cavernous sinus, and then grow peripherally along division 3 of the trigeminal nerve. Preoperative MRI imaging of MAC should be considered for long-standing or recurrent tumors, especially post-radiation recurrences, and any tumor that demonstrates signs or symptoms of perineural disease.

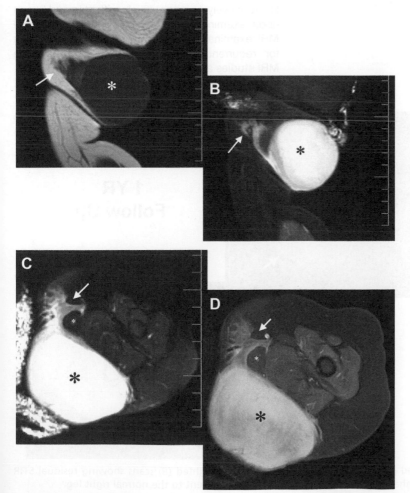

Fig. 16. (*A, B*) MRI sagittal T1 without gadolinium (*A*) and STIR (*B*) sequences showing well-circumscribed tumor mass (*asterisk*) and infiltrative component (*arrow*). (*C, D*) MRI axial STIR (*C*) and postgadolinium fat-suppressed T1-weighted (*D*) sequences showing tumor mass (*large asterisk*) and infiltrative component (*arrow*) wrapping around the gracilis muscle (*small asterisk*) and saphenous vein. The high water content of the tumor, as well as the diaper, are responsible for the high signal (*C*). (*C, D: From* Thornton S, Reid J, Papay FA, Vidimos AT. Childhood dermatofibrosarcoma protuberans: role of preoperative imaging. J Amer Acad Dermatol 2005;53:76–83; with permission.)

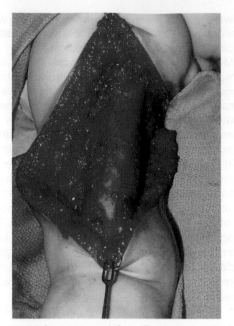

Fig. 17. Mohs surgery defect illustrating extent of tumor resection corresponding to the extent of tumor infiltration seen preoperatively on MRI.

Case 5: Dermatofibrosarcoma Protuberans

An 8-month-old Caucasian girl presented with her parents for a second opinion for a slowly enlarging mass of the left medial proximal thigh since age 4 months. Outside MRI was interpreted as a hemangioma. Physical examination revealed an 8-cm tumor of the medial and proximal aspect of the left thigh (Fig. 15). No lymphadenopathy was detected. Incisional biopsy revealed a derma-tofibrosarcoma protuberans (DFSP). An MRI was ordered to assess the extent of tumor infiltration. MRI revealed a solid tumor of the left medial thigh with tumor infiltration in a honeycomb pattern into the fat, wrapping around the gracilis muscle and saphenous vein (Fig. 16A, B).

Mohs micrographic surgery was performed under general anesthesia in concert with a pediatric surgeon and plastic surgeon. Two layers were required to achieve a tumor-free plane (Fig. 17). The anatomic extent of tumor infiltration at the time of surgery mirrored the MRI findings. The wound was repaired with rotation flaps and a split-thickness skin graft. The patient was followed closely postoperatively with skin and lymph node examinations every 6 months and annual MRI examinations for the first 3 years to assess for recurrence. The postoperative surveillance MRI studies at 1 and 2 years are shown, which revealed scar tissue, but no evidence of recurrent

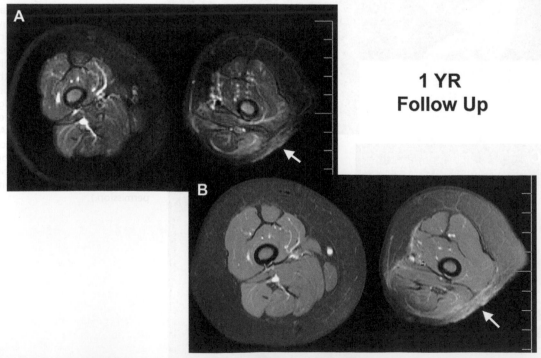

1 YR
Follow Up

Fig. 18. (A, B) Axial STIR (A) and postgadolinium fat-suppressed T1-weighted (B) scans showing residual STIR hyperintense and gadolinium enhancing scar (arrow) in the left leg adjacent to the normal right leg.

DFSP (**Figs. 18** and **19**). It has been 6 years since the surgery and there is no clinical evidence of recurrence and she is able to run and dance without difficulty.

This case is one of 10 cases of pediatric DFSP reported by Thornton and colleagues[46] in 2005. MRI imaging was used in 5 of the 10 cases in this series to assess depth and extent of tumor infiltration prior to surgery in the large tumors and those with a suspected deeper component to assist in preoperative planning and consultation, and for follow-up in this case.

MRI was initially shown to be helpful in assessing DFSP preoperatively by Kransdorf and Meis-Kindblom[47] and Torreggiani and colleagues.[48] Most of these tumors were superficially located and well demarcated. Torreggiani and colleagues recommended the following 3 sequence MRI protocol to optimally image DFSP: T1-weighted and T2-weighted spin-echo or fast spin echo and STIR; they do not recommend routine use of gadolinium. Subsequently, Mendenhall and colleagues[49] and McArthur[50] reported on the

2 YR Follow Up

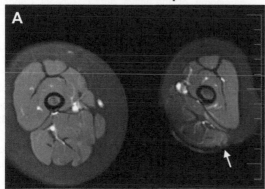

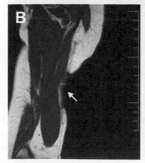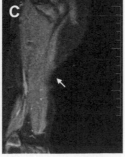

Fig. 19. (A) Axial fat-suppressed postgadolinium T1-weighted scan showing continued reduction of scar enhancement at 2-year follow-up. (B, C) Sagittal T1-weighted scan without gadolinium (B), sagittal STIR (C) showing some return of subcutaneous fat high T1 signal in the area of resection, and no residual STIR hyperintensity at 2-year follow-up (*arrows*).

advisability of preoperative MRI for DFSP to determine deep surgical margins. The management of DFSP located on the face should include preoperative imaging with MRI to optimize surgical cure but spare vital structures, if possible.[51,52] Bony invasion by a primary DFSP of the leg has been demonstrated on MRI by Garg and colleagues.[53] Intracranial infiltration by recurrent DFSPs of the scalp were demonstrated on MRI in 3 subjects reported by Kim and colleagues,[54] Marakovic and colleagues,[55] and Abe and colleagues.[56]

DFSP of the breast has been characterized on ultrasound and mammography as well as MRI.[57,58] On mammography, the DFSPs were skin based or intramammary in location, oval, well-circumscribed masses with subtle areas of microlobulation or spiculation evident only on magnification. On ultrasound examination, the DFSPs were either broad-based abutting the dermis or lying subcutaneously without visible connection to the skin, predominantly well circumscribed, with hypoechoic and hyperechoic areas. Shin and colleagues[59] illustrated that the hypoechoic areas exhibit high cellularity with spindle cells arranged in a distinct storiform pattern, and the hyperechoic areas represented mixtures of tumor cells and fibrous tissue infiltrating the subcutaneous fat. Finally, intraoperative MRI using a special open machine along with MRI-compatible titanium surgical instruments has been used for the excision of 3 DFSPs, using a STIR sequence in the axial and sagittal planes.[60] Histologic clearance was confirmed, although no long-term follow-up was reported.

SUMMARY

The majority of cutaneous nonmelanoma skin cancers treated by dermatologists do not require radiologic evaluation. However, tumors that are large, recurrent, fixed, deeply invasive, or accompanied by clinical signs or symptoms of perineural involvement warrant radiologic evaluation to assess the primary tumor site. Tumors at risk for regional or distant metastases also merit radiologic evaluation. MRI provides superior soft-tissue resolution to CT, but is less sensitive for subtle bone erosion, as cortical bone shows a signal void on MRI. Gross bone destruction and replacement by abnormal soft tissue is clearly visible on MRI and CT. Subtle marrow infiltration without appreciable bone destruction is more easily visualized on MRI. Typically, this visibility is related to replacement of high T1 signal fatty marrow by lower T1 signal tumor. Postgadolinium images can make tumor infiltration of bone less conspicuous, as the enhancing tumor is closer in signal to fatty marrow. MRI is also superior to CT to identify subtle intracranial extension of the tumor, including meningeal involvement. Identification of early perineural involvement by tumor is problematic, as the bulk of neoplasm necessary for visualization on MRI indicates gross disease. Microscopic involvement is below the detection threshold for CT or MRI. Nonetheless, perineural pathology on imaging is relevant to overall staging and treatment planning, and currently is optimally detected with MRI. CT has been considered superior for detecting skull base invasion, central nodal necrosis, extracapsular spread, subtle bone erosion or more extensive bone destruction, and cartilage involvement, but with advances in MRI technology, including faster scan times, higher field magnets, and soft copy interpretation, MRI has taken on a larger role in sorting out complex lesions.

The sensitivity and specificity of PET/CT in staging and follow-up for aggressive nonmelanoma skin cancers remains to be elucidated; however, the available data from head and neck cancers illustrate the utility in assessing patients with an unknown primary tumor, detection of recurrent disease, and distant metastases. Although routine surveillance of the neck, chest, and abdomen are commonly accomplished with CT, concerns regarding radiation exposure, wide availability of MRI, and the potential for clinical PET-MRI scanners may eventually lead to MRI taking over in this role.

In general, ultrasound is the least costly modality, followed by CT, MRI, and PET-CT in increasing order. Information yield at initial staging and restaging should be the primary factor considered. For routine follow-up, the cost gap between routine CT and MRI has narrowed, and so likewise, the information yield for the specific issue is the main consideration.

REFERENCES

1. Krug B, Crott R, Lonneux M, et al. Role of PET in the initial staging of cutaneous malignant melanoma: a review. Radiology 2008;3:836–44.
2. Solomon SB, Silverman SG. Imaging in interventional oncology. Radiology 2010;3:624–40.
3. Hounsfield GN. Computerized transverse axial scanning (tomography): part I: description of system. Br J Radiol 1973;46:1016–22.
4. Hounsfield GN. Computed medical imaging. Nobel lecture December 8, 1979. J Comput Assist Tomogr 1980;4:568–86.
5. Katzberg RW. Urography into the 21st century: new contrast media, renal handling, imaging characteristics, and nephrotoxicity. Radiology 1997;204:297–312.
6. Shellock FG, Spinazzi A. MRI safety update 2008: part 1, MRI contrast agents and nephrogenic systemic fibrosis. AJR Am J Roentgenol 2008;191: 1129–39.
7. Yousem DM, Som PM, Hackney DB, et al. Central nodal necrosis and extracapsular neoplastic spread in cervical lymph nodes. MR imaging vs CT. Radiology 1992;182:753–9.
8. Brenner DJ, Hall EJ. Computed Tomography — an increasing source of radiation exposure. N Engl J Med 2007;357:2277–84.
9. Jambusaria-Pahlajani A, Schmults CD, Miller CJ, et al. Test characteristics of high resolution ultrasound in the preoperative assessment of margins of basal and squamous cell carcinoma in patients undergoing Mohs micrographic surgery. Dermatol Surg 2009;35:9–15.
10. Marmur ES, Berkowitz EZ, Fuchs BS, et al. Use of high frequency, high resolution ultrasound before Mohs surgery. Dermatol Surg 2010;36:841–7.
11. Land R, Herod J, Moskovic E, et al. Routine computerized tomography scanning, groin ultrasound with or without fine needle aspiration cytology in the surgical management of primary squamous cell carcinoma of the vulva. Int J Gynecol Cancer 2006;16:312–7.
12. Van Overhagen H, Brakel K, Heijenbrok M, et al. Metastases in supraclavicular lymph nodes in lung cancer: assessment with palpation, US, and CT. Radiology 2004;232:75–80.
13. Lyshchik A, Higashi T, Asato R, et al. Cervical lymph node metastases: diagnosis at sonoelastography– initial experience. Radiology 2007;243: 258–67.
14. Hany T, Steinert H, Goerres G, et al. PET diagnostic accuracy: improvement with in-line PET-CT system: initial results. Radiology 2002;225:575–81.
15. Gaa J, Rummeny E, Seeman M, et al. Whole body imaging with PET/MRI. Eur J Med Res 2004;9: 309–12.
16. Judenhofer M, Wehrl H, Newport D, et al. Simultaneous PET-MRI: a new approach for functional and morphological imaging. Nat Med 2008;14(4): 459–65.
17. Bailet JW, Abemayor E, Jabour BA, et al. Positron emission tomography: a new, precise imaging modality for detection of head and neck tumors and assessment of cervical adenopathy. Laryngoscope 1992;102:281.
18. Fosko SW, Weimin H, Cook TF, et al. Positron emission tomography for basal cell carcinoma of the head and neck. Arch Dermatol 2003;139:1141.
19. Beer K, Waibel J. Recurrent basal cell carcinoma discovered using positron emission tomography scanning. J Drugs Dermatol 2008;7:879.

20. Boswell JS, Flam MS, Tashjian DN, et al. Basal cell carcinoma metastatic to cervical lymph nodes and lungs. Dermatol Online J 2006;12:9.

21. Conrad GR, Sinha P, Holzhauer M. Perineural spread of skin carcinoma to the base of the skull: detection with FDG PET and CT fusion. Clin Nucl Med 2004;29:717.

22. Cho SB, Chung WG, Yun M, et al. Fluorodeoxyglucose positron emission tomography in cutaneous squamous cell carcinoma: retrospective analysis of 12 patients. Dermatol Surg 2005;31:442.

23. Leach BC, Kulbersh JS, Day TA, et al. Cranial neuropathy as a presenting sign of recurrent aggressive skin cancer. Dermatol Surg 2008;34:483.

24. Roh JL, Moon BJ, Kim JS, et al. Use of f-fluorodeoxyglucose positron emission tomography in patients with rare head and neck cancers. Clin Exp Otorhinolaryngol 2008;1:103–9.

25. Rudmik L, Lau HY, Matthews TW, et al. Clinical utility of PET/CT in the evaluation of head and neck squamous cell carcinoma with unknown primary: a prospective clinical trial. Head Neck 2010. [Epub ahead of print].

26. Kao J, Vu HL, Genden EM, et al. The diagnostic and prognostic utility of positron emission tomography/computed tomography-based follow-up after radiotherapy for head and neck cancer. Cancer 2009; 115:4586–94.

27. Gourin CG, Watts T, Williams HT, et al. Identification of distant metastases with PET/CT in patients with suspected recurrent head and neck cancer. Laryngoscope 2009;119:703–6.

28. Ginsberg LE. MR imaging of perineural tumor spread. Magn Reson Imaging Clin N Am 2002;10:511.

29. Nemzek WR, Hecht S, Gandour-Edwards R, et al. Perineural spread of head and neck tumors: how accurate is MR imaging? AJNR Am J Neuroradiol 1998;19:701–6.

30. Chen AY, Zirwas MJ, Heffernan MP. Nephrogenic systemic fibrosis: a review. J Drugs Dermatol 2010; 9:829.

31. Altun E, Martin DR, Wertman R, et al. Nephrogenic systemic fibrosis: change in incidence following a switch in gadolinium agents and adoption of a gadolinium policy- report from two U.S. universities. Radiology 2009;3:689–96.

32. Shellock FG. Reference manual for magnetic resonance safety, implants, and devices. Los Angeles (CA): Biomedical Research Publishing Group; 2010.

33. Mohs FE, Lathrop TG. Modes of spread of cancer of skin. AMA Arch Derm Syphilol 1952;66:427.

34. Niazi ZB, Lamberty BG. Perineural infiltration in basal cell carcinomas. Br J Plast Surg 1993;46:156.

35. Brown CI, Perry AE. Incidence of perineural invasion in histologically aggressive types of basal cell carcinoma. Am J Dermatopathol 2000;22:123.

36. Goepfert H, Dichtel WJ, Medina JE, et al. Perineural invasion in squamous cell carcinoma of the head and neck. Am J Surg 1984;148:542.

37. Mohs FE. Chemosurgery: microscopically controlled surgery for skin cancer. Springfield (IL): Charles C. Thomas; 1978. p. 262.

38. Cottell WI. Perineural invasion by squamous cell carcinoma. J Dermatol Surg Oncol 1982;8:589.

39. Mendenhall WM, Parsons JT, Mendenhall NP, et al. Carcinoma of the head and neck with perineural invasion. Head Neck Surg 1989;11:301.

40. Gulya AJ, Scher R, Schwartz A, et al. Facial and trigeminal neural dysfunction by a primary cutaneous squamous cell carcinoma: MRI and clinicopathologic correlates. Am J Otol 1992;13:587.

41. Veness MJ. Treatment recommendations in patients diagnosed with high-risk cutaneous squamous cell carcinoma. Australas Radiol 2005;49:365–76.

42. Ballantyne AJ, McCarten AB, Ibanez ML. The extension of cancer of the head and neck through peripheral nerves. Am J Surg 1963;106:651.

43. Williams LS, Mancuso AA, Medenhall WM. Perineural spread of cutaneous squamous and basal cell carcinoma: CT and MR detection and its impact on patient management and prognosis. Int J Radiat Oncol Biol Phys 2001;49:1061.

44. Galloway TJ, Morris CG, Mancuso AA, et al. Impact of Radiographic findings on prognosis for skin carcinoma with clinical perineural invasion. Cancer 2005; 103:1254–7.

45. Li C, Jiang XZ, Zhai YF. Connection of trigeminal nerve and facial nerve branches and its clinical significance. Shanghai Kou Qiang Yi Xue 2009;18: 545 [in Chinese].

46. Thornton S, Reid J, Papay FA, et al. Childhood dermatofibrosarcoma protuberans: Role of preoperative imaging. J Am Acad Dermatol 2005;53: 76–83.

47. Kransdorf MJ, Meis-Kindblom JM. Dermatofibrosarcoma protuberans: radiologic appearance. AJR Am J Roentgenol 1994;163:391–4.

48. Torreggiani WC, Al-Ismail K, Munk PL, et al. Dermatofibrosarcoma protuberans: MR imaging features. AJR Am J Roentgenol 2002;178:989–93.

49. Mendenhall WM, Zlotecki RA, Scarborough MT. Dermatofibrosarcoma protuberans. Cancer 2004;101: 2503–8.

50. McArthur G. Dermatofibrosarcoma protuberans: recent clinical progress. Ann Surg Oncol 2007;14: 2876–86.

51. Bryar P, Sun R, Ebroon D. Nasolacrimal duct obstruction secondary to dermatofibrosarcoma protuberans. Ophthalmology 2004;111:1398–400.

52. Maggoudi D, Vahtesevanos K, Psomaderis K, et al. Dermatofibrosarcoma protuberans of the face: report of 2 cases and an overview of recent literature. J Oral Maxillofac Surg 2006;64:140–4.

53. Garg MK, Yadav MK, Gupta S, et al. Dermatofibro-sarcoma protuberans with contiguous infiltration of underlying bone. Cancer Imaging 2009;9:63–6.

54. Kim SD, Park JY, Choi WS, et al. Intracranial recurrence of the scalp dermatofibrosarcoma. Clin Neurol Neurosurg 2007;109:172–5.

55. Marakovic J, Vilendecic M, Marinovic T, et al. Intracranial recurrence and distant metastasis of scalp dermatofibrosarcoma protuberans. J Neurooncol 2008;88:305–8.

56. Abe T, Kamida T, Goda M, et al. Intracranial infiltration by recurrent scalp dermatofibrosarcoma protuberans. J Clin Neurosci 2009;16:1358–60.

57. Djilas-Ivanovic D, Prvulovic N, Bogdanovic-Stojanvic D, et al. Dermatofibrosarcoma protuberans of the breast: mammographic, ultrasound, MRI and MRS features. Arch Gynecol Obstet 2009;280: 827–30.

58. Lee SJ, Mahoney MC, Shaughnessy E. Dermatofibrosarcoma protuberans of the breast: imaging features and review of the literature. AJR Am J Roentgenol 2009;193:W64–9.

59. Shin YR, Kim JY, Sung MS, et al. Sonographic findings of dermatofibrosarcoma protuberans with pathologic correlation. J Ultrasound Med 2008;27: 269–74.

60. Gould SWT, Agarwal T, Benoist S, et al. Resection of soft tissue sarcomas with intraoperative magnetic resonance guidance. J Magn Reson Imaging 2002; 15:114–9.

Histologic Pitfalls in the Mohs Technique

Navid Bouzari, MD[a,b], Suzanne Olbricht, MD[a,b],*

KEYWORDS

- Mohs • Skin cancer • Histology • Skin surgery

The Mohs micrographic surgical procedure is an important modality that achieves the highest cure rate for most common skin cancers using an intraoperative stepwise histologic evaluation of surgical margins. The success of the procedure is inherently tied to the reliability of each of many steps that make up the technique. Pitfalls in histologic preparation of the tissue specimens may occur during debulking, excising, orienting, creating the map, sectioning, inking, tissue flattening and freezing, cutting, slide fixation, staining, and mapping the tumor. Challenges are also present in the interpretation of the slides. This article discusses some of the histologic pitfalls of the Mohs technique.

TECHNICAL PITFALLS

Because Mohs surgery involves many steps between taking the tissue from the patient and having the slides ready for interpretation, there are many chances for human error and technical problems (**Table 1**).

Debulking

Mohs surgeons typically use curettage for tumor debulking to remove friable tumor-infiltrated dermis, thereby more accurately defining the tumor margins. Whether preoperative curettage can offer a more precise first-stage excision without compromising tissue conservation remains a subject of debate.[1] Some researchers argue that preoperative curettage may remove normal, healing, and/or actinically damaged skin, creating an unnecessary larger wound that subsequently requires fewer Mohs stages for tumor

clearance.[2,3] In contrast, some researchers have shown that preoperative curettage may be tumor-specific and potentially assists in delineating the subclinical extensions of the tumors.[4,5] Because there is no evidence-based recommendation regarding preoperative curettage, at present, the decision to perform preoperative curettage rests largely on an individual surgeon's preferences and personal experience. Mohs surgeons should be aware of several pitfalls encountered during pre-Mohs curettage. The curette may not remove tissue in a uniform fashion with smooth sharply defined borders. If curettage yields jagged edges, it is difficult to take a uniformly narrow specimen during Mohs' surgery. In addition, curettage can create shearing forces in the surrounding epidermis, which may lead to epidermal loss during tissue processing. Curetting severely photodamaged skin in areas such as the forearm and cheek may sometimes create overhanging pieces of epidermis at the edges.[3,6] Furthermore, preoperative curettage may increase the incidence of floaters (**Fig. 1**).[7]

Excising

To achieve a flat pancakelike Mohs layer the optimum bevel angle is from 30° to 45°. A bevel angle less than 15° increases the chance of cutting into the cancerous skin thereby increasing the number of Mohs layers and the diameter of the defect. On the other hand, a bevel angle greater than 45° interferes with proper tissue flattening for optimal sectioning. Specimens that are cut thickly or with tall 90° edges do not lie flat on their own. In such circumstances, there is a higher

---

[a] Department of Dermatology, Lahey Clinic, Burlington, MA, USA
[b] Department of Dermatology, Harvard Medical School, Boston, MA, USA
* Corresponding author. Lahey Clinic, 41 Mall Road, Burlington, MA 01805.
E-mail address: Suzanne.m.olbricht@lahey.org

Dermatol Clin 29 (2011) 261–272
doi:10.1016/j.det.2011.01.002
0733-8635/11/$ – see front matter © 2011 Elsevier Inc. All rights reserved.

derm.theclinics.com

Table 1
Potential technical pitfalls in Mohs surgery

	Potential Pitfall	Recommendation
Debulking	Curettage may create jagged borders, epidermal loss, or induce floater	Curettage when indicated instead of routinely doing it, saline irrigation after excision
Excising	Cutting into cancerous tissue if bevel angle <15°; thick and tall edges if bevel angle >45° Cutting marginal surfaces when making relaxing incisions	Bevel angle of 30° to 45°, use relaxing incisions when tissue doesn't lie flat Make the relaxing incisions close to the center of the specimen
Orienting	Tissue rotation Introducing floaters when making the hash marks	Double-hash at one point, asymmetric hash marks, saline irrigation
Mapping	Inaccurate mapping	Consistency regardless of the mapping method
Sectioning	Inducing tissue lacerations which may be mistaken for hash marks	Controversial whether Mohs surgeon or histotechnician should do the sections. Number of tissue sections are a matter of debate as well
Inking	Placing it in the wrong margin, inadequate inking, ink running over the wrong sections	Controversial whether Mohs surgeon or histotechnician should do the inking. High-quality ink, appropriate amount of ink
Tissue Flattening and Freezing	Ice crystal formation if frozen too slowly leading to cracks and holes in the specimen; curling the tissue if blades are not cold enough	Appropriate temperature from −22°C to −30°C. Cold cutting blades
Cutting	Tearing or curling the tissue with dull blades; tear in the tissue if nicks on the blade; thick specimen with loose screws; inducing floaters	Use sharp blades; check blades for nicks; try to achieve the thinnest sections possible; check the screws; clean the blades
Slide Fixation	Artifact due to short time dehydration; tissue doesn't attach due to defects on the slides; errors in labeling	Appropriate dehydration time; check for defects on the slide; proper labeling
Staining	Artifacts if not long enough time for dehydration; floaters if staining solution is contaminated	Complete dehydration, change staining solution frequently

chance of losing epidermal and/or dermal margins. It is therefore necessary to make relaxing incisions to improve tissue flattening. A potential pitfall is to cut the marginal surface while making the relaxing incisions,[8] which can confuse the orientation as well as interrupt the continuity of the margin. Pitfalls can also occur when taking additional layers for second and subsequent Mohs stages. These sections can be rectangular or crescent shaped. Some investigators think that when a rectangular specimen is taken, tumor may hide in the part of the margin at the end, distal to the acute margin. To avoid a false-negative view, relaxing cuts need to be made in a way such that the 90° angle of the vertical edges is converted to a curved line. This cut can be difficult

to perform, especially in narrow specimens. Therefore, some investigators suggest using crescent-shaped sections instead of rectangular sections.[9]

Orienting

The surgeon has many ways of marking the tissue for orientation. Most surgeons create hash marks (nicks) cutting into both the specimen and the edge of the wound simultaneously. Frequently, a nick is created at the 6- and 12-o'clock (or 3- and 9-o'clock) positions in anticipation of a bisected specimen. A potential pitfall for this method is that the tissue may be rotated from the time it is excised to the time it gets to the laboratory. To avoid this rotation, some Mohs surgeons

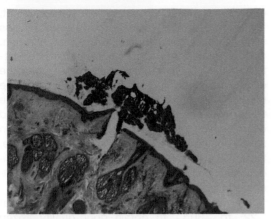

Fig. 1. Floaters can be introduced during curettage, as well as while making nicks, cutting, and staining.

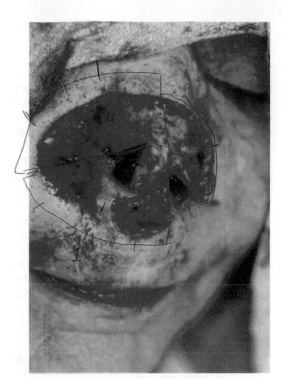

Fig. 2. A printed digital photograph that is available intraoperatively for mapping produces a detailed representation of the defect.

make asymmetric nicks (eg, at the 3- and 12-o'clock positions) or a double nick at 1 point (eg, at the 12-o'clock position). Asymmetric nicks can, however, lead to distortion on the maps in bisected specimens because the bisected line is the result of estimating the half of the specimen. Regardless of the method used by the surgeon, consistency of the orienting method helps to minimize the errors because it provides the ability to the surgeon, the histotechnician, and all the assistants to predict and then identify the right orientation of the tissue without difficulty. Another pitfall that Mohs surgeons should be aware of is that when the tissue is scored from the surface to the depth, a floater can be introduced by forcing tissue at the surface down to the base, producing a false-positive margin (see **Fig. 1**).

Creating the Map

Inaccurate mapping results in false-negative subsequent layers and failure of the technique and may account for some tumor recurrences.[10] There is variability in mapping methods used by Mohs surgeons. Silapunt and colleagues[11] showed in a survey that most of the Mohs surgeons prepare tissue maps themselves using hand-drawn pictures to map and orient specimens. This method is fast and inexpensive. Hand-drawn pictures, however, cannot provide the exact size and shape of the excised area; therefore, these investigators suggest the use of digital and Polaroid photographs, which can produce detailed representations of defects, the excised tissue, and their interrelationship (**Fig. 2**). There are other methods for mapping, such as using preprinted maps or cartoons of anatomic sites. There is no study to show which mapping method is superior in preventing errors. However, consistency of mapping by whichever method

used allows for predictability and thus better accuracy.

Sectioning

Many Mohs surgeons cut the tissue into 2 pieces in the first stage. However, the first-stage tissue may be divided into 3 or 4 pieces in certain circumstances. Cutting into more pieces is more expensive and time consuming but may provide better sections for evaluating epidermal margins.[11] However, there is a higher chance of mislabeling or mixing up the specimens or mismapping positive margins when there are more pieces. Another problem with multiple small sections is the higher likelihood of folding at the epidermal edges, which may lead to false-positive results. In addition, the technician may assume tissue lacerations as hash marks and may make incorrect sections. Hence, some Mohs surgeons section the specimen in the procedure room to reduce the chance of incorrect cuts and inaccurate mapping. However, other surgeons consider that sectioning and grossing by the histotechnician under magnified light allows for better tissue preparation. Still other surgeons prefer that the first stage be processed as 1 piece (pac-man technique), so that orientation cannot be misconstrued. This option works only for relatively small pieces and requires exceptional skill on the part of the person using the cryotome to section the tissue.[12]

Inking

Inking can be done by the surgeon in the procedure room or by the histotechnician. Some Mohs surgeons prefer to do the inking in the procedure room to reduce the chance of placing ink on the wrong margins. This procedure can, however, be more time consuming for the surgeon, as well as increase the expense because it requires multiple magnifiers and inking equipment in each room. Furthermore, the surgeon should be well acquainted with sectioning because after inking he/she cannot further cut the tissue if the specimen is too large. Inking is most helpful when the ink is placed along a significant portion of the surgical margin rather than just as an orienting dot at the specimen pole (**Fig. 3**). If the specimen is inked along the entire margin, missing ink indicates that a margin is not fully evaluable. On the other hand, if too much ink is used, ink may inadvertently run over and confuse the margins. The same problem can also occur if the specimen is too wet. Quality of the ink is important too. Poor-quality ink may be washed off during the tissue preparation.[13,14]

Tissue Flattening and Freezing

This step is critical for achieving sections in which it is possible to examine the complete en face outer margin of a specimen. Proper flattening makes it possible to section the complete undersurface, the sidewall, and the epidermal margin in a single piece. Several methods are used for flattening: heat-extractor flattening with optimal

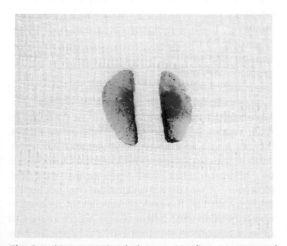

Fig. 3. Inking is optimal along a significant portion of the surgical margin rather than just as an orienting dot at the specimen pole.

cutting temperature (OCT) medium in the cryostat, tissue cuts or slits, aerosol freezing on a glass slide, mechanical flattening with liquid nitrogen, or different combinations of these methods.[11] Flattening the tissue can be challenging when the edges are vertical, requiring relaxing cuts to be made. If there is inadequate relaxation of the tissue, peripheral margins may not be teased down, which results in missing epidermis.[15] In some anatomic areas such as periocular tissue, flattening and embedding can be difficult, because delicate periocular tissue may fold easily before embedding.

The tissue should be kept adequately frozen, at −22° to −30°C, to obtain good-quality frozen sections. Colder temperatures of −28° to −32°C may be required for fat-containing tissue. If tissue is frozen too slowly, ice crystals can leave holes in the tissue. Condensate that accumulates in humid conditions can also result in ice crystal formation that causes cracks and holes in the specimen. If the cutting blade in the cryostat is not cold enough, either the sections tend to attach to the blade or the tissue may curl during the cutting. High humidity in the room can also lead to curling of the specimen.[8,14]

Cutting

Blades are either permanent or disposable. Dull blades may cause tearing or curling of the tissue, or sometimes cause chatter lines in the tissue as they cut. It is therefore important to sharpen the permanent blades and to move the disposable blades along the blade holder over the course of the day. It is also important to check the blade for nicks. A small microscopic nick in the edge of the blade can create a large tear in the tissue.

The goal in cutting is to achieve the thinnest sections possible because this promotes ease in having the entire epidermis visible on the slide. However, it is difficult to obtain sections thinner than 3 to 4 μm. Thick sections are also difficult to read because some of the cellular details may be obscured (**Fig. 4**). If the knife or chuck screws are loose, the sections may be cut thin in one section and thick in another. Thin sections may make it difficult to cut fat, and holes or tears may be visible. For this reason, thicker sections may be cut. Because the evaluation of both fat and epidermis/dermis is important, alternating thicker and thinner sections may be optimal.[8] Another potential pitfall during cutting is the introduction of a floater from the blade. In this case, the fragment may be visualized on multiple cuts on the slide and may be directly continuous with the true specimen (in contrast to the floaters from

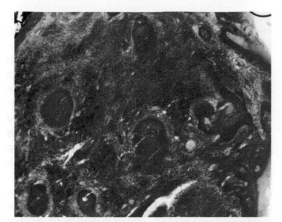

Fig. 4. Cellular details are obscured in thick section (hematoxylin and eosin, original magnification ×2).

the contaminated staining well; see later discussion). The Mohs histotechnician can minimize the potential for introducing floaters by ensuring that the cutting surface and cryostat blade are cleaned between the cases and that the staining solutions are changed frequently.[7] Challenges also occur when the section is slid from the blade onto the slide. After placing each section on the slide, the extra OCT medium around it should be wiped off the glass slide before placing the subsequent specimen. If the subsequent section is placed over the OCT medium, it may not adhere properly during the fixation and as a result it can be washed off the slide during staining. The space between the specimens on the glass slide should be wide enough to avoid overlapping OCT medium with the tissue sections. In addition, if the OCT medium covers the tissue, it may interfere with proper tissue staining.

Slide Fixation

Slide fixation involves the use of chemicals or heat to adhere the tissue to the slide before staining. Mohs laboratories typically use 10% neutral buffered formalin, alcoholic formalin, alcohol, or acetone as a fixative for frozen section slides before staining. Alcohol seems to be the most popular choice, especially because the other 3 agents require the use of a hood. If the slides are removed too quickly from the fixative, they will not have enough time for dehydration, which affects the staining quality (see **Fig. 3**). Another potential pitfall in the slide fixation process is a flaw with the glass slide. If glass slides have any defects or are dirty, tissue may not adhere properly to them. Slides can have frosted or unfrosted ends. The frosted end in slides is usually used to identify the first section that is cut. So slides with a frosted end are preferred because

they decrease the chance of confusing the sections. Proper labeling is of utmost importance. Typically, slide labels should include the patient's last name, stage of the surgery, section and level cut, date, and the histotechnician's initials.[16]

Staining

Most Mohs surgeons use hematoxylin-eosin (H&E) for staining. Maintaining quality with H&E staining can be difficult. The staining steps are postfixation preparation, nuclear staining, cytoplasm staining, dehydration, clearing, and cover slipping. Of note, stains are particularly subject to pH changes.[8] Dehydration is also very important to the final outcome. Unless all water is removed, the final slides will have artifact and be difficult to read (**Fig. 5**). Some Mohs surgeons prefer toluidine blue staining.[17] Toluidine blue stains the mucin bright red and, therefore, attracts the eyes to the potential tumor sites. However, mucopolysaccharides can sometimes be abundant around normal adnexal structures, so the bright red color is not specific for tumor. In addition, toluidine blue is not ideal for staining squamous cell carcinomas (SCCs), which have little or no mucopolysaccharides. Another potential pitfall in staining is the introduction of a floater to the slide from a contaminant in the staining solution well. This floater would be expected at only a single locus and at a random orientation to the surgical specimen. The staining solutions should be changed frequently to minimize the risk of introducing floaters.[7]

Mapping Tumor

The surgeon's task of sitting at the microscope and accurately mapping tumor seen on the slides depends on the reliability of the preparation steps

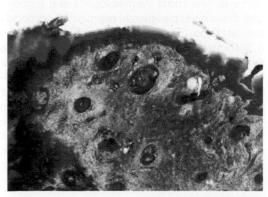

Fig. 5. A thick specimen that is incompletely dehydrated demonstrates low-quality staining and artifact formation (hematoxylin and eosin, original magnification ×2).

detailed so far. Good communication with the histotechnicians as well as daily quality assessment of at least 1 set of slides will facilitate improvement in suboptimal preparation. Specific details of orientation or problems during embedding for unusual specimens can be discussed during handoff of the slides from the histotechnician to the surgeon and may be important and/or time saving during examination of the slides. The surgeon must verify that the slides are matched with the appropriate map and that the pieces are accurately labeled and appropriately represented on the map. Generally, the Mohs surgeon scans the slide first to make sure that the epidermis, dermis, and subcutaneous fat are fully represented; the color of the staining is interpretable; and the ink is visible. Nicks are located on the section, and the location is confirmed on the map. Magnification with a ×2 objective allows the surgeon to easily scan an entire section in 1 power field. Once the tumor has been identified and confirmed with a higher-power lens, the surgeon may then review its location using a ×2 lens to facilitate accurate mapping.

DIAGNOSTIC PITFALLS

A critical component of Mohs technique is the surgeon's skill in interpreting histologic specimens (**Table 2**). Fellowship-trained Mohs surgeons spend much of their time at the microscope acquiring dermatopathology expertise, which improves steadily in relation to the number of cases. Murphy and colleagues[18] showed that more than 1300 Mohs surgery cases and more than 6 months of fellowship training were required before reducing errors to a minimum acceptable level of less than 1 critical error per 100 cases read. Frozen section slides may be more difficult to interpret than formalin-fixed permanent sections, and most dermatologists and pathologists have no experience in examining horizontally cut sections. The Mohs surgeon must follow a systematic, comprehensive, and reproducible system for evaluation of the frozen section slides, correlating the findings observed with the 3-dimensional specimen represented by sequential cuts. There are many challenging situations in which Mohs surgeons must be able to decide whether what they see is a malignant process or a benign structure such as an adnexal structure. Inflammatory cells can both be mistaken for a malignant process or obscure malignant cells.

Floater

If a Mohs surgeon does not accurately identify a floater, an unnecessary excision of normal tissue

may ensue. Floaters are extraneous tissue fragments found on a slide in addition to the intended section (see **Fig. 1**).[7] As discussed in the "Technical Pitfall" section, they can be introduced onto the slide at any time during tissue handling and processing. Mohs surgeons may suspect floaters when the visualized tumor differs from the suspected pathologic condition. Location of ink may also help in identification of a floater, in that if the tissue lies outside the ink margin, it is likely to be a floater. The assumption in this case is that the floater is detached from other parts of the specimen and is not located at the true margin. If the origin of the floater is in doubt, another Mohs stage is generally warranted. The occurrence of floaters can be minimized by implementing the preventive methods explained earlier (see the "Technical Pitfalls" section).

Inflammation Versus Tumor

Inflammation may be mistaken for tumor or may obscure an underlying malignancy (**Fig. 6**). Katz and colleagues[19] investigated whether inflammation could mask basal cell carcinoma (BCC). In almost half of the cases, tumor was present in the immediate vicinity of the inflammation. Inflammation can also obscure or resemble SCC, although lymphocytes tend to be smaller and more rounded than epitheloid cells (**Fig. 7**). Some Mohs surgeons stress that prominent aggregates of inflammatory cells may indicate that tumor is nearby, indicating the need for an additional stage of surgery. Using immunohistochemistry, Zachary and colleagues[20] showed single cells or small clumps of SCC in areas in which H&E staining only showed inflammation. However, finding inflammatory cells does not necessarily indicate the presence of tumor. Inflammation can also occur in areas of ulceration or previous biopsy sites.[21] Obtaining a deeper section from the block or having a deeper section cut more thinly may identify if tumor is actually present.

BCC Versus Benign Conditions

A common diagnostic difficulty in histology of skin is distinguishing tangentially sectioned hair follicles from BCC (**Fig. 8**). There are several features that help differentiate the 2, including cleft formation (separation artifact), palisading, mitotic figures, and apoptotic cells that are present around or in BCC nests. Hair follicles are usually surrounded by a fibrous sheath.[22] BCCs that invade deeply into the side of the face or neck may invade into the parotid gland. Mohs surgeons must differentiate the tumor from the blue glandular cells of the parotid (**Fig. 9**). Examining the

Table 2
Potential diagnostic pitfalls in Mohs surgery

	Potential Pitfall	Recommendation
Floater	Floater may be introduced during curettage, making nicks, cutting, and staining	Irrigate with Saline after excision, keep the blades clean, change staining solution frequently
Inflammation vs Tumor	Inflammation can obscure or resemble the tumor	Examine another section from deeper in the block. Immunohistochemistry may be helpful
BCC vs Benign Conditions	Tangentially sectioned hair follicles can be mistaken for BCC	Examine relevant location in multiple sections
BCC vs Other Neoplasms	Trichoepithelioma, spiradenoma, cylindroma, MAC, and metastatic breast cancer may resemble BCC	Examine multiple sections, thaw the block and send for permanent sections. Immunohistochemistry may be helpful
AK vs SCC In Situ vs SCC	Misreading AK for SCC, vice versa, missing SCC clumps in the dermis	Define AK and SCC in situ and make consistent diagnosis. Evaluate the dermis carefully for small clumps of SCC cells. Immunohistochemistry may be helpful
SCC vs Benign Conditions	Healing wound and biopsy sites may be mistaken for SCC. Tangential sectioning of epidermis may resemble SCC	Identify biopsy site grossly and microscopically. Examine multiple sections for lumina, fragments of hair and papillae
SCC vs Other Neoplasms	Inflamed seborrheic keratoses and wart can be mistaken for SCC; adnexal tumors may resemble SCC	Examine multiple sections, thaw the block and send for permanent sections. Immunohistochemistry may be helpful
Perineural Invasion	Missing perineural invasion; Confusing with peritumoral fibrosis, re-excision perineural invasion, reparative perineural proliferation, and epithelial sheath neuroma	Have high index of suspicion in invasive SCC; Examine multiple sections; May need final full margin taken and send for permanent sections and special stains
Melanoma	Hard to recognize melanocytes in frozen section specimen; Inferior quality of frozen section regarding cellular detail	MART-1 staining may be helpful; good communication and close working relationship with dermatopathologist is optimal
Other Tumors	Skip areas in Merkel cell carcinoma, Paget disease, and sebaceous carcinoma; scar may be mistaken for DFSP; normal pilar apparatus may resemble leiomyosarcoma	Be aware of the potential false negative clear margin in multifocal tumors; consider an additional excision of margins for processing as formalin-fixed sections

Abbreviations: AK, actinic keratosis; BCC, basal cell carcinoma; DFSP, dermatofibrosarcoma protuberans; MAC, microcystic adnexal carcinoma.

suspicious area on multiple sections often clarifies confusing histologic results.

BCC Versus Other Neoplasms

Sometimes benign appendageal tumors such as trichoepitheliomas can be confused with BCC. Although trichoepitheliomas characteristically have horn cysts, fibrous stroma, and clusters of mesenchymal cells, in some cases, it is impossible to differentiate them from BCC. Other tumors with blue cells such as poroma, spiradenoma, cylindroma, and metastatic breast carcinoma may resemble BCC. Poromas usually have broadbase connections to the epidermis. Spiradenomas usually have no connection to the surface and make a rosette pattern. Metastatic breast cancer is typically seen in a patient with a history of breast cancer, and commonly in skin of the chest wall. Microcystic adnexal carcinoma is frequently misdiagnosed as BCC, but the appearance of tadpolelike extensions and an increased number of

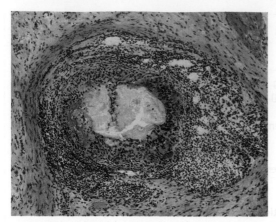

Fig. 6. Inflammation and giant cell reaction around a hair follicle may be confused with tumor (hematoxylin and eosin, original magnification ×10).

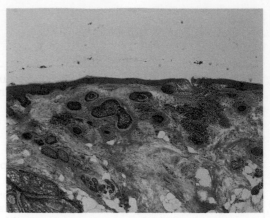

Fig. 8. Tangentially sectioned hair follicle may resemble BCC. Note hair fragments and lack of palisading and retraction artifact. Examination of adjacent sections verified the diagnosis of hair follicle without tumor (hematoxylin and eosin, original magnification ×2).

glandular structures should help the Mohs surgeon make the correct diagnosis.[21] Examining multiple sections often assists in making an accurate diagnosis. In addition, the block can be thawed and sent for preparation as formalin-fixed paraffin-embedded permanent sections, vertically cut for the dermatopathologist to review.

Actinic Keratosis Versus SCC In Situ Versus Invasive SCC

This diagnostic spectrum has long been a topic of debate within dermatopathology. Distinguishing changes along the actinic damage spectrum is challenging for both clinicians and dermatopathologists (see **Fig. 7**; **Fig. 10**). Some pathologists think that no fundamental difference exists between actinic keratosis (AK) and SCC but that it is rather a progression along a spectrum.[23,24]

Studies have shown that up to 60% of SCCs begin as AKs and that there is histologic evidence of contiguous AK in 97% of SCC lesions that arise on sun-damaged skin.[25,26] Furthermore, AKs demonstrate features of malignancy from their inception, from both a cytologic and a molecular biologic perspective. They share genetic tumor markers and have *p53* gene mutations identical with SCCs that involve the dermis.[27] In fact, if cells of an AK could be artificially transplanted into the dermis, the histologic and molecular features would be identical to those of SCC.[23] Invasive disease underlying AK-SCC in situ histology can also be missed. The underlying dermis should be evaluated carefully for nests and cords of atypical squamous cells. It is especially easy to miss small clumps or single cells of SCC in areas of inflammation. Immunostaining using cytokeratin is helpful to

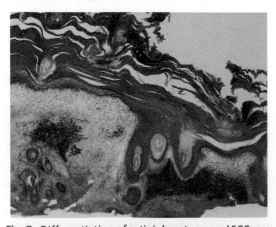

Fig. 7. Differentiation of actinic keratoses and SCC may sometimes be difficult, especially when there is a dense inflammation obscuring the underlying dermis (hematoxylin and eosin, original magnification ×2).

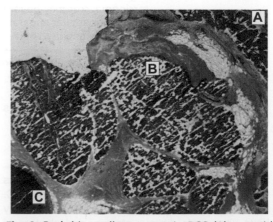

Fig. 9. Dark blue cells are seen in BCC (A), parotid gland cells (B), and lymphocytes in a lymph node (C) (hematoxylin and eosin, original magnification ×2).

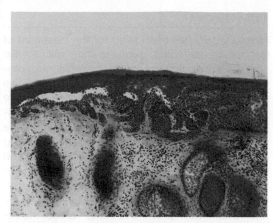

Fig. 10. Distinguishing between actinic keratoses, SCC in situ, and SCC can be challenging, causing disagreement between the Mohs surgeon and the pathologist (hematoxylin and eosin, original magnification ×2).

detect the squamous cells but has the disadvantages of being time consuming and expensive. Moreover, globular material in the papillary dermis may falsely be stained and mistaken for SCC.[28,29] Considering the differences in their treatments, it is important to differentiate AK, SCC in situ, and SCC. Presence of AK in the Mohs sections does not warrant further excision. However, if the Mohs surgeon decides that the extent of atypia is enough to diagnose SCC in situ, it is advisable in most situations to excise another tissue specimen. The threshold for diagnosis of SCC in situ may vary between Mohs surgeons or between Mohs surgeons and dermatopathologists; however, in more than 95% of cases, Mohs surgeons and dermatopathologists agree on the diagnosis as shown in a study by Mariwalla and colleagues.[30]

SCC Versus Benign Conditions

Hair follicles and sweat glands in healing wounds and biopsy sites may show metaplastic changes that can resemble SCC. Keratin pearls, cytologic atypia, and mitoses are all seen in healing wounds and biopsy sites. Helpful clues to differentiate these conditions from SCC are the presence of lumina in the sweat ducts and fragments of hair in the follicles, as well as fibrosis and inflammation at wounded sites. A major difficulty, however, is that SCCs can also exhibit fibrosing inflamed stroma. Tangential sectioning of the epidermis, which is usual in Mohs sections, can produce the appearance of a thickened epidermis resembling SCC. The presence of dermal papillae within the epidermis and the absence of parakeratosis are helpful clues that the diagnosis is not SCC.[21,31]

SCC Versus Other Neoplasms

A variety of benign and malignant neoplasms can be mistaken for SCC. Seborrheic keratoses and warts can show cytologic atypia when irritated. They may have keratin pearls, which are also seen in SCC. Adnexal tumors can also resemble SCC: trichoadenomas usually have numerous horn cysts, sebaceous carcinomas usually arise on the eyelid, and proliferating trichilemmal cysts are commonly seen on the scalp.[21] As with the diagnosis of BCC, examining multiple sections often assists in making an accurate diagnosis. In addition, the block can also be thawed and sent for preparation as permanent sections, vertically cut for the dermatopathologist to review.

Perineural Invasion

Perineural invasion is claimed to occur in approximately 1% of all cases of BCC and in 3% of all cases of SCC (**Fig. 11**).[32] Both Mohs surgeons and pathologists are expected to be able to accurately diagnose perineural invasion. This diagnosis is especially important for Mohs surgeons because studies have shown that the survival rates of patients with SCC complicated by perineural invasion that is cleared by Mohs surgery are better than any other treatment or combination of treatments.[33] Perineural disease can have skip lesions histologically, so that once it is diagnosed, a larger than normal next stage might be performed. Also, if perineural disease is diagnosed, consideration should be given to recommending extensive surgery, such as a parotidectomy for a perineural tumor deep in the cheek, or adjuvant therapy, such as radiotherapy. Although it is important not to miss the perineural invasion, confusing it with other benign conditions may lead to unnecessary Mohs stages and adjuvant

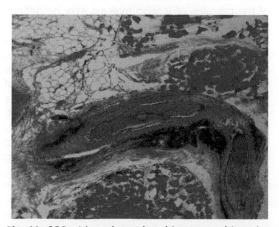

Fig. 11. SCC with perineural and intraneural invasion (hematoxylin and eosin, original magnification ×5).

therapies. In case of a novice, a hair follicle transected through the dermal papilla or an arrector pili muscle surrounded by inflammation could be confused with perineural invasion. Other conditions such as peritumoral fibrosis, reexcision perineural invasion, reparative perineural proliferation, and epithelial sheath neuroma could be challenging for even more-experienced Mohs surgeons.[32,34] Multiple sections must be thoroughly reviewed, and consideration should be given to excising a large complete margin for processing as a permanent section with special stains.

Melanoma

The use of Mohs technique in the treatment of melanoma, compared with nonmelanoma skin cancer, is more complicated, and its role in the management of melanoma has been controversial. Although there is mounting evidence to support the use of Mohs technique for melanoma, there are several pitfalls that Mohs surgeons should be aware of. It has been stressed that frozen section quality is inferior to paraffin-embedded sections, especially with regard to cellular detail. Identification of melanocytes is easier when the tissue is processed in formalin-fixed paraffin-embedded sections. During the formalin fixation process, a clear halo is produced in melanocytes as an artifact of the fixation process because of perinuclear cytoplasmic retraction. This artifact allows for easier identification of single melanocytes in formalin-fixed sections compared with frozen sections because it is not present in the latter. Another disadvantage of the Mohs technique is that horizontal sectioning does not allow for evaluation of the growth characteristics of the central tumor mass or its progression toward the margin, or measurement of the maximal Breslow depth.[35] In addition, evaluation of the margins of lentigo maligna may be difficult because sun-damaged skin often contains atypical melanocytes as a baseline and not a manifestation of cancer or a precancerous lesion. Mohs surgeons should decide whether to consider single atypical melanocytes as an indicator of positive margin. The biologic behavior of these single atypical melanocytes is difficult to predict, but some studies suggest that their removal may be unnecessary and may lead to increased surgical morbidity.[36–38] Although immunostaining with MART-1 has shown to be helpful in diagnosis, there is still a significant amount of discrepancy in diagnoses among Mohs surgeons and dermatopathologists. In some reports, the Mohs sections had unacceptably high false-negative results, 47% in one study.[39,40]

Other Tumors

Mohs surgery has been used for the treatment of dermatofibrosarcoma protuberans, microcystic adnexal carcinoma, sebaceous carcinoma, leiomyosarcoma, and atypical fibroxanthoma, as well as extramammary Paget disease. In some cases, it may be beneficial to work with dermatopathologists, and sometimes modifications of the Mohs technique are necessary, such as using paraffin-embedded sections instead of frozen sections when cellular detail is important. For tumors such as Paget disease, Merkel cell carcinoma, and sebaceous carcinoma, which can be multifocal with prominent skip areas, false-negative clear margins may be seen in the Mohs sections,[14] and it may be advisable to take an extra full margin for examination, either as frozen Mohs sections or as permanent sections in the dermatopathology laboratory. For Merkel cell carcinoma in particular, differentiation of cancer from a small focus of inflammation can be difficult using frozen sections. Another diagnostic challenge is to differentiate the tumor from normal tissue. For example, a scar with reactive fibroblast proliferation may be mistaken for dermatofibrosarcoma protuberans. Leiomyosarcomas must be distinguished from normal pilar apparatus. The presence of mitosis, atypical nuclei, and necrosis favors malignancy. For spindle cell tumors, some investigators advise to take an additional Mohs layer for permanent formalin-fixed sections even after Mohs surgeons are convinced that they have achieved clear margins.[41]

SUMMARY

The reliability of the Mohs procedure in curing skin cancers rests on the accuracy with which tissue is excised, oriented, prepared for slide examination, and evaluated by the surgeon. The technique requires time, teaching, and a sufficient quantity of cases from which to learn, as well as continuous attention to the pitfalls that can occur with the processing and interpretation of the histologic appearance of the specimens. Errors of any kind can lead to cancer persistence and local recurrence. Previous studies have shown that technical and interpretational errors are the most important factors affecting recurrence rate of cancer after Mohs surgery[10] and that a significant number of cases and at least 6 months of training under direct supervision are required to reach to an acceptable level of accuracy.[18] The authors also believe that extended time with both direct and indirect mentoring is essential in developing expertise in both the technical and histopathologic aspects of Mohs surgery.

REFERENCES

1. Ratner D, Lee DA. Economic impact of preoperative curettage before Mohs micrographic surgery for basal cell carcinoma. Dermatol Surg 2006;32: 916–23.
2. Huang CC, Boyce S, Northington M, et al. Randomized, controlled surgical trial of preoperative tumor curettage of basal cell carcinoma in Mohs micrographic surgery. J Am Acad Dermatol 2004;51: 585–91.
3. Jih MH, Friedman PM, Goldberg LH, et al. Curettage prior to Mohs' micrographic surgery for previously biopsied nonmelanoma skin cancers: what are we curetting? Retrospective, prospective, and comparative study. Dermatol Surg 2005;31:10–5.
4. Chung VQ, Bernardo L, Jiang SB. Presurgical curettage appropriately reduces the number of Mohs stages by better delineating the subclinical extensions of tumor margins. Dermatol Surg 2005; 31(9 Pt 1):1094–9.
5. Ratner D, Bagiella E. The efficacy of curettage in delineating margins of basal cell carcinoma before Mohs micrographic surgery. Dermatol Surg 2003; 29:899–903.
6. Miller SJ. Commentary. Dermatol Surg 2000;26:165–6.
7. Walling HW, Swick BL. Identifying a tissue floater on Mohs frozen sections. Dermatol Surg 2009;35: 1009–10.
8. Nguyen DH, Siegel DM, Zell D, et al. Quality assurance. In: Morgan MB, Hamill JR, Spencer JM, editors. Atlas of Mohs and frozen section cutaneous pathology. New York: Springer; 2009. p. 9–14.
9. Yu Y, Finn DT. Crescent versus rectangle: is it a true negative margin in second and subsequent stages of Mohs surgery? Dermatol Surg 2010;36:171–6.
10. Hruza GJ. Mohs micrographic surgery local recurrences. J Dermatol Surg Oncol 1994;20:573–7.
11. Silapunt S, Peterson SR, Alcalay J, et al. Mohs tissue mapping and processing: a survey study. Dermatol Surg 2004;30(6):961.
12. Gross KG, Steinman HK, Rapini RP. Mohs surgery: fundamentals and techniques. St Louis (MO): Mosby; 1999. p. 86–9.
13. Rapini RP. Comparison of methods for checking surgical margins. J Am Acad Dermatol 1990;23: 288–94.
14. Rapini RP. Pitfalls of Mohs micrographic surgery. J Am Acad Dermatol 1990;22:681–6.
15. McColloch M, Geddis C, Hetzer MR, et al. Embedding techniques. In: Fish FS, editor. Manual of frozen section processing for Mohs micrographic surgery. Milwaukee (WI): ACMMSCO; 2008. p. 601–88.
16. Geddis C, Keating J. Slide fixation and clearing agents. In: Fish FS, editor. Manual of frozen section processing for Mohs micrographic surgery. Milwaukee (WI): ACMMSCO; 2008. p. 901–3.
17. Hetzer MR. The Mohs laboratory. In: Snow SN, Mikhail GR, editors. Mohs micrographic surgery. London: The University of Wisconsin Press; 2004. p. 329–38.
18. Murphy ME, Brodland DG, Zitelli JA. Errors in the interpretation of Mohs histopathology sections over a 1-year fellowship. Dermatol Surg 2008;34(12):1637–41.
19. Katz KH, Helm KF, Billingsley EM, et al. Dense inflammation does not mask residual primary basal cell carcinoma during Mohs micrographic surgery. J Am Acad Dermatol 2001;45:231–8.
20. Zachary CB, Rest EB, Furlong SM, et al. Rapid cytokeratin stains enhance the sensitivity of Mohs micrographic surgery for squamous cell carcinoma. J Dermatol Surg Oncol 1994;20:509–10.
21. Rapini RP. Basal cell carcinoma and squamous cell carcinoma in Mohs sections. In: Gross KG, Steinmann HK, Rapini RP, editors. Mohs surgery fundamentals and techniques. St Louis (MO): Mosby; 1999. p. 161–91.
22. Smith-Zagone MJ, Schwartz MR. Frozen section of skin specimens. Arch Pathol Lab Med 2005;129: 1536–43.
23. Fu W, Cockerell CJ. The actinic (solar) keratosis: a 21st-century perspective. Arch Dermatol 2003; 139(1):66–70.
24. Ackerman AB. Solar keratosis is squamous cell carcinoma. Arch Dermatol 2003;139(9);1216–7.
25. Marks R, Renne G, Selwood TS. Malignant transformation of solar keratosis to squamous cell carcinoma. Lancet 1988;1:795–7.
26. Hurwitz RM, Monger LE. Solar keratosis: an evolving squamous cell carcinoma: benign or malignant? Dermatol Surg 1995;21:184.
27. Brash DE, Ziegler A, Jonason AS, et al. Sunlight and sunburn in human skin cancer: p53, apoptosis, and tumor promotion. J Investig Dermatol Symp Proc 1996;1:136–42.
28. Thosani MK, Marghoob A, Chen CS. Current progress of immunostains in Mohs micrographic surgery: a review. Dermatol Surg 2008;34(12):1621–36.
29. El Tal AK, Abrou AE, Stiff MA, et al. Immunostaining in Mohs micrographic surgery: a review. Dermatol Surg 2010;36(3):275–90.
30. Mariwalla K, Aasi SZ, Glusac EJ, et al. Mohs micrographic surgery histopathology concordance. J Am Acad Dermatol 2009;60:94–8.
31. Grunwald MH, Lee JY, Ackerman AB. Pseudocarcinomatous hyperplasia. Am J Dermatopathol 1988; 10:95–103.
32. Hassanein AM, Proper SA, Depcik-Smith ND, et al. Peritumoral fibrosis in basal cell and squamous cell carcinoma mimicking perineural invasion: potential

pitfall in Mohs micrographic surgery. Dermatol Surg 2005;31(9 Pt 1):1101–6.

33. Lawrence N, Cottel WI. Squamous cell carcinoma of the skin with perineural invasion. J Am Acad Dermatol 1994;31:30–3.

34. Dunn M, Morgan MB, Beer TW. Perineural invasion: identification, significance, and a standardized definition [review]. Dermatol Surg 2009;35(2):214–21.

35. Whalen J, Leone D. Mohs micrographic surgery for the treatment of malignant melanoma. Clin Dermatol 2009;27:597–602.

36. Bricca GM, Brodland DG, Ren D, et al. Cutaneous head and neck melanoma treated with Mohs micrographic surgery. J Am Acad Dermatol 2005; 52:92–100.

37. Bienert TN, Trotter MJ, Arlette JP. Treatment of cutaneous melanoma of the face by Mohs micrographic surgery. J Cutan Med Surg 2003;7:25–30.

38. Bhardwaj SS, Tope WD, Lee PK. Mohs micrographic surgery for lentigo maligna and lentigo maligna melanoma using Mel-5 immunostaining: University of Minnesota experience. Dermatol Surg 2006;32: 690–6.

39. Zitelli JA. Accuracy of en face frozen sections for diagnosing margin status in melanocytic lesions. Am J Clin Pathol 2004;121:937–8.

40. Cohen LM, McCall MW, Hodge SJ, et al. Successful treatment of lentigo maligna and lentigo maligna melanoma with Mohs' micrographic surgery aided by rush permanent sections. Cancer 1994;73: 2964–70.

41. Siegel DM. Mohs surgery for large and difficult tumors and in special clinical situations. In: Gross KG, Steinmann HK, Rapini RP, editors. Mohs surgery fundamentals and techniques. St Louis (MO): Mosby; 1999. p. 231–8.

Special Stains in Mohs Surgery

Christopher J. Miller, MD[a,*], Joseph F. Sobanko, MD[a],
Xiaodong Zhu[a], Terri Nunnciato[a],
Christopher R. Urban, MD[b]

KEYWORDS

- Mohs surgery • Immunostains • Melanoma • MART-1
- MITF • AE1/AE3 • CD34

The excellent cure rates associated with Mohs micrographic surgery depend on accurate interpretation of high-quality microscopic frozen sections that allow examination of 100% of the microscopic margin. Reliable interpretation of microscopic slides is only possible if the surgeon can distinguish tumor cells from surrounding normal tissue. Although routine hematoxylin and eosin (H&E) frozen sections are usually sufficient, tumor cells can be difficult to detect on even the highest-quality H&E frozen sections if the cancer is poorly differentiated; if the tumor exhibits single cell spread; if tumor is surrounded by a dense inflammatory infiltrate; if tumor tracks along nerves, vessels, or fascial planes; if tumor is embedded in fibrotic tissue or connective tissue; or if there is pagetoid distribution of tumor. By highlighting tumor cells with a chromogen that is visible on light microscopy, immunostaining allows the Mohs surgeon to distinguish tumor from normal cells in these challenging scenarios. Several excellent comprehensive reviews of immunostaining in Mohs surgery have recently been published.[1–3] This article focuses on practical aspects involving the most commonly used immunostains in dermatologic surgery, including MART-1 for melanocytic neoplasms, cytokeratin stains for keratinocytic neoplasms, and CD34 stains for dermatofibrosarcoma protuberans.

HISTORY OF IMMUNOSTAINING IN MOHS MICROGRAPHIC SURGERY

Immunostaining in Mohs surgery has evolved rapidly. In 1984, Robinson and Gottschalk[4] published the first report of immunoperoxidase staining with cytokeratin antibodies on frozen sections during Mohs surgery for basal cell cancer (BCC) and squamous cell cancer (SCC). Although their immunostaining technique allowed improved identification of tumor cells with growth patterns that were challenging to detect on H&E slides, their complicated protocol required more than 24 hours to complete. Approximately one decade later, 2 groups independently reported successful treatment of BCCs and SCCs with anticytokeratin immunostaining protocols that required fewer than 90 minutes to complete.[5,6] As immunostaining kits became commercially available and immunostaining protocols required fewer than 2 hours on frozen sections, surgeons expanded application of immunostains of Mohs frozen sections to other tumors, such as extramammary Paget disease,[7] dermatofibrosarcoma protuberans,[8] and melanoma.[9,10]

Despite the proliferation of reports of immunostaining of Mohs frozen sections during the 1990s, only 13 of 108 laboratories run by members of the American College of Mohs Surgery reported

The authors have nothing to disclose.
a Department of Dermatology, Perelman Center for Advanced Medicine, University of Pennsylvania, 3400 Civic Center Boulevard, Suite 1-330S, Philadelphia, PA 19104, USA
b Department of Medicine, Pennsylvania Hospital, 800 Spruce Street, Philadelphia, PA 19107, USA
* Corresponding author.
E-mail address: christopher.miller@uphs.upenn.edu

Dermatol Clin 29 (2011) 273–286
doi:10.1016/j.det.2011.01.003

the use of immunostains in a survey sent in 2000.[11] The cost of reagents, the additional time required for both physicians and histotechnologists, and the additional expertise required for the application and interpretation of the stains may have deterred many Mohs surgeons from employing immunostains in their laboratories.

During the last 10 years, the number of reports of immunostains during Mohs surgery has proliferated, as documented by several excellent recent review articles.[1–3] Bricca's publication of a 1-hour protocol for immunostaining of melanoma frozen sections has inspired numerous investigators to innovate increasingly quicker protocols, including a 19-minute protocol for both cytokeratin and MART-1 immunostaining.[12–14] As the time required to complete immunostains has decreased and immunostaining kits have become commercially available, Mohs surgeons can integrate immunostains into their practice with relative ease.

CONTROVERSIES REGARDING THE USE OF FROZEN VERSUS PERMANENT SECTIONS

Due to the wealth of data confirming superior cure rates when examining 100% of the microscopic margin, Mohs surgery with frozen sections has emerged as the gold standard compared with less thorough conventional methods of tissue processing in the treatment of BCC and SCC. While immunostaining may improve accuracy in the interpretation of frozen section microscopic margins, the percentage of BCCs and SCCs requiring immunostaining is relatively small. Consequently, scant data examine the efficacy of immunostaining in the treatment of these nonmelanoma skin cancers. Nevertheless, because the Mohs technique has proved so effective in the treatment of these tumors, little controversy arises with the addition of immunostaining to enhance the already excellent cure rates achieved with frozen section interpretation and H&E sections.

By contrast, the use of frozen sections to treat melanoma ignites considerable controversy. In comparison with BCCs and SCCs, immunostaining offers value and a practical advantage for the vast majority of melanomas. Distinguishing melanocytes from keratinocytes in the epidermis can be very challenging, especially if there is single cell proliferation and pagetoid spread of melanocytes or if there are surrounding atypical keratinocytes. Although melanocytes and keratinocytes have defining characteristics visible on H&E frozen sections, immunostaining offers more rapid and reliable identification of melanocytes at scanning magnification as compared with the H&E sections alone.

Perhaps because immunostains are a practical necessity for a higher percentage of melanocytic neoplasms, the volume of literature dedicated to frozen sections and immunostains for melanoma is much greater than for any other cutaneous neoplasm. Framing the controversies about frozen section immunostains for melanoma highlights several key points that apply to the treatment of many cutaneous neoplasms. First, many melanocytic tumors have microscopic extension that is not clinically visible. Second, if clinical examination is unreliable to determine tumor extent, then surgical margins based on clinical parameters are unreliable. Third, microscopic examination is the gold standard both to diagnose skin cancer and to determine margin status after excision. Fourth, the more thorough the examination of the microscopic margin, the more accurate the interpretation of margins status will be. Finally, microscopic examination is reliable only if tumor cells are clearly visible. Immunostains facilitate the identification of subtle tumor.

Substantial evidence demonstrates that clinical parameters are not sufficient in the diagnosis and treatment of melanoma. Because multiple benign pigmented lesions (eg, solar lentigines and atypical nevi) share clinical characteristics with melanoma and because a subset of melanomas defy clinical diagnostic criteria (such as the ABCDE criteria and the "ugly duckling" sign), diagnosis of melanoma is a complex process.[15,16] In fact, the naked eye correctly diagnoses melanoma in only about 60% of cases.[17–20] Another indication of the inaccuracy of naked eye examination is that dermatologists biopsy 18 benign nevi for every 1 melanoma.[21] Microscopic examination is a practical necessity for the diagnosis of melanoma.

Surgical margins based on clinically visible parameters of melanoma are not reliable. Clinical and microscopic margins do not correlate in 90% of melanoma excisions.[22] Sixty percent of the time, the true microscopic margin is less than the margin that the surgeon intended, based on clinical examination. Thirty percent of the time, the true microscopic margin is greater than the margin that the surgeon intended, based on clinical examination.[22] Determining surgical margins is especially challenging on the head and neck, where the melanoma often arises in sun-damaged skin with multiple adjacent lentigines and keratinocytic growths. The high rates of positive margins and high recurrence rates after conventional surgical excision emphatically demonstrate that melanoma is a microscopic disease for which clinical parameters alone are insufficient to determine surgical margins. One out of 4 conventional wide local excisions on head and neck melanomas has positive microscopic margins, usually due to occult in situ melanoma.[23] Recurrence rates after conventional excision of melanoma in situ on the head and neck range from 9% to 13%.[24] The recurrence rates after conventional excision of lentigo maligna are even higher, ranging from 8% to 20%.[25]

Compared with conventional excision, Mohs micrographic surgery offers superior local cure rates for melanoma. For melanoma in situ on the head and neck, multiple investigators have published local recurrence rates of only 0% to 2% after Mohs surgery.[24,26] These superior local cure rates result because Mohs surgery allows examination of 100% of the microscopic margin, compared with examination of less than 1% of the microscopic margin with conventional methods of tissue processing. The consistently excellent local cure rates after Mohs surgery provide the greatest evidence of the accuracy of the technique. Nevertheless, opponents argue that frozen section examination of melanocytic lesions is inaccurate. Immunostains vastly improve one's ability to detect melanoma, either with frozen or permanent sections.

It is important first to emphasize that Mohs surgery usually does not involve the diagnosis of the original tumor. Rather, the diagnosis is usually made via permanent sections prior to Mohs surgery. Therefore, the Mohs surgeon's primary task is to determine whether tumor is present at the margin of the excision. The challenges of interpreting margin status for melanoma in situ apply to both frozen and permanent sections alike. When determining the presence or absence of melanoma in situ on H&E permanent sections, skilled dermatopathologists have only moderate agreement.[27] Interpretation of melanoma margins poses similar challenges for both permanent and frozen sections.

Previous investigators have demonstrated that interpretation of melanoma margins using the highest-quality frozen sections is accurate in comparison with paraffin-embedded sections. Bienert and colleagues[28] treated 97 patients with melanoma in situ or invasive melanoma of the face. In 25 patients, 117 tissue margins, which were defined as negative for melanoma at the time of H&E frozen sections, were reevaluated on H&E stains after formalin-fixation and paraffin-embedded tissue processing. There was 100% concordance between the negative status of the frozen and permanent sections in all 117 tissue margins. There were no cases of local recurrence in any of the 92 patients followed for a mean of 33 months. Similarly, Zitelli and colleagues[29] demonstrated the reliability of using H&E-stained

frozen sections to assess the margin status of 59 patients with lentigo maligna and melanoma. The investigators thawed 221 frozen sections from the 59 patients for paraffin sectioning. The H&E frozen sections had 100% sensitivity (ie, there were no cases where melanoma was detected on paraffin sections but not on frozen sections). There was 90% specificity of the H&E frozen section interpretation. In 4 patients, the specimens were read as melanoma or regressing melanoma by frozen sections, but paraffin sections showed only sun-induced epidermal atypia without melanoma.

Interpretation of margin status of melanoma by H&E sections alone is challenging, in part because melanoma in situ has some features in common with melanocytic hyperplasia in sun-damaged skin.[30] Pagetoid spread, exocytosis of lymphocytes, and keratinocytic atypia make it especially difficult to distinguish between keratinocytes and melanocytes in the epidermis. Immunostains facilitate identification of melanocytes.

Immunostains in frozen sections allow detection of melanocytes as accurately as permanent section immunostains. Cherpelis and colleagues[13] used a 19-minute MART-1 immunostaining protocol to compare melanoma-associated antigen recognized by T cells (MART-1) immunostained frozen and permanent sections. A board-certified dermatopathologist who was blinded to tissue preparation examined the slides. No significant difference was found in any of the following measurements: number of keratinocytes at dermal-epidermal junction, nuclear diameter of keratinocytes, numbers of melanocytes, melanocyte nucleus diameter, and melanocyte cytoplasm diameter. No significant difference was found in contiguity, pagetoid spread, melanocyte nesting, or atypical melanocytes. Because no statistically significant differences were observed in the measured variables between frozen sections and permanent sections, the investigators concluded that MART-1 immunostaining of frozen tissues is a reliable and useful technique with which to supplement Mohs micrographic surgery. Kelley and Starkus[31] also found 100% correlation between frozen and paraffin-embedded sections of lentigo maligna stained with MART-1. Whether treating melanoma or other tumors, immunostains serve as a valuable adjunct to routine H&E-stained sections.

APPLYING IMMUNOSTAINS IN THE MOHS LABORATORY
Cutting and Mounting

The application of immunostains in the Mohs laboratory requires considerable expertise and dedication from both the histotechnologist and the Mohs surgeon. Regardless of variations in immunostaining protocols, any laboratory employing immunostains must produce meticulous frozen sections. Sections of 4 μm are ideal. Thicker sections can mask cellular detail, due to overlap of keratinocytes and melanocytes. Thinner sections are more difficult to handle and often stain with less intensity than thicker sections. Cutting 4-μm sections without tissue fallout, freeze artifact, or folding requires considerable practice and experience, and is an absolute necessity for high-quality immunostains. Such thin sections require optimal equipment, including high-grade cryostats and very sharp cryostat blades. Mounting the thin section to silanized glass slides can help to prevent tissue folding or freeze artifact.

The Basic Steps of Immunostaining

The indirect, or amplifying, method has emerged as the dominant method of immunohistochemistry (**Fig. 1**). Indirect immunohistochemical staining requires a general sequence of steps (**Box 1**). First, frozen sections are incubated with a primary antibody that links to the epitope on the target cell type. The tissue is then rinsed to remove excess antibody before incubating with a secondary antibody conjugated to a labeling enzyme, such as peroxidase. Next, a chromogen is added and the conjugated labeling enzyme reacts to form an insoluble colored deposit, which is visible on light microscopy.[1,32]

Choosing an Immunostain

The most commonly used antibodies are commercially available in kits that provide all the necessary reagents (**Table 1**). The ideal immunostain targets the desired antigen, is inexpensive, and can be applied to frozen sections in an efficient manner with a consistent and predictable result. To interpret the immunostains accurately, the Mohs surgeon must know the antigen targeted by each immunostain and all the cells that contain the antigen (**Table 2**). Whereas the ideal immunostain would highlight only the cells of interest, most immunostains have a balance between sensitivity and specificity. For example, S-100 has excellent sensitivity for most melanocytic neoplasms, but it has poor specificity because it highlights many different cell types.

Troubleshooting

While manufacturers of immunostains provide useful guidelines for reagent dilutions and tissue preparation, each laboratory must dedicate considerable effort to develop protocols that reliably produce high-quality microscopic sections. The multitude of publications with increasingly shorter protocols demonstrates the wide variation possible with individual immunostains.[13,14] The Mohs surgeon must be prepared to troubleshoot common problems.

The most common problems result from ineffective tissue cutting and mounting. Uniform cutting of 4-μm sections is the first step toward successful immunostaining. Tissue with a lot of

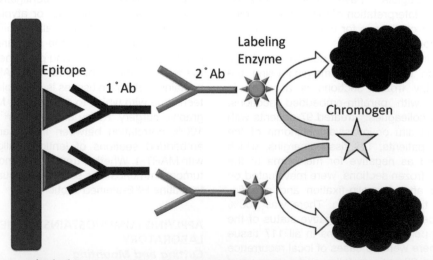

Fig. 1. Indirect method of immunostaining. The primary antibody (1° Ab) binds to the epitope on the cell. The secondary antibody (2° Ab) binds to the primary antibody. The labeling enzyme is conjugated to secondary antibody. The chromogen reacts with the labeling enzyme to form an insoluble color deposit.

Box 1
Basic steps for indirect method of immunostaining

1. Cut complete frozen sections ranging from 4 to 6 μm

2. Mount sections onto positively charged slides to enhance tissue adhesion

3. Air dry slides at room temperature

4. Fix in acetone

5. Rehydrate slides in Tris-buffered saline

6. Apply blocking diluent, then shake off

7. Apply primary antibody (eg, MART-1)

8. Rinse slides in Tris-buffered saline

9. Apply the secondary antibody that is already conjugated to an enzyme (eg, peroxidase)

10. Rinse sections in Tris-buffered saline

11. Apply chromogen to stimulate color production

12. Rinse slides in distilled water

13. Dip in counterstain (eg, hematoxylin), then immediately rinse in water

14. Dehydrate slides in reagent grade alcohol

15. Clear slides with xylene

16. Apply mounting media

fat is particularly challenging to cut into complete sections without holes. Grossly sectioning the epidermis and dermis from the fat and/or grossly sectioning tissue into 1- to 2-cm pieces will help the histotechnician to cut complete 4-μm sections. Incomplete sections risk fallout of tumor in holes of the section. When the sections are too thick, there is frequently nonspecific bleeding of the stain that makes it more difficult to determine individual cell outline, or there is cell overlap that masks individual cell details. If the sections are too large, tissue folding is more common. Mounting the tissue sections on silanized slides facilitates accurate transfer of the tissue from the cryostat to the slides without tissue folding.

Problems associated with the staining itself usually result from human error, ineffective titrations of antibody, or suboptimal exposure times for each step. To minimize human error, Mohs surgeons may want to automate the immunostaining process (Table 3). However, autostainers are expensive and most laboratories will justify purchasing this equipment only if they perform a high volume of immunostains. As laboratories modify their immunostaining protocols, they will experiment with different antibody titers and times for each step of the staining process. These changes can affect slide quality. For example, high titers of antibody can rapidly drive the reaction, but increase background and nonspecific staining. Practicing the immunostaining on normal tissue is advisable before using immunostains on patients' tumors.

For all cases, positive and negative controls are recommended. The positive control is achieved by performing the immunostaining on archived tissue of the same tumor type. For example, when treating a melanoma one should consider staining archived melanoma tissue simultaneously. The negative control may be achieved by performing all steps of the staining process on the tissue, except for addition of the primary antibody. These negative control slides help to identify nonspecific staining that does not represent tumor.

Costs, Billing, and Coding

The Current Procedural Terminology (CPT) designates 88342 as the code for immunostaining section in Mohs surgery. The surgeon should bill the 88342 according to the number slides in the Mohs case. For example, when treating a melanoma grossly sectioned into 5 pieces processed on 5 different Mohs slides, the surgeon would bill 88342 × 5. The Medicare reimbursement is approximately $100. The current estimate of cost per slide is between $20 and $25.[1]

Table 1
Examples of commercially available immunostaining kits

Primary Antibody	Manufacturer	Location	Product Cost (US$)	Slide Volume	Cost Per Slide (US$)
MART-1 (Melan-A)	Thermo scientific	Fremont, CA, USA	200 μg/ml concentrate 457.08	4 μl/slide	1.83
Multi-Cytokeratin (AE1/AE3)	Leica Microsystems	Bannockburn, IL, USA	128.51 μg/ml concentrate 373.00	4 μl/slide	1.49
Endothelial Cell Marker (CD34)	Leica Microsystems	Bannockburn, IL, USA	45 μg/ml concentrate 385.00	4 μl/slide	1.54

Table 2
Characteristics of common antibodies used for immunostaining of cutaneous neoplasms

Antibodies	Cellular Epitope	Staining Pattern	Stained Cells	Pearls	Pitfalls
Human melanoma, black-45 (HMB-45)	30–35 kDa cytoplasmic melanosome-associated glycoprotein	Cytoplasmic	Melanocytes; cells containing melanosomes (eg, retinal epithelium)	Aids detection of melanoma and nevi Stains mainly intraepidermal and superficial dermal component of compound nevi Does not stain keratinocytes	Desmoplastic melanoma-negative or with much lower rates of positivity (better to use S-100) Rarely reported to have a positive granular, perinuclear stain in nonmelanomatous tumors or normal skin
Melanoma antigen recognized by T cells (Melan-A, MART-1)	22 kDa cytoplasmic melanosome-associated glycoprotein	Cytoplasmic	Melanocytes; cells containing melanosomes (eg, adrenal cortex)	Aids detection of melanoma and nevi Intensity of staining directly proportional to positivity of tumor	Limited value in spindle and desmoplastic melanoma Risk of false-positive MIS with pigmented AKs
S-100	Intracellular calcium (also with variable affinities for zinc and manganese)	Nuclear/Cytoplasmic	Melanocytes; Langerhans cells; eccrine glands; Schwann cells; chondrocytes; adipose tissue	Aids detection of melanoma and nevi Most reliable marker for identifying the spindled component of a melanoma	High sensitivity, low specificity Will occasionally stain liposarcomas and breast carcinomas
Microphthalmia transcription factor (MITF)	DNA	Nuclear	Melanocytes; retinal epithelium; cervical cancer cells; PEComas; melanocytic schwannomas	Aids detection of melanoma and nevi Does not stain dendritic processes, common in melanocytes present in chronic sun-damaged skin	Limited value in spindle and desmoplastic melanoma
Mel-5	Gp75 melanosome-associated sialated glycoprotein	Cytoplasmic	Melanocytes; cells containing melanosomes	Aids detection of melanoma and nevi Stains black and sun-damaged skin more prominently than white skin because of the increased density of melanosomes	Poor sensitivity and specificity Limited value in amelanotic or desmoplastic melanoma

Cytokeratin (CK-Pan = AE1/AE3)	Intermediate filaments	Cytoplasmic	All normal epithelium and epithelial-derived tumors (epidermis, sebaceous glands, hair follicles); rare mesenchymal-derived tumors	Aids detection of SCC Predominant expression of stratified-epithelial CKs ("high molecular weight"), such as CK5 is helpful for the recognition of poorly differentiated, nonkeratinizing SCC	May also stain germ cell tumors and sarcomas
CD34 (myeloid progenitor cell antigen)	Transmembrane glycoprotein	Cytoplasmic	Dermal, periadnexal, and endoneural fibroblast-like dendritic cells; endothelia; bone marrow precursor cells	Invariably found in DFSP and solitary fibrous tumors Reliable for vascular tumors, hematogenous tumors, and GI stromal tumors	Variable expression of CD34 in nodular areas of DFSP, making excision difficult
Carcinoembryonic antigen (CEA)	Glycocalyx of cells	Cytoplasmic	Eccrine and apocrine structures	Useful for extramammary Paget disease	Will stain other neoplasms such as adnexal neoplasms, adenocarcinomas (colon, lung, breast, stomach, pancreas), epithelioid sarcomas
CK7	Intermediate filament	Cytoplasmic	Ductal, glandular, and transitional epithelia (does not react with stratified squamous epithelia)	Sensitive and specific for detecting extramammary Paget disease Also detects ovarian, breast, and lung adenocarcinoma	Infrequently stains Bowen disease

Abbreviations: AK, actinic keratosis; DFSP, dermatofibrosarcoma protuberans; GI, gastrointestinal; MIS, melanoma in situ; PEComa, perivascular epithelioid cell tumor; SCC, squamous cell cancer.

IMMUNOSTAINS FOR MELANOMA

Several immunostains identify melanocytes, including include S-100, HMB-45, MEL-5, MART-1, and MITF (see **Table 2**). Although previous investigators have demonstrated the utility of each of these stains in frozen sections for Mohs surgery, MART-1 has emerged as the most useful stain for the majority of melanomas. Therefore, this article focuses on the utility of MART-1 stains in frozen sections. Readers should be aware that early data suggest that MITF may also be helpful, because it stains the nucleus of melanocytes, eliminating the diffuse staining that can occur with cytoplasmic staining of dendrites.[33] S-100 remains the immunostain of choice for desmoplastic and spindle cell melanomas.

Melan-A antigen or Melanoma antigen recognized by T cells (MART-1) is a melanocyte differentiation antigen and a 22 kDa cytoplasmic melanosome-associated glycoprotein.[34] It is present in most melanomas, resting adult melanocytes, and nevus cells located in both the epidermis and dermis.[34] It is also present in pigmented cells of the retina, adrenal cortex, ovaries and testes, and in rare tumors including angiomyolipomas, lymphangiomatosis, and clear cell "sugar tumors."[34] Blessing and colleagues[35] found 97% positivity for MART-1 in primary melanomas, while in metastatic melanomas Jungbluth and colleagues[36] reported 81% positivity and Cormier and colleagues[37] reported 89% positivity. Busam and Jungbluth[38] report that MART-1 is recognized by cytotoxic T cells, and may be associated with the endoplasmic reticulum and melanosomes.

Of all the melanocytic immunostains, MART-1 is regarded as the most accurate and reliable (**Figs. 2–4**).[34,39] Zalla and colleagues[34] compared the effectiveness of different melanocytic immunostains in the excision of melanoma. This study used a 64-minute staining protocol and employed 4 immunostains: HMB-45, MEL-5, MART-1, and S-100. Sixty-eight patients were treated, including 46 with malignant melanoma in situ (MMIS) and 22 with invasive melanoma. Sixty-two of the lesions were located on the head or neck. Interpretation

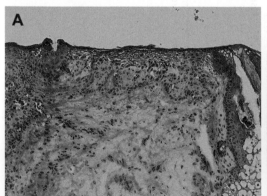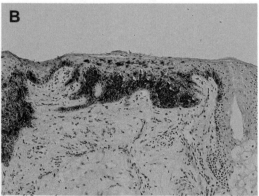

Fig. 2. Hematoxylin and eosin (H&E)-stained frozen sections of melanoma in situ. (*A*) Melanocytic nests, characterized by a granular, gray cytoplasm, are clearly visible in lower half of epidermis. Some atypical melanocytes, most notably along the basal layer on the left side of the photomicrograph, exhibit retraction from neighboring keratinocytes. The superior half of epidermis demonstrates frozen section artifact, making it difficult to distinguish cytology (original magnification ×20). (*B*) MART-1–stained frozen section corresponding to A. MART-1 immunostain highlights the proliferation of melanocytes in the lower half of the epidermis, which was also clearly visible on the H&E-stained section in A. The MART-1 section also allows visualization of high-level pagetoid spread, which was not distinguishable on the corresponding frozen section H&E stain (original magnification ×20).

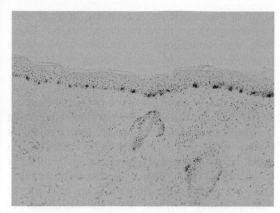

Fig. 3. Sample negative margin in sun-damaged skin. The hallmark of normal skin is regularly spaced melanocytes limited to the basal layer. Atypical melanocytes, which are noted on the right half of the photomicrograph, are common in sun-damaged skin (original magnification ×10).

of frozen sections stained with H&E was described as slow and laborious when compared with immunostained frozen sections. HMB-45 stained 50 of 59 tumors and produced false negatives in 2 of 2 desmoplastic, neurotropic malignant melanomas (DNMM). With HMB-45 staining, there were fewer equivocal sections because keratinocytes did not stain. Despite this benefit, positive staining was observed in only 85% of cases, so it was necessary to have a positive control tumor on each slide to confirm stain quality. Staining with HMB-45 was noted to be less uniform and intense when compared with MART-1. S-100 was positive in 5 of 5 cases, including 1 of 1 DNMM, but staining was less crisp and exhibited more background staining than the other stains. MEL-5 staining

was positive in 12 of 13 cases (one DNMM failed to stain), but was less intense and crisp and had more background staining than MART-1. MART-1 successfully stained 26 of 27 tumors and 1 of 2 DNMM. Zalla and colleagues concluded that MART-1 was the superior immunostain because it provided the most reliable epidermal staining and was the simplest to interpret. Its use greatly facilitated the identification of melanocytes and evaluation of tissue margins. Patients were followed for an average of 16 months with a range of 1 to 32 months, and no recurrences were reported.

Albertini and colleagues[39] published another study in 2002 comparing different melanocytic immunostains during Mohs micrographic surgery for the treatment of melanoma. In 10 consecutive cases consisting of 7 in situ melanomas and 3 invasive melanomas, different immunostains were compared. Sections of 8 μm were stained with MART-1, HMB-45, and S-100 using positive and negative controls processed with each layer. One dermatopathologist and one Mohs surgeon graded each specimen as good, fair, or poor based on intensity of melanocytic staining compared with background stain. Permanent sections from debulking specimens confirmed the staging in each case, and no tumors were either upgraded or downgraded after review. In the comparison of immunostains, MART-1 was used for diagnosis in every case because it was consistently superior and showed the most clear and crisp melanocyte staining. Although HMB-45 controls were good, they failed to show many groups of melanocyte proliferation visible with MART-1. S-100 was the least useful and produced poor controls in frozen tissue, although it had

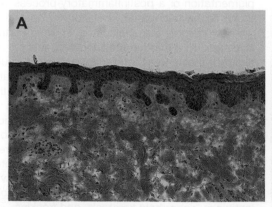

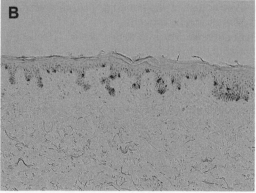

Fig. 4. Sample H&E and MART-1 frozen sections of lentigo at a Mohs margin. (*A*) H&E section with epidermal budding typical of benign lentigo. Slightly increased density of melanocytes and hyperpigmentation are present (original magnification ×10). (*B*) MART-1 frozen section corresponding to *A* demonstrates slight increase in melanocyte density with architecture typical of a benign lentigo. Correlation with H&E sections is helpful in interpreting MART-1 sections (original magnification ×10).

excellent performance on permanent sections. Even the 6 S-100 specimens with good controls failed to highlight melanoma and melanocytic hyperplasia in all cases on frozen sections. When treating a desmoplastic melanoma for which S-100 is the preferable stain, the investigators suggest that it may be beneficial to prepare permanent sections. Albertini and colleagues[39] also report that MART-1 can be used to identify junctional melanocytic proliferations such as melanoma in situ, describing a case in which an H&E-stained biopsy showed a lentiginous keratocytic proliferation consistent with a solar lentigo and HMB-45 showed no melanocytic proliferation. This lesion went on to develop into a deeply invasive melanoma. When the original biopsy tissue block was retrieved and stained with MART-1, it revealed both a junctional melanocytic proliferation and a focal dermal proliferation of melanocytes that was missed on HMB-45. Albertini and colleagues concluded that the use of MART-1 immunostaining can help clearly identify melanocytes on frozen sections during Mohs surgery.

Multiple investigators have described rapid MART-1 immunostaining protocols for frozen sections. Bricca and colleagues[12] published a study in 2004 describing a shortened 1-hour protocol for immunostaining with MART-1. The investigators shortened the protocol time by deleting the linking step and shortening the protein blocking step. This shortened blocking step used an agent containing high quantities of nonspecific IgG molecules to saturate other binding sites, which allowed the primary antibody to specifically bind the melanoma antigen and the secondary antigen to specifically bind the primary. Their 1-hour MART-1 immunostaining protocol stained melanocytes brightly and specifically on all melanoma sections and positive controls, and improved logistics for patients, histotechnicians, and dermatologic surgeons.

Subsequent investigators have published increasingly shorter protocols. Kimyai-Asadi and colleagues[40] published an ultra-rapid 20-minute MART-1 immunostaining protocol to treat 30 consecutive malignant melanomas. Frozen section slides were cut at 4 μm and stained with both H&E and the 20-minute MART-1 protocol. The normal staining of background melanocytes was used as an internal control. Specific staining of melanocytes was observed on every slide, allowing the identification of normal melanocytes, melanocyte hyperplasia from sun damage, and malignant melanoma. MART-1 staining increased sensitivity by allowing the detection of small foci of melanoma, and increased specificity by ruling out melanoma in areas with atypical clear cells

such as freeze artifact, spongiosis, and pagetoid keratocytic atypia. As mentioned earlier, Cherpelis and colleagues[14] published a 19-minute MART-1 immunostaining protocol, and demonstrated that MART-1–stained frozen sections allow detection of melanocytes as accurately as MART-1–stained permanent sections.

The major limitation with MART-1 staining is that it does not distinguish benign from malignant melanocytes. When interpreting margins in patients with severely sun-damaged skin or surrounding keratocytic neoplasms, inflammation, or benign pigmented lesions, the risk of calling falsely positive margins increases. El Shabrawi-Caelen and colleagues[41] report that in 10 unequivocal cases of pigmented actinic keratosis, the immunostaining with MART-1 was much larger than with S-100, HMB-45, and tyrosinase. In addition, in 4 cases clusters of MART-1–positive cells near the pigmented actinic keratosis resembled melanocytic nests. Beltraminelli and colleagues[42] reported that inflammation can lead to damage of the epidermis that may falsely label keratocytes and other cells with MART-1. Three cases were reported in which patients with sun-damaged skin were diagnosed with melanoma in situ because MART-1 staining showed single cells in small nests along the dermoepidermal junction. Further clinical examination showed that lichenoid dermatitis was responsible for the lesions. This phototoxic reaction could easily be misinterpreted as melanoma with MART-1 staining alone. For this reason the investigators express concern about using MART-1 immunostaining in cases with lichenoid tissue reaction on chronic sun-damaged skin. Maize and colleagues[43] also reported a case in which a biopsy stained with MART-1 for what was thought to be drug-induced hyperpigmentation or a postinflammatory process was found to have apparent melanocytic nests that were worrisome for melanoma in situ. Further investigation with other melanocyte stains did not highlight these areas, and the diagnosis was ultimately decided to be discoid lupus erythematosus. Maize and colleagues[43] proposed that this disease process may have led to damage of melanocytes at the dermal-epidermal junction, resulting in their breakdown. Melanocytic debris engulfed by macrophages could explain the presence of antigen in these areas. Other pigmented lesions that may make slide interpretation with MART-1 staining more challenging include solar lentigines, seborrheic keratosis, and freckles.

Because many melanomas, especially those on the head and neck, present with surrounding lesions that may make slide interpretation difficult, the Mohs surgeon must have deep understanding of melanocyte distribution patterns in sun-damaged skin. In 2006 Hendi and colleagues[30] published a study to explore the characteristics of normal melanocytes stained by MART-1 in long-standing sun-exposed skin. One-hundred and forty-nine patients undergoing Mohs surgery for BCCs and SCCs of the face and neck were randomly selected as subjects in the study. The mean number of melanocytes per high-power field and confluence of adjacent melanocytes were measured to determine the level of normal melanocyte hyperplasia in sun-exposed skin. The investigators reported an average of 15 to 20 melanocytes per high-power field in sun-exposed skin. Confluence of up to 9 adjacent melanocytes and extension along hair follicles are also normal in sun-exposed skin. Nesting and pagetoid spread were not observed in normal sun-exposed skin. Barlow and colleagues[44] also published a study to clarify the density and distribution patterns of melanocytes adjacent to skin cancers. One hundred and eighty patients were enrolled, with nearly 59% of cancers being located on the face and neck. This group reported an overall melanocyte density of 7.97 melanocytes per millimeter of epidermis, with a broad variation between individual cases. Findings of melanocytic hyperplasia and contiguous melanocytes can be normal in skin bordering melanomatous and nonmelanomatous skin cancers. Therefore findings of increased melanocyte density, moderate confluence, and presence of melanocytes along follicular epithelium are not enough to make the diagnosis of melanoma in sun-exposed skin. Instead features such as nesting, vertical stacking, or pagetoid spread should be present to warrant taking further Mohs layers.

After overcoming the technical and logistical barriers to integrate immunostains in the Mohs laboratories, the greatest challenges lie in slide interpretation. Mohs surgeons should seek mentorship from other surgeons or pathologists skilled in the interpretation of these difficult cases.

IMMUNOSTAINS FOR BASAL AND SQUAMOUS CELL CANCER

It is well established that Mohs micrographic surgery is the most effective treatment for poorly differentiated and recurrent keratinocytic tumors.[45,46] However, BCC and SCC with poor differentiation, dense inflammation, tracking along nerves, vessels, or fascial planes, or spread in fibrotic tissue or connective tissue can be difficult to detect on H&E sections alone. In these instances, immunohistochemical stains can improve detection of BCCs and SCCs.[1]

Supplementary immunohistochemical staining of nonmelanocytic tumors during Mohs surgery was first published in 1984, and revealed that antibodies to cytokeratin could delineate specific tumor cells derived from the epidermis.[4] By distinguishing epidermal-derived keratinocytic tumor cells from mesodermal cells devoid of keratin proteins, the immunohistochemical stain helped to visualize tumor. This seminal study also revealed that, among other things, polyclonal antibodies targeting the numerous fibrous keratin epitopes provided the highest sensitivity of tumor detection. In fact, monoclonal antibodies were unable to detect poorly differentiated SCCs. The benefit of targeting multiple cellular epitopes was further documented in a follow-up study by the same author.[47] In this latter study it was revealed that use of a broad-staining cocktail such as AE1/AE3 outperformed other more single-target specific antibodies when staining BCCs and SCCs, particularly when the neoplasms became more histologically aggressive.

AE1/AE3 is a commercially available immunostain that is useful for the treatment of BCCs and SCCs. AE1/AE3 has an affinity for a variety of cytokeratins, essentially allowing for all epithelial-derived tissue to be stained. AE1 recognizes cytokeratins 9, 10, 13, 14, 15, 16, and 19, while AE3 detects cytokeratins 1 to 8. Cytokeratins are intermediate filament proteins specific for epithelial cells. Approximately 20 different types of cytokeratins exist as heterodimeric acid-base pairs. Acidic cytokeratins (type I: CK9-20) and basic cytokeratins (type II: CK1-8) join in tandem, with each cell expressing between 2 and 10 different types of cytokeratin. The levels of expression are determined by the type of epithelium and differentiation. BCCs express cytokeratins 5, 14, 15, and 17, and cutaneous SCCs express cytokeratins 5, 6, 8, 14, 17, and 18.[48,49] Targeting these epitopes with stains during Mohs surgery helps distinguish BCC and SCC cells from nonepithelial derived tissue.

The use of cytokeratin staining during Mohs surgery has evolved over time. In 1994 Zachary and colleagues[6] demonstrated the effectiveness of cytokeratin stain when used during Mohs surgery to stain SCCs. Tumor otherwise indistinguishable on H&E, due to being masked within inflammation, infiltrating along nerve or among muscle fibers, was readily visualized with the stain and allowed for complete tumor extirpation. A year later, Jimenez and colleagues[5] published a staining protocol for AE1/AE3 that decreased the waiting time for immunohistochemistry slides. By decreasing the protocol to 1 hour and maintaining the efficacy of the technique, implementation of this method became quite practical for many

Mohs surgeons. More recently, Cherpelis and colleagues[14] further decreased the turnover time of AE1/AE3-stained frozen sections while giving results equivalent to sections submitted for permanent processing. Their ultra-rapid protocol mimicked many of the steps used for staining melanocytes with MART-1.[13]

The advantages of supplementing Mohs H&E-stained frozen sections with broad cytokeratin-targeted immunostains are many. Cytokeratin-staining antibodies enhance the visualization of tumor, thus facilitating more precise tumor extirpation in situations that are notoriously difficult for the Mohs surgeon to call "clear." Slides with suspected nonmelanocytic neoplasms that are recurrent, poorly differentiated, suspected of having perineural invasion, believed to have invaded the adipose tissue, or are clouded with dense inflammation can be more easily evaluated with stains such as AE1/AE3. Moreover, the addition of immunostains also facilitates the tissue-sparing principles of Mohs surgery by decreasing the number of stages performed in ambiguous situations. If cytokeratin-stained slides fail to reveal tumor, the Mohs surgeon may be more confident of clear margins.

One point to note is that use of a broad-spectrum antibody cocktail is important because SCCs will variably express cytokeratins depending on their level of differentiation. For example, poorly differentiated, nonkeratinizing SCCs are known to predominantly express CK5 (and CK13 to a lesser extent).[50] Cytokeratin-specific antibodies lacking CK5 may fail to stain such a neoplasm.[6] Other antibodies such as TNKH1,[51] Ber-EP4,[52,53] and anti-dsg[54] have also demonstrated varying amounts of success when used on frozen sections to stain keratinocytic tumors. Undoubtedly this technique of enhancing evaluation of BCC and SCC specimens during Mohs surgery will continue to grow, and will likely aid in preventing locoregional recurrence and tumor spread.

IMMUNOSTAINS FOR DERMATOFIBROSARCOMA PROTUBERANS

Dermatofibrosarcoma protuberans (DFSP) is a fibrohistiocytic, spindled-cell neoplasm that arises in the dermis and has the ability to invade deeper tissues. This neoplasm has recurrence rates as high as 30% to 60% when excised with margins less than 3 cm, due to an ability to mimic scarring and a proclivity to dissect between collagen bundles and into deeper tissues such as fascia and muscle.[55,56] Mohs micrographic surgery has evolved as the standard of care for treating DFSP, due to its precise evaluation of surgical margins.

In fact, the recurrence rates for DFSP are as low as 2% when treated with Mohs surgery.[57]

Because distinguishing DFSP from scar tissue and normal fibroblasts can be so challenging, immunohistochemical staining can be invaluable when treating DFSP with Mohs surgery. CD34 is found in multiple cell types, including hematopoietic stem cells, endothelium, and dendritic cells of the dermal, periadnexal, and endoneuronal varieties.[1] Staining with CD34 helps distinguish DFSP from keloids, dermatofibroma, and atypical fibroxanthoma, and can aid in demarcating the surgical margins. To date, 3 reports of Mohs surgery supplemented with CD34 staining have been published.[8,58–60] As increasing numbers of Mohs surgeons employ immunostains, future studies will likely demonstrate an improved ability to detect DFSP using frozen sections stained with CD34.

SUMMARY

Many advances have been made in the development and application of immunostains for Mohs micrographic surgery. Using these techniques has great potential to improve cure rates for subtle tumors that are difficult to detect on routine H&E frozen sections.

REFERENCES

1. El Tal AK, Abrou AE, Stiff MA, et al. Immunostaining in Mohs micrographic surgery: a review. Dermatol Surg 2010;36(3):275–90.
2. Thosani MK, Marghoob A, Chen CS. Current progress of immunostains in Mohs micrographic surgery: a review. Dermatol Surg 2008;34(12):1621–36.
3. Stranahan D, Cherpelis BS, Glass LF, et al. Immunohistochemical stains in Mohs surgery: a review. Dermatol Surg 2009;35(7):1023–34.
4. Robinson JK, Gottschalk R. Immunofluorescent and immunoperoxidase staining of antibodies to fibrous keratin. Improved sensitivity for detecting epidermal cancer cells. Arch Dermatol 1984;120(2):199–203.
5. Jimenez FJ, Grichnik JM, Buchanan MD, et al. Immunohistochemical techniques in Mohs micrographic surgery: their potential use in the detection of neoplastic cells masked by inflammation. J Am Acad Dermatol 1995;32(1):89–94.
6. Zachary CB, Rest EB, Furlong SM, et al. Rapid cytokeratin stains enhance the sensitivity of Mohs micrographic surgery for squamous cell carcinoma. J Dermatol Surg Oncol 1994;20(8):530–5.
7. Harris DW, Kist DA, Bloom K, et al. Rapid staining with carcinoembryonic antigen aids limited excision of extramammary Paget's disease treated by Mohs surgery. J Dermatol Surg Oncol 1994;20(4):260–4.

8. Jimenez FJ, Grichnik JM, Buchanan MD, et al. Immunohistochemical margin control applied to Mohs micrographic surgical excision of dermatofibrosarcoma protuberans. J Dermatol Surg Oncol 1994;20(10):687–9.

9. Griego RD, Zitelli JA. Mohs micrographic surgery using HMB-45 for a recurrent acral melanoma. Dermatol Surg 1998;24(9):1003–6.

10. Gross EA, Andersen WK, Rogers GS. Mohs micrographic excision of lentigo maligna using Mel-5 for margin control. Arch Dermatol 1999;135(1):15–7.

11. Robinson JK. Current histologic preparation methods for Mohs micrographic surgery. Dermatol Surg 2001; 27(6):555–60.

12. Bricca GM, Brodland DG, Zitelli JA. Immunostaining melanoma frozen sections: the 1-hour protocol. Dermatol Surg 2004;30(3):403–8.

13. Cherpelis BS, Moore R, Ladd S, et al. Comparison of MART-1 frozen sections to permanent sections using a rapid 19-minute protocol. Dermatol Surg 2009; 35(2):207–13.

14. Cherpelis BS, Turner L, Ladd S, et al. Innovative 19-minute rapid cytokeratin immunostaining of nonmelanoma skin cancer in Mohs micrographic surgery. Dermatol Surg 2009;35(7):1050–6.

15. Marghoob AA, Scope A. The complexity of diagnosing melanoma. J Invest Dermatol 2009;129(1): 11–3.

16. Demierre MF, Chung C, Miller DR, et al. Early detection of thick melanomas in the United States: beware of the nodular subtype. Arch Dermatol 2005;141(6): 745–50.

17. Riker AI, Glass F, Perez I, et al. Cutaneous melanoma: methods of biopsy and definitive surgical excision. Dermatol Ther 2005;18(5):387–93.

18. Curley RK, Cook MG, Fallowfield ME, et al. Accuracy in clinically evaluating pigmented lesions. BMJ 1989;299(6690):16–8.

19. Grin CM, Kopf AW, Welkovich B, et al. Accuracy in the clinical diagnosis of malignant melanoma. Arch Dermatol 1990;126(6):763–6.

20. Wolf IH, Smolle J, Soyer HP, et al. Sensitivity in the clinical diagnosis of malignant melanoma. Melanoma Res 1998;8(5):425–9.

21. Carli P, De Giorgi V, Crocetti E, et al. Improvement of malignant/benign ratio in excised melanocytic lesions in the 'dermoscopy era': a retrospective study 1997–2001. Br J Dermatol 2004;150(4): 687–92.

22. Clausen SP, Brady MS. Surgical margins in patients with cutaneous melanoma–assessing the adequacy of excision. Melanoma Res 2005;15(6):539–42.

23. Berdahl JP, Pockaj BA, Gray RJ, et al. Optimal management and challenges in treatment of upper facial melanoma. Ann Plast Surg 2006;57(6):616–20.

24. Bricca GM, Brodland DG, Ren D, et al. Cutaneous head and neck melanoma treated with Mohs micrographic surgery. J Am Acad Dermatol 2005; 52(1):92–100.

25. Bub JL, Berg D, Slee A, et al. Management of lentigo maligna and lentigo maligna melanoma with staged excision: a 5-year follow-up. Arch Dermatol 2004; 140(5):552–8.

26. Clark GS, Pappas-Politis EC, Cherpelis BS, et al. Surgical management of melanoma in situ on chronically sun-damaged skin. Cancer Control 2008; 15(3):216–24.

27. Florell SR, Boucher KM, Leachman SA, et al. Histopathologic recognition of involved margins of lentigo maligna excised by staged excision: an interobserver comparison study. Arch Dermatol 2003; 139(5):595–604.

28. Bienert TN, Trotter MJ, Arlette JP. Treatment of cutaneous melanoma of the face by Mohs micrographic surgery. J Cutan Med Surg 2003;7(1):25–30.

29. Zitelli JA, Moy RL, Abell E. The reliability of frozen sections in the evaluation of surgical margins for melanoma. J Am Acad Dermatol 1991;24(1): 102–6.

30. Hendi A, Brodland DG, Zitelli JA. Melanocytes in long-standing sun-exposed skin: quantitative analysis using the MART-1 immunostain. Arch Dermatol 2006;142(7):871–6.

31. Kelley LC, Starkus L. Immunohistochemical staining of lentigo maligna during Mohs micrographic surgery using MART-1. J Am Acad Dermatol 2002; 46(1):78–84.

32. Mondragon RM, Barrell TL. Current concepts: the use of immunoperoxidase techniques in Mohs micrographic surgery. J Am Acad Dermatol 2000; 43(1 Pt 1):66–71.

33. Glass LF, Raziano RM, Clark GS, et al. Rapid frozen section immunostaining of melanocytes by microphthalmia-associated transcription factor. Am J Dermatopathol 2010;32(4):319–25.

34. Zalla MJ, Lim KK, Dicaudo DJ, et al. Mohs micrographic excision of melanoma using immunostains. Dermatol Surg 2000;26(8):771–84.

35. Blessing K, Sanders DS, Grant JJ. Comparison of immunohistochemical staining of the novel antibody melan-A with S100 protein and HMB-45 in malignant melanoma and melanoma variants. Histopathology 1998;32(2):139–46.

36. Jungbluth AA, Busam KJ, Gerald WL, et al. A103: an anti-melan-a monoclonal antibody for the detection of malignant melanoma in paraffin-embedded tissues. Am J Surg Pathol 1998;22(5):595–602.

37. Cormier JN, Hijazi YM, Abati A, et al. Heterogeneous expression of melanoma-associated antigens and HLA-A2 in metastatic melanoma in vivo. Int J Cancer 1998;75(4):517–24.

38. Busam KJ, Jungbluth AA. Melan-A, a new melanocytic differentiation marker. Adv Anat Pathol 1999; 6(1):12–8.

39. Albertini JG, Elston DM, Libow LF, et al. Mohs micrographic surgery for melanoma: a case series, a comparative study of immunostains, an informative case report, and a unique mapping technique. Dermatol Surg 2002;28(8):656–65.

40. Kimyai-Asadi A, Ayala GB, Goldberg LH, et al. The 20-minute rapid MART-1 immunostain for malignant melanoma frozen sections. Dermatol Surg 2008; 34(4):498–500.

41. El Shabrawi-Caelen L, Kerl H, Cerroni L. Melan-A: not a helpful marker in distinction between melanoma in situ on sun-damaged skin and pigmented actinic keratosis. Am J Dermatopathol 2004;26(5): 364–6.

42. Beltraminelli H, Shabrawi-Caelen LE, Kerl H, et al. Melan-a-positive "pseudomelanocytic nests": a pitfall in the histopathologic and immunohistochemical diagnosis of pigmented lesions on sun-damaged skin. Am J Dermatopathol 2009;31(3):305–8.

43. Maize JC Jr, Resneck JS Jr, Shapiro PE, et al. Ducking stray "magic bullets": a Melan-A alert. Am J Dermatopathol 2003;25(2):162–5.

44. Barlow JO, Maize J Sr, Lang PG. The density and distribution of melanocytes adjacent to melanoma and nonmelanoma skin cancers. Dermatol Surg 2007;33(2):199–207.

45. Rowe DE, Carroll RJ, Day CL Jr. Mohs surgery is the treatment of choice for recurrent (previously treated) basal cell carcinoma. J Dermatol Surg Oncol 1989; 15(4):424–31.

46. Ratner D, MacGregor JL. Mohs surgery. In: MacFarlane D, editor. Skin cancer management: a practical approach. New York: Springer; 2010. p. 143–52.

47. Robinson JK. Expression of keratin proteins in deeply invasive basal and squamous cell carcinoma: an immunohistochemical study. J Dermatol Surg Oncol 1987;13(3):283–94.

48. Alessi E, Venegoni L, Fanoni D, et al. Cytokeratin profile in basal cell carcinoma. Am J Dermatopathol 2008;30(3):249–55.

49. Perkins W, Campbell I, Leigh IM, et al. Keratin expression in normal skin and epidermal neoplasms demonstrated by a panel of monoclonal antibodies. J Cutan Pathol 1992;19(6):476–82.

50. Moll R, Franke WW, Schiller DL, et al. The catalog of human cytokeratins: patterns of expression in normal epithelia, tumors and cultured cells. Cell 1982;31(1):11–24.

51. Setoyama M, Hashimoto K, Dinehart SM, et al. Immunohistochemical differentiation of basal cell epithelioma from cutaneous appendages using monoclonal anti-glycoprotein antibody TNKH1. Its application in Mohs' micrographic surgery. Cancer 1990;66(12):2533–40.

52. Kist D, Perkins W, Christ S, et al. Anti-human epithelial antigen (Ber-EP4) helps define basal cell carcinoma masked by inflammation. Dermatol Surg 1997; 23(11):1067–70.

53. Jimenez FJ, Burchette JL Jr, Grichnik JM, et al. Ber-EP4 immunoreactivity in normal skin and cutaneous neoplasms. Mod Pathol 1995;8(8):854–8.

54. Krunic AL, Garrod DR, Madani S, et al. Immunohistochemical staining for desmogleins 1 and 2 in keratinocytic neoplasms with squamous phenotype: actinic keratosis, keratoacanthoma and squamous cell carcinoma of the skin. Br J Cancer 1998;77(8): 1275–9.

55. Gloster HM Jr. Dermatofibrosarcoma protuberans. J Am Acad Dermatol 1996;35(3 Pt 1):355–74 [quiz: 375–6].

56. Gloster HM Jr, Harris KR, Roenigk RK. A comparison between Mohs micrographic surgery and wide surgical excision for the treatment of dermatofibrosarcoma protuberans. J Am Acad Dermatol 1996; 35(1):82–7.

57. Ratner D, Thomas CO, Johnson TM, et al. Mohs micrographic surgery for the treatment of dermatofibrosarcoma protuberans. Results of a multiinstitutional series with an analysis of the extent of microscopic spread. J Am Acad Dermatol 1997; 37(4):600–13.

58. Garcia C, Clark RE, Buchanan M. Dermatofibrosarcoma protuberans. Int J Dermatol 1996;35(12): 867–71.

59. Garcia C, Viehman G, Hitchcock M, et al. Dermatofibrosarcoma protuberans treated with Mohs surgery. A case with CD34 immunostaining variability. Dermatol Surg 1996;22(2):177–9.

60. Young CR 3rd, Albertini MJ. Atrophic dermatofibrosarcoma protuberans: case report, review, and proposed molecular mechanisms. J Am Acad Dermatol 2003;49(4):761–4.

The Role of Radiation Therapy in the Management of Skin Cancers

Rohun Hulyalkar[a], Tina Rakkhit, MD[b],
Jorge Garcia-Zuazaga, MD, MS[b,c],*

KEYWORDS

- Radiation therapy • Basal cell carcinoma
- Squamous cell carcinoma • Malignant melanoma
- Merkel cell carcinoma • Sebaceous carcinoma
- Angiosarcoma

The administration of radiation therapy for the treatment of skin cancers spans several decades.[1] In the context of more effective and efficient surgical methods, such as Mohs micrographic surgery and advances in reconstructive techniques, radiation is less frequently used in the management of skin cancer.[2–4] However, radiation therapy remains a very useful tool both as a primary treatment and as an adjunctive treatment to enhance cure, specifically for skin cancers of the head and neck.[2] Radiation can also be helpful in palliation for symptomatic relief of incurable skin cancer.[5] This article reviews the current evidence on the use of radiation therapy for the treatment of skin cancer and describes the recommendations of the National Comprehensive Cancer Network (NCCN). Nonmelanoma skin cancers for which radiotherapy can play a role in treatment include basal cell carcinoma, squamous cell carcinoma, Merkel cell carcinoma (MCC), angiosarcoma, dermatofibrosarcoma protuberans, and sebaceous carcinoma.

TECHNIQUES OF RADIATION THERAPY

Radiation therapy can be administered to a cutaneous lesion through a variety of techniques. However, 3 specific methods have been used to deliver radiation to tissue. The first method, orthovoltage radiation, is preferred for more superficial lesions, whereas megavoltage electron beam technology is preferred for reaching deeper tissue. Also, brachytherapy can be used in the interest of delivering radiation directly to the cancer, while sparing noncancerous surrounding tissue.

Orthovoltage X-rays, also known as superficial X-rays, usually range from 75 to 125 kV.[3] Orthovoltage X-rays are the usual choice for radiating lesions thinner than 5 mm, because the X-rays interact maximally with the skin at the surface, before losing strength as they penetrate downward and are attenuated rapidly by interactions with atoms in the tissues traversed.[1,3] Orthovoltage rays lose 10% of their strength every 0.5 cm that they travel, even when a filter is used.[1] As such, a 100 kV superficial X-ray would diminish to only 90 kV after passing through 0.5 cm of tissue.[1]

Because most cutaneous tumors lie within a few millimeters of the skin surface, superficial X-rays have favorable beam characteristics to more than adequately penetrate such neoplasms. However, some tumors are too thick to be irradiated in this manner.[1] Because of the limited

The authors have nothing to disclose.
[a] School of Humanities and Sciences, Stanford University, Stanford, CA, USA
[b] Department of Dermatology, Case Western Reserve University, 11100 Euclid Avenue, Lakeside Building, 3rd Floor, Cleveland, OH 44106, USA
[c] Department of Dermatology, Mohs Micrographic Surgery and Cutaneous Oncology, University Hospitals Westlake Medical Center, 11100 Euclid Avenue, Lakeside Building, 3rd Floor, Cleveland, OH 44106, USA
* Corresponding author. 950 Clague Road, Building B, Suite 104, Westlake, OH 44124.
E-mail address: Jorge.Garcia-Zuazaga@uhhospitals.org

Dermatol Clin 29 (2011) 287–296
doi:10.1016/j.det.2011.01.004
0733-8635/11/$ – see front matter © 2011 Elsevier Inc. All rights reserved.

derm.theclinics.com

applicability of orthovoltage X-rays for treatment of other cancers, many radiation therapy departments have phased it out in favor of other modes of radiation therapy.[3]

In the place of orthovoltage X-rays, megavoltage electron beam technology has emerged as a more widely available radiotherapy option.[3] This type of radiation is produced by devices known as linear accelerators, which afford clinicians the advantage of being able to generate radiation of variable energy.[3] Electron beams range in strength from 6 to 20 MeV and can reach tissue up to approximately 6 cm deep, radiating the tissue in a relatively even manner.[3] The electron beams provide homogenous tissue coverage to a known depth and then dissipate rapidly. One disadvantage of megavoltage electron beam radiation is the significantly lower than maximum dose delivered at the surface of an air-tissue interface in a low-energy electron beam. The peak energy is delivered below the skin, resulting in a weaker dose being administered to the surface than to underlying tissues. This issue is typically corrected by placing skin-equivalent material on the skin surface to achieve the strongest possible surface dose.[3] In addition, the clinician must take into account the presence of structures, such as the nose or the ears, that have an uneven contour; specific techniques are applied to compensate for such contours when delivering electron beam radiation to preserve the homogeneity of the radiation.[3]

Also, brachytherapy, also known as interstitial therapy, is useful in treating small accessible skin cancers by allowing the delivery of large doses of radiation directly to the lesion.[3] This technique relies on the insertion of radioactive material, usually in the form of iridium 192 seeds, into the tumor to treat the cancer.[3] This insertion is accomplished by placing the seeds in nylon ribbons, which introduce the radioactive seeds manually into the lesion so that they are spaced 1 cm apart.[3] The radiation dose delivered by an interstitial source declines proportionally to the inverse square of the distance from the source. Because of this physical property, very high radiation doses can be delivered close to the source, and the dose declines rapidly with distance. Brachytherapy spares much of the surrounding normal tissue that would otherwise be radiated with electron beam or orthovoltage radiation.[1] The tumor is irradiated continuously for 4 to 6 days, which may be a theoretical advantage because tumor proliferation during the radiation course is limited. Some of the notable disadvantages of brachytherapy include the necessity for the patient to remain hospitalized in isolation during treatment and the

insertion of radiation sources under general anesthesia.[3] Thus, external beam therapy is generally more practical.

In treating tumors of the skin with radiotherapy, 2 concepts are fundamental. The first is the half-dose depth, the tissue depth at which half of the surface dose is delivered. Because superficial X-rays penetrate the skin, interaction with atoms in the tissues through which they travel attenuates them, and at a certain depth, only 50% of the surface dose is delivered. If 50% of the surface energy reaches the base of a given tumor, the normal tissues directly deep to the tumor receive 50% of the surface dose, and radiation damage to the normal tissue is limited. Therefore, careful calculation of the radiation dose is imperative to ensure that the amount of radiation delivered to the tumor base and the tissue beneath it is approximately 50% of the dose delivered to the skin surface.[1]

The second concept, known as the 90% isodose concept, relates to electron beam radiation. This type of radiation can be used to treat a tumor homogeneously with the same dose, with less than 10% variation. The base of the tumor receives no less than 90% of its surface radiation dose. As a result, the normal tissue underlying a cancer receives more radiation.[1]

Fractionation of the radiation dose is another important concept in optimizing the cosmetic outcome and minimizing side effects of radiation therapy at the treatment site. By dividing the total radiation dose into fractions that are delivered at intervals over several days or weeks, the side effects of a single large dose are mitigated. The total radiation dose is modified according to the size of each fraction.

BASAL CELL CARCINOMAS AND SQUAMOUS CELL CARCINOMAS

According to the most recent NCCN guidelines of 2010, approximately 1 million cases of basal and squamous cell carcinoma are diagnosed every year, with squamous cell cancers (SCCs) accounting for approximately 300,000 cases and basal cell cancers (BCCs) constituting the remaining cases.[6] According to a recent survey, radiation is used as a first-line treatment for only 8% of BCCs in the United Kingdom and 2% in the Netherlands.[1] Surgical treatments, such as Mohs micrographic surgery or standard surgical excision, are typically the initial treatments for most BCCs and provide histologic evidence of tumor clearance, excellent cure rates, as well as cosmetic and functional preservation. However, because basal and SCCs are relatively radioresponsive, radiotherapy can be used as a primary modality with a curative intent, a preoperative or postoperative adjunctive modality, or as a palliative treatment. NCCN guidelines for treatment of basal and squamous cell carcinomas are helpful in determining when to consider radiation therapy and are described later.[6] Of note, the NCCN guidelines for the use of radiotherapy in management of skin cancers are category 2B, indicating that they are based on a lower level of evidence and nonuniform consensus but without major disagreements among the experts involved in formulating the guidelines. Because of the lack of controlled prospective studies, there are no consensus recommendations for the use of radiation for SCCs of the skin.

Primary Treatment

When surgical excision of a cancer may result in functional or aesthetic compromise, radiation therapy may be the optimal primary treatment, even for superficial lesions such as Bowen disease (cutaneous SCC in situ).[2,6] Radiotherapy is also suitable as the primary treatment of extensive tumors that are surgically unresectable, such as inaccessible tumors located at the skull base.[5] Deep lesions at the cranial nerve foramina or in the brain are most effectively radiated with electron beam radiation that can deliver radiation dose to a depth of 6 cm.[5] Radiation therapy becomes the primary treatment of choice for patients who are poor surgical candidates; patient preference may also lead to selection of radiation therapy as the primary treatment.[6]

Scouting biopsies around the site of the cutaneous malignancy can help to determine the extent of the cancer and the size of the radiation field when the cancer is ill defined or extensive. The radiation field includes the area involved by the cancer and a margin around it.[7]

Adjuvant Radiotherapy

Adjuvant radiation therapy can be used preoperatively to reduce the extent of a tumor in an effort to make it resectable.[8] In clinical settings where extended surgical excision to obtain negative margins with Mohs micrographic surgery might involve sacrificing major nerve structures and cause significant functional and cosmetic morbidity, adjuvant radiotherapy is a valuable tool. In such a scenario, further excision may be deferred to preserve vital structures, and radiation therapy is added to treat the residual skin cancer. The role of adjuvant radiation in the management of perineurally invasive skin cancer is discussed separately later. Postoperative adjunctive radiation is used when there remains residual cancer after inadequate excision and reexcision is not

possible or there is a high likelihood of residual disease after excision and the probability of successful treatment of a recurrence is modest. Tumors excised with positive margins, multiply recurrent tumors, and those with perineural or bony invasion are indications for postsurgical adjunctive radiation.[2,5]

Management of regional lymph nodes

Elective radiation of clinically uninvolved nodes is performed when there is a high probability ($\geq$20%) of subclinical disease as might be expected in the presence of multiple high-risk features and proximity to the parotid gland.[2,9] The presence of tumor in palpable regional lymph nodes must be confirmed by fine needle aspiration or lymph node biopsy.[6] Imaging studies help to rule out distant disease in addition to determining the number, size, and location of involved nodes.[6] Lymphadenectomy is sufficient for a solitary cervical lymph node, less than 3 cm, without extracapsular extension. For more advanced disease with larger nodes, multiple nodes, or bilateral nodal involvement, postoperative radiation should be strongly considered and is recommended by some radiation oncologists.[2,6] Preoperative radiation may be used before lymph node dissection for borderline unresectable clinically positive disease in the neck.[2,8] Radiation alone is used for unresectable lymph node disease or for patients who are medically inoperable.[2]

Palliative Radiotherapy

Palliative radiotherapy may be helpful in managing symptomatic basal and squamous cell carcinomas in terminally ill patients. The discussion of this subset of patients is beyond the scope of this article.

Perineural Invasion

The histologic finding of perineural invasion (PNI) by cancer cells is associated with aggressive tumor behavior in both basal and SCCs.[5] PNI may be categorized as either microscopic or macroscopic (clinical). It is estimated that approximately 60% to 70% of all PNIs are microscopic, in that they only affect smaller nerves (<1 mm in diameter in the reticular dermis).[5] The remaining 30% to 40% of PNIs manifests with clinical signs or symptoms and involve larger nerves of diameters greater than or equal to 1 mm.[5] Most cases of PNI occur in SCCs, which have a 2.5% to 14% risk of becoming perineurally invasive. However, BCCs may also exhibit such behavior and carry a 1% risk of developing PNI.[5]

A review of the data on the behavior of cutaneous SCC (cSCC) and BCC, described later, demonstrates the role and significance of adjuvant radiotherapy in improving outcomes. PNI carcinomas tend to be larger and have greater subclinical extension and a higher risk of recurrence than those without PNI.[10] In one study, Leibovitch and colleagues[10] reported a 5-year recurrence rate after Mohs surgery for BCCs with PNI of 7.7%, compared with 2.4% for BCCs without PNI. Evidence from many studies suggests that the size of involved nerves in cases of perineurally invasive squamous cell carcinoma can serve as an important prognostic indicator. In a small retrospective cohort study of 48 patients, Ross and colleagues[11] noted rates of local recurrence of 50%, nodal metastases of 38%, distant metastases of 32%, disease-specific death of 32%, and all-cause death of 48% for patients presenting with macroscopic PNI, involving nerves 1 mm or more in diameter. These rates were significantly higher than the 9% local recurrence rate, 0% nodal metastasis rate, 0% distant metastasis rate, 0% disease-specific death rate, and 17% all-cause death rate associated with microscopic PNI, which involved nerves measuring less than 0.1 mm in diameter.[11] In another study, conducted by Mendenhall and colleagues,[7] it was observed that patients presenting with incidental PNI had higher rates of local control over the course of 5 years at 79% when compared with their counterparts who presented with clinical PNI and had a 5-year local control rate of 53%. Hence, adjuvant radiation therapy is recommended for cSCC with extensive perineural disease, even if the margins of resection are tumor free.[6]

The association between PNI and tumor recurrence, as well as the role of adjuvant radiotherapy in the treatment of perineurally invasive disease, has been the subject of several studies.[5] Early detection followed by complete surgical resection provides for the best chance of local and eventual cure.[8] Han and Ratner[5] observed in a 2007 study that the cure rate for cSCCs with microscopic PNI treated with Mohs surgery with or without radiation was 92% to 100%, compared with cure rates of 38% to 100% for those treated with standard excision with or without adjunctive radiotherapy. These findings emphasize the importance of complete excision of the cancer. However, because of the more aggressive biologic behavior and poorer outcomes of cSCC with PNI, adjuvant radiation to the site of the primary cancer may be helpful in achieving better cure rates. Adjuvant radiation may be considered after Mohs surgery in the presence of PNI because of the belief that "skip areas" beyond an excision site may exist, creating a false-negative margin.[5] Many recommendations for radiation therapy are based on retrospective studies of both BCCs and SCCs and do not separately identify recommendations for BCCs.[8] The role of adjuvant radiotherapy for microscopic PNI is not as well defined in the literature as it is for extensive PNI.[5] Total tumor doses of 75 Gy with an altered-fractionation schedule are recommended for tumors with clinical PNI.[8]

Because of the risk of incomplete excision and local recurrence, postoperative radiotherapy is often recommended after standard excision for SCC with PNI.[5] Retrospective data show that radiation therapy to the site of the SCC reduces the risk of local, regional, and distant recurrence, especially for tumors with PNI.[8] Mendenhall and colleagues[4] recommended that most patients with PNI undergo radiation therapy as an adjuvant to surgery in an effort to prevent local and regional recurrence. Local control rates achieved with surgery, with or without adjuvant radiation, in different studies of cSCC with PNI, are summarized in **Table 1**. **Table 2** compares the local recurrence rate and disease-free survival in patients treated with surgery alone and those treated with surgery plus adjuvant radiation.

Elective radiation of clinically normal regional lymph nodes in patients with PNI has been shown to be important in preventing regional recurrences.[8] In a retrospective study of skin cancers (including both BCCs and SCCs) with PNI conducted by Garcia-Serra and colleagues[8] in 2003, the regional (lymph node) recurrence rate in patients with clinical PNI was 5%, compared with 14% in those with microscopic PNI. The difference was attributed to the fact that twice as many patients in the clinical PNI group had been given elective radiation of the regional lymph nodes when compared with those in the microscopic PNI group. This observation underscores the value of elective irradiation of regional lymph nodes in the setting of PNI. These data imply that microscopic metastases may already be present in the lymph nodes and become clinically apparent even though the tumor has been completely excised. Because 15% to 20% of patients with clinically negative nodes are likely to have subclinical disease, Mendenhall and colleagues[4] further recommended that such patients undergo elective radiation therapy to the regional lymph nodes. There is general agreement that adjuvant radiation therapy is warranted in cases of PNI involving larger named nerves. However, adjuvant radiotherapy seldom leads to improvement in cranial nerve deficits, with improvement in symptoms in only 7% of patients without local recurrence.[8]

Table 1
Local control rates in perineurally invasive cutaneous BCCs and SCCs treated with surgical excision and/or radiotherapy

Author	Year	No. of Patients	Treatment	5-year (Unless Noted Otherwise) Local Control Rate
Ampil et al[29]	1995	9 SCC	Surgery ± radiation therapy	3-y local control rate: 66.7%,
Mendenhall et al[7]	2002	46 SCC 16 BCC	Radiation therapy ± surgery	Microscopic PNI: 79% Clinical PNI: 50%
Garcia-Serra et al[8]	2003	135 BCC and SCC	Radiation therapy ± surgery	Microscopic PNI: 87% Clinical PNI: 55%
Leibovitch et al[10]	2005	70 SCC	MMS ± radiation therapy	Microscopic and clinical PNI: 92%

In a multivariate analysis, Ross and colleagues[11] did not observe involved nerve diameter as a significant risk factor in their small study. Only tumor size and patient age were found to be meaningful predictors of survival. Therefore, they only recommended the use of adjuvant radiation therapy when other high-risk factors associated with poor outcomes are also present in addition to PNI (**Box 1**). They did, however, acknowledge the necessity of larger prospective studies to confirm this conclusion.

The role of radiotherapy in the treatment of non-melanoma skin cancers was the most controversial among the panel of experts in the NCCN.[6] Complex tumors with high-risk features or PNI benefit from a discussion at a multispecialty tumor board, including Mohs surgeons, radiation oncologists, and head and neck surgeons, to determine

the utility of radiotherapy based on tumor and host characteristics, dosage, and the mode of radiation.

Contraindications

Radiation therapy is contraindicated for the treatment of skin cancers in patients with basal cell nevus syndrome and xeroderma pigmentosum because of the impaired DNA repair mechanisms in these conditions that predispose them to radiation-induced skin cancers. Radiation is generally not used in young patients because the cosmetic outcome gradually deteriorates over many years.[2,3,5] It is also avoided because of the risk of developing radiation-induced malignancy several years later.[2,5] Radiotherapy is also contraindicated in patients with connective tissue

Table 2
Results of surgery versus surgery and adjuvant radiotherapy for SCC with PNI

Author	Year	No. of Patients	Treatment	Outcome (5-year)
Veness et al[9]	2007	167	Surgery (21)	Local recurrence rate: 43% Disease-free survival rate: 54%
			Surgery + ART (146)	Local recurrence rate: 20% Disease-free survival rate: 73%
Jambusaria-Pahlajani et al[30]	2009	28	Surgery alone (9)	Local recurrence rate: 0% Disease-free survival rate: 100%
			Surgery + ART (19)	Local recurrence rate: 0% Disease-free survival rate: 74%

Abbreviation: ART, adjuvant radiation therapy.

> **Box 1**
> **Non-PNI features associated with high-risk SCC for which radiation therapy should be considered**
>
> Features:
>
> Diameter greater than 2 cm
>
> Ill-defined margins
>
> Recurrence
>
> Location on areas such as lip and ear
>
> Depth 4 mm or more or infiltration into deep reticular dermis or fat (Clark level IV, V)
>
> Poor differentiation; adenoid, adenosquamous, or desmoplastic histology
>
> Site of chronic inflammation
>
> Rapid growth
>
> Immunosuppression of host

diseases such as scleroderma.[6] The NCCN guidelines[6] exclude verrucous carcinoma because several reports have documented an increased risk of metastases after radiation. The genitalia, hands, and feet are also excluded.[6]

MCC

MCC is a rare neuroendocrine cancer of the sun-exposed skin, typically observed in elderly patients.[12] Its incidence has tripled in the last 15 years.[13] The cause-specific mortality rate from this cancer is between 30% and 38% at 5 years.[13,14] The increase in annual incidence, exceeding 1000 cases per year in the United States, makes MCC the second most common cause of nonmelanoma skin cancer–associated death. Therapeutic recommendations are based on data from retrospective studies of relatively few patients and vary widely.[12] MCC is a radiosensitive tumor. A combination of surgical excision and radiotherapy forms the mainstay of treatment of primary and regional lymph node disease. There is agreement that wide excision with 2 to 3 cm margins, when possible, is the first step in treatment. However, it is often impossible to excise MCC of the head and neck with wide margins. Therefore, adjuvant radiation of 5500 to 6000 cGy over 6 weeks may be added.[12] However, when coupled with adjunctive radiation therapy to the tumor site, a decrease in local recurrences as much as 4-fold has been observed in multiple retrospective studies.[13] Regional recurrences are also diminished (23% vs 56%) by local adjuvant irradiation.[13] These data strongly support a role for local adjuvant radiation therapy in the management of MCC. A trend to improved cause-specific survival was also noted in an analysis of retrospective studies.[13] A similar result is observed in MCC treated with Mohs micrographic surgery. With Mohs excision alone, a higher rate of both local and regional lymph node recurrence is observed. When Mohs surgery was complemented by postoperative adjuvant radiation to the site of the primary cancer, with or without the regional lymph nodes, there were no recurrences at the local site or in the regional lymph nodes.[12] Thus, local adjuvant irradiation seems to contribute to improved outcomes for patients with MCC.

The most important prognosticator in MCC is the stage of the disease at the time of diagnosis.[12] Sentinel lymph node (SLN) biopsy is a valuable tool in staging MCC. About 25% of patients with MCC have metastasis in the SLN (stage 2 disease). Although survival benefit has never been documented, a complete lymphadenectomy is recommended if an SLN biopsy result is positive.[12] Adjuvant irradiation of the nodal bed after complete lymphadenectomy for a positive SLN result is usually not recommended.[12] However, in patients with large regional metastases or with extracapsular extension, adjuvant irradiation after complete lymphadenectomy may improve regional control. If SLN biopsy tests negative for metastasis (stage I disease), adjuvant radiation to the regional lymph node basin is a consideration, as discussed previously.

MALIGNANT MELANOMA

Malignant melanoma may occur as melanoma in situ (MIS), also known as lentigo maligna, or as an invasive melanoma. Lentigo maligna occurs on sun-exposed areas, predominantly on the head and neck. Over the last 20 years, the incidence of MIS has increased significantly. In 1992, the National Institutes of Health consensus statement established the standard of care for MIS as surgical excision with 5 mm margins. However, this approach is associated with a 6% to 20% recurrence rate, and 58% of lentigo maligna melanomas require surgical margins greater than 5 mm for complete excision, because of subclinical extension.[15] The prevalence of lentigo maligna on the head and neck poses a challenge to the surgeon in preserving cosmetic and functional outcomes. The elderly patients who usually develop lentigo maligna often have co-morbidities that make them poor surgical candidates. These circumstances have led to the exploration of radiation therapy as a treatment option. Radiotherapy, with Grenz rays or soft X-rays using the Meischer technique, has been used as a primary treatment of lentigo maligna in small studies, with cure rates ranging from 86% to 95% at 2 to 5 years after treatment. Because of the limited evidence regarding the long-term efficacy of radiation therapy for lentigo maligna, it is generally reserved for patients with unresectable lesions and those who are poor surgical candidates.[15]

Invasive malignant melanomas are notable for being more aggressive. Surgery has remained the principal treatment of invasive melanomas. About 80% of patients present with localized disease that, most of the time, can be cured with surgical excision. Surgical treatment can achieve very high cure rates for melanomas less than 1 mm thick, exceeding 90%, at 5 years.[16] As tumors enlarge, the risk of local and regional recurrence as well as distant metastases increases. Surgery remains a mainstay of treatment of advanced melanomas, but adjuvant therapy, including radiation, becomes more important. Radiation therapy plays a role in optimizing cure rates in melanomas that are greater than 1 mm in Breslow depth. Historically, melanomas were thought to be radioresistant. However, more recent investigations have shown heterogeneity in the response of melanoma cells to radiotherapy.[17] The response rate of melanoma to radiation depends on the fraction size, with complete response in 57% of tumors with fractions more than 4 Gy, compared with a 23% complete response rate with fractions less than 4 Gy in one study.[16]

Radiation therapy in the treatment of melanoma can be adjunctive or palliative. Melanomas more than 2 mm thick have a 20% or greater chance of a positive SLN biopsy result. Patients with positive nodes have a 20% to 80% risk of regional recurrence.[18,19] However, when adjuvant radiation therapy is administered, in addition to surgical resection, to both the primary site and, if necessary, the regional lymph nodes, the risk of local or regional recurrence declines significantly, with control rates of at least 85% to 90%.[18,19] Fenig and colleagues[17] observed a local and regional control rate of 87% in a study in which conventional fractions of adjuvant radiation were given to patients presenting with cutaneous malignant melanoma.

The 2010 NCCN guidelines suggest that radiation should be used to treat patients with stage III in-transit disease as an alternative to complete excision. Furthermore, the NCCN guidelines recommend the use of palliative radiation therapy for patients with unresectable stage IV disease, metastatic to the brain. Radiation therapy may also be used in patients with recurrent in situ, stage I, or stage II disease as an adjunctive

treatment to surgical resection. These recommendations are based on a lower level of evidence and nonuniform consensus without major disagreements, which classifies them as category 2B. Surgery alone has been proven to be insufficient in treating advanced melanoma, leaving the patient at a high risk for local or regional recurrence.[18] In addition, it has been demonstrated that the effect of radiotherapy in the treatment of metastatic melanomas is mainly palliative. Radiation successfully eased the more agonizing symptoms of 50% of patients in one study, although its actual impact on patient survival is deemed insignificant.[1,18] Shuff and colleagues[16] reported that, despite its demonstrated success in local control, radiotherapy can do little more than palliate after melanoma has begun to systematically spread throughout the body.

ANGIOSARCOMA

Arising from vascular endothelial cells, angiosarcoma occurs commonly in older white men, on the head, neck, limbs, and chest wall.[20] Angiosarcomas are characterized by high rates of local recurrence and metastasis and reported 5-year survival rates ranging from 12% to 41%.[20] For these reasons, early detection is essential to effective management.[21] Although angiosarcomas are known to be fairly radioresponsive, surgery has been the mainstay of therapy.[1] Once a diagnosis of angiosarcoma is established, aggressive surgical treatment, such as wide excision, with either preoperative or postoperative high-dose radiation therapy, is undertaken.[20]

Ward and colleagues[20] reported on a group of 25 patients with angiosarcoma and noted that more aggressive surgical resection with wide margins, and radiation doses higher than 61.5 Gy were associated with better survival. Another study reported that radiation doses of less than 45 Gy achieved a local control rate of 25%, whereas doses greater than 50 Gy resulted in a local control rate of 68%.[22] Accelerated hyperfractionation, with a radiation dose of 1 Gy given 3 times a day, is now being used to achieve better success in the treatment of angiosarcomas.[20]

In the study by Ward and colleagues,[20] the only statistically significant variable predicting absolute survival was the anatomic location of the cancer. All patients with lesions of the scalp died of their disease. Many angiosarcomas are large at the time of clinical diagnosis, often making adjuvant radiation therapy necessary to preserve function and cosmesis. For tumors less than 5 cm, in which negative margins can be achieved, surgical removal followed immediately by postoperative radiation is recommended. When tumor size is larger than 5 cm, or when wide margins would compromise function or cosmesis, preoperative radiation generally precedes resection. With large tumors, consideration should be given to radiation of regional lymph nodes. The predominant pattern of recurrence is local. Thus, local therapies must not be delayed or compromised. Patients with metastatic angiosarcoma were treated with palliative radiation, and all died of their disease in less than 6 months.

DERMATOFIBROSARCOMA PROTUBERANS

Although dermatofibrosarcoma protuberans (DFSP) is the world's most common cutaneous sarcoma, it remains one of the less common types of skin cancer.[23] Similar to angiosarcomas, they are observed more frequently in men and are usually found on the trunk but have also been reported on the extremities, head, and neck of patients.[24] Ugurel[23] reported that most DFSPs occur superficially and have a diameter of less than 5 cm. The tumors are indolent, inflicting significant damage on surrounding tissues, but metastasizing in 5% or fewer cases. When recognized and treated in the early stages, radiation therapy is usually not necessary, with most clinicians opting for either excision with wide margins or Mohs micrographic surgery.[25] Surgical treatment modalities result in local control rates around 90%.[26] However, if tumor is present close to or at the margins are after excision, adjuvant radiotherapy of approximately 50 or 60 Gy is usually recommended.[25,26] Radiation, when delivered either before or after surgery, can help to minimize the risk of local recurrence.[25,26] In one study, adjuvant radiation achieved local control rates of at least 85%.[26] Palliative radiotherapy can be used for surgically incurable or metastatic DFSP.[23] Although DFSPs are radioresponsive, there is insufficient evidence to support the use of radiation as a primary treatment, and further study remains necessary.[24,26]

SEBACEOUS CARCINOMA

Sebaceous carcinomas of the skin are rare, arising from the epithelial cells of sebaceous glands.[27] Often misdiagnosed as BCCs or SCCs, they occur most commonly in hair-covered regions of the head and neck, and are most common among women aged between 60 and 80 years. Sebaceous carcinomas can be divided into 2 different subtypes. Periorbital sebaceous carcinoma is the more common of the 2, accounting for 70% of the cases and occurring approximately 3 times more frequently than extraorbital sebaceous carcinoma.[27] Periorbital sebaceous carcinomas are noted for their aggressive behavior, frequent metastasis, and treatment refractory nature, whereas extraorbital cancers are more locally aggressive and rarely metastasize.[27,28] A 1974 study of 59 patients with extraorbital sebaceous carcinoma reported a 19% recurrence rate and a 14% metastasis rate.[27] A 5-year mortality rate of 20% for periorbital sebaceous carcinomas has also been reported.[27] Thus, an excision with wide margins is usually conducted to ensure complete resection of the tumor.[27] Radiation therapy is also used in specific cases as the preferred primary modality of treatment.[27]

COMPLICATIONS OF RADIATION THERAPY

The incidence of complications associated with radiation therapy is related to the maximum dose administered. The potential side effects are also related to anatomic location. Adverse effects from radiation to head and neck sites include dry desquamation, wet desquamation, alopecia, dyspigmentation, atrophy, telangiectasia, mucositis, parotiditis, soft tissue necrosis, bone exposure, osteoradionecrosis, hearing loss, ocular damage, transient central nervous system syndrome, and fistula formation.[8,16] Radiation to the axillary or inguinal lymph node basins may result in prolonged edema of the upper and lower extremities, respectively.[16] In patients who may benefit from treatment with radiation therapy, the risk of potential side effects must be weighed against the potential benefits of treatment. In addition, the incidence of complications can be reduced by careful fractionation of the radiation dose.

SUMMARY

In sum, the role of radiation therapy in the treatment of skin cancers is still highly controversial and remains the largest source of disagreement among NCCN experts. However, reflection on the reports of previous studies may provide reliable guidelines for management. BCC and SCC without PNI are usually treated without the use of radiation therapy. In the presence of microscopic PNI associated with other high-risk features, local and regional radiotherapy are helpful in providing a higher cure rate. Clinical manifestations of PNI should prompt consideration of adjuvant radiation to optimize tumor control. MCCs are best treated with a combination of wide surgical excision and local adjuvant radiation to achieve optimal control. Melanomas are optimally controlled with surgical excision. However, adjuvant or palliative radiation may be useful for more aggressive disease. Angiosarcomas are generally best treated with an aggressive primary surgical excision accompanied by high-dose radiation therapy to avoid recurrent lesions. DFSP, while widely accepted as radioresponsive, is not yet treated primarily with radiation in the absence of sufficient data to support its use. Instead, DFSP is commonly treated by excision with wide margins or Mohs surgery. Adjuvant radiotherapy may be considered in the presence of tumor close to or at the margins. Sebaceous carcinoma is most optimally treated with wide local excision, but radiation presents an effective alternative when anatomic location precludes such an excision. In the future, larger, randomized, prospective studies comparing the outcomes of surgical resection and both primary and adjunctive radiation therapy in treating melanoma and nonmelanoma skin cancers will be useful in better defining the therapeutic role and survival benefit, if any, of radiation.

REFERENCES

1. Cooper Jay S. Radiation therapy in the treatment of skin cancers. Philadelphia (PA): Elsevier; 2005.

2. Mendenhall WM, Amdur RJ, Hinerman RW, et al. Radiotherapy for cutaneous squamous and basal cell carcinomas of the head and neck. Laryngoscope 2009;119:1994–9.

3. Morrison WH, Garden AS, Ang KK. Radiation therapy for nonmelanoma skin carcinomas. Clin Plast Surg 1997;24:719–29.

4. Mendenhall WM, Amdur RJ, Hinerman RW, et al. Skin cancer of the head and neck with perineural invasion. Am J Clin Oncol 2007; 30(1):93–6.

5. Han A, Ratner D. What is the role of adjuvant radiation therapy in the treatment of cutaneous squamous cell cancer with per neural invasion? Cancer 2007; 109:1053–9.

6. National Comprehensive Cancer Network Clinical Practice Guidelines in Oncology. Basal cell and squamous cell skin cancers. V.1.2010. Available at: http://www.nccn.org.

7. Mendenhall WM, Amdur RJ, Williams LS, et al. Carcinoma of the skin of the head and neck with perineural invasion. Head Neck 2002;24:78–83.

8. Garcia-Serra A, Hinerman RW, Mendenhall WM, et al. Carcinoma of the skin with perineural invasion. Head Neck 2003;25:1027–33.

9. Veness MJ. High-risk cutaneous squamous cell carcinoma of the head and neck. J Biomed Biotechnol 2007;2007(3):80572.

10. Leibovitch I, Huilgol SC, Selva D, et al. Basal cell cancer treated with Mohs surgery in Australia III. Perineural invasion. J Am Acad Dermatol 2005; 53(3):458–63.

11. Ross AS, Whalen FM, Elenitsas R, et al. Diameter of involved nerves predicts outcomes in cutaneous squamous cell carcinoma with perineural invasion: an investigator-blinded retrospective cohort study. Dermatol Surg 2009;35:1859–66.

12. Brady MS. Current management of patients with Merkel cell carcinoma. Dermatol Surg 2004;30: 321–5.

13. Garneski KM, Nghiem P. Merkel cell carcinoma adjuvant therapy: current data support radiation but not chemotherapy. J Am Acad Dermatol 2007;57(1): 166–9.

14. Lewis KG, Weinstock MA, Otley CC. Adjuvant local irradiation for Merkel cell carcinoma. Arch Dermatol 2006;142(46):771–4.

15. Erickson C, Miller SJ. Treatment options in melanoma in situ: topical and radiation therapy, excision and Mohs surgery. Int J Dermatol 2010;49(5):482–91.

16. Shuff JH, Siker ML, Daly MD, et al. Role of radiation therapy in cutaneous melanoma. Clin Plast Surg 2010;37:147–60.

17. Fenig E, Eidelvich E, Njuguna E, et al. Role of radiation therapy in the management of cutaneous malignant melanoma. Am J Clin Oncol 1999;22:184–6.

18. Mendenhall WM, Amdur RJ, Grobmyer ST, et al. Adjuvant radiation therapy for cutaneous melanoma. Cancer 2008;112:1189–96.

19. National Comprehensive Cancer Network. Melanoma Clinical Practice Guidelines in Oncology, V.2. 2010. Available at: http://www.nccn.org.

20. Ward JR, Feigenberg SJ, Mendenhall NP, et al. Radiation therapy for angiosarcoma. Head Neck 2003; 25:873–8.

21. Donghi D, Kerl K, Dummer R, et al. Cutaneous angiosarcoma: own experience over 13 years. Clinical features, disease course and immunohistochemical profile. J Eur Acad Dermatol Venereol 2010;24(10): 1230–4.

22. Mark RJ, Poen JC, Tran LM, et al. Angiosarcoma. A report of sixty-seven patients and a review of the literature. Cancer 1996;77:2400–6.

23. Ugurel S. Dermatofibrosarcoma protuberans. Hautarzt 2008;59:933–9.

24. Ballo MT, Zagars GK, Pisters P, et al. The role of radiation therapy in the management of dermatofibrosarcoma protuberans. Int J Radiat Oncol Biol Phys 1998;40:823–7.

25. Fattoruso SI, Visca P, Lopez M. Molecular approach in treatment of dermatofibrosarcoma protuberans. Clin Ter 2008;159(5):361–7 [in Italian].

26. Mendenhall WM, Zlotecki RA, Scarborough MT dermatofibrosarcoma protuberans. Cancer 2004;101: 2503–8.

27. Dowd MB, Kumar RJ, Sharma R, et al. Diagnosis and management of sebaceous carcinoma: an Australian experience. ANZ J Surg 2008;78: 158–63.

28. Pickford MA, Hogg FJ, Fallowfield ME, et al. Sebaceous carcinoma of the periorbital and extraorbital regions. Br J Plast Surg 1995;48(2): 93–6.

29. Ampil FL, Hardin JC, Peskind SP, et al. Perineural invasion of skin cancers of the head and neck: a review of nine cases. J Oral Maxillofac Surg 1995;53(1):34–8.

30. Jambusaria-Pahlajani A, Miller CJ, Quon H, et al. Surgical monotherapy versus surgery plus adjuvant radiotherapy in high-risk cutaneous squamous cell carcinoma: a systematic review of outcomes. Dermatol Surg 2009;35(4):574–85.

Nonsurgical Treatment of Nonmelanoma Skin Cancer

Edward M. Galiczynski, DO[a],*, Allison T. Vidimos, RPh, MD[b]

KEYWORDS

- Nonmelanoma skin cancer • Tropical therapies
- Electrodessication and curettage • Cryotherapy
- Radiotherapy • PDT • Intralesional therapies

Nonmelanoma skin cancer (NMSC) is the most common type of cancer in humans, accounting for more than 1 million new cases in the United States in 2009. The increased incidence of primary cutaneous malignancies has led to the need for multiple treatment options. Surgery remains the mainstay of treatment of NMSC and should be the preferred method of treatment in many circumstances (**Box 1**). However, it is essential for the dermatologic surgeon to have a thorough understanding of the various nonsurgical modalities (**Box 2**) for the treatment of NMSC. This information is equally important to patients in order for them to make the most informed decision in the treatment of their malignancy.

NONSURGICAL PHYSICAL MODALITIES
Electrodessication and Curettage

Electrodessication and curettage (ED&C) is one of the most widely used methods used in the treatment of basal cell carcinoma (BCC), squamous cell carcinoma in situ (SCCIS), and squamous cell carcinoma (SCC). Electrodessication uses markedly damped, high-voltage, low-amperage current to produce superficial tissue destruction. ED&C is performed by first marking an outline of the tumor margins and anesthetizing the area

around the lesion with lidocaine with epinephrine. The tumor is then curetted in a checkerboard pattern until the lesion is removed. The lesion is touched with the tip of the electrode until a grayish, superficial charred layer covers the lesion. The charred debris is removed from the treated lesion with a curette. The process is repeated 2 to 3 times until the tumor has been eradicated. The success rate of ED&C is operator dependent because the surgeon must be able to detect subclinical tumor using the curette. Low-risk areas with a thick underlying dermis such as the trunk and extremities are ideal locations for ED&C. The treatment of lesions in these areas usually leads to rapid healing and high cure rates. If the tumor extends into the subcutaneous fat, the procedure should be abandoned and an excision performed. In patients with implantable cardioverter-defibrillators or cardiac pacemakers, electrocautery should be used instead. Proper tumor and patient selections are crucial to achieve complete tumor clearance and to avoid recurrence. Primary tumors with distinct clinical borders located on sites, such as non–H zone regions of the face, trunk, and extremities, or of superficial or nodular histologic subtype with a diameter of less than 1 cm on the face and less than 2 cm on the trunk and extremities can be treated effectively with ED&C. Treatment sites can

The authors have nothing to disclose.

[a] Department of Dermatology, A-61, Cleveland Clinic Foundation, 9500 Euclid Avenue, Cleveland, OH 44195, USA

[b] Section of Dermatologic Surgery and Cutaneous Oncology, Department of Dermatology, Cleveland Clinic Foundation, 9500 Euclid Avenue, Cleveland, OH 44195, USA

* Corresponding author.

E-mail address: galicze@ccf.org

Dermatol Clin 29 (2011) 297–309
doi:10.1016/j.det.2011.01.011
0733-8635/11/$ – see front matter. Published by Elsevier Inc.

Box 1
Circumstances in which surgery is the preferred method of treatment

Recurrent tumor

Tumors with aggressive histologic features (perineural, deeply invasive, poorly differentiated)

High-risk locations (periorificial, embryonic fusion planes, mucosal)

Tumor arising adjacent to a scar

Box 3
Risk of recurrence by area

High

Nose

Nasolabial folds

Ear

Chin

Periorificial

Medium

Other facial sites not included in high risk areas

Low

Trunk

Extremities

---

be divided into low-, medium-, and high-risk areas (**Box 3**). Several large retrospective studies have shown that the 5-year recurrence rate for primary BCC's less than 1 cm in diameter treated with ED&C ranges from 3.3% to 5.7%.[1,2] The 5-year recurrence rates of SCC treated with ED&C are similar. One study found no difference in the recurrence rates of SCC and BCC.[1,3] A prospective study comparing ED&C with cryotherapy showed a lower recurrence rate with ED&C (12% vs 50%). The ED&C cohort also had shorter healing times (median of 36 days and 46 days, respectively).[4]

Box 2
Nonsurgical modalities for the treatment of NMSC

Traditional nonsurgical modalities

Electrodessication and curettage

Cryosurgery

Radiotherapy

Topical modalities

Imiquimod

5-Fluorouracil (5-FU)

Diclofenac

Retinoids

   Newer agents

Ingenol mebutate

Resiquimod

Emerging nonsurgical modalities

Chemical peels

Laser ablation

Intralesional therapy

   5-FU

   Bleomycin

   Interferon-α

Photodynamic therapy

Oral capecitabine

Risk factors of ED&C include hypopigmentation, hypertrophic scars and keloids, depressed or atrophic scars, and tissue contracture.[3] Cosmetic outcome of ED&C is site dependent. On the face, ED&C usually heals with a thin white plaque that may be depressed or indurated. In general, surgical excision is superior to ED&C when treating lesions on the face because it often leads to a better cosmetic outcome. On areas such as the trunk and extremities, as well as concave areas, ED&C may provide a good cosmetic result. ED&C is an efficient cost-effective procedure that has consistently shown high cure rates and should be considered as an alternative first-line treatment of small primary, nonaggressive BCC and SCC.

Cryosurgery

Cryosurgery is a cost-effective and versatile modality used in the treatment of benign, premalignant, and malignant skin lesions. A cryogen, most commonly liquid nitrogen (boiling point −195.6°C), is applied to the skin using a handheld device using an open spray technique or probe. Tissue injury is caused by 2 mechanisms: ice crystal formation within the cells and vascular thrombosis during freezing followed by vascular stasis after thawing. This injury ultimately leads to ischemic necrosis of the tissue. A pyrometer-thermocouple device may be used to monitor tissue temperature and depth of freezing. A final tissue temperature of −50°C to −60°C is needed for destruction of malignant lesions. Pulsing, or intermittent spray technique, is recommended when treating malignant lesions. Using this method, the "ice ball" will have a greater depth while minimizing lateral spread. The maximum depth of penetration is 10 mm. On the contrary, when treating superficial lesions, a continuous spray technique can be used to limit the depth of penetration. Premalignant lesions such as actinic keratoses (AKs) usually require 1 or 2 freeze-thaw cycles of 5 to 7 seconds with a lateral spread to the edge of the lesion. When treating malignant tumors, the goal is to destroy the same amount of tissue that would be removed during an excision of the same lesion. Therefore, it is essential that an adequate margin be frozen around the area of the tumor. The lateral spread should form a 3- to 5-mm halo around the lesion. Malignant tumors require 2 to 3 freeze-thaw cycles. Larger lesions should be curetted and debulked before freezing, which enables the lesion to be frozen more rapidly. The halo time, or the duration of thawing of the marginal surface around the lesion, should be longer than 60 seconds. The total thaw time for the lesion should exceed 90 seconds. Although cryosurgery is an efficient and effective treatment option in many cases, cryosurgery is not recommended for treatment of ill-defined lesions, tumors with an aggressive histologic subtype, or lesions that are deeply invasive.

Common postoperative symptoms include pain, swelling, tenderness, and redness. Blisters and crusting may occur when treating malignant lesions with longer freeze times with deep depth of penetration. Patients can be given a sterile 22-gauge needle to drain the blister or bullae. Complications of cryosurgery include hypopigmentation or hyperpigmentation, blister or bullae formation, nerve damage, and secondary infection. Caution must be taken not to damage surrounding structures, such as hair follicles (alopecia), superficial cutaneous nerves (dysesthesia), nail matrix (onychodystrophy), and cartilage (notching of the nose or ear). Occasionally, hypertrophic and keloid scars may form. Cosmetically, cryosurgery is comparable to radiotherapy but worse than photodynamic therapy (PDT) and surgical excision.[5–8] In studies comparing cryotherapy with PDT, cosmetic outcomes were rated as good or excellent in 89% to 94% of patients treated with PDT versus 50% to 66% in patients treated with cryotherapy.[5,9,10] In a prospective study comparing cosmetic outcomes of surgical excision and cryosurgery, both patients and clinical professionals preferred surgical excision to cryosurgery. In addition, cryosurgery may be associated with longer healing times and more discomfort than other nonsurgical modalities.[4,5,10] With superior cosmesis and lower recurrence rates, surgical excision remains the treatment of choice when practical.

Radiotherapy

Radiation therapy is a valuable alternative to surgical management of SCC and BCC, especially in patients with inoperable tumors and in those with significant comorbidities who would have a difficult time undergoing an extensive surgery. For further discussion of radiotherapy for the treatment of NMSC, see article by Hulyalkar and colleagues elsewhere in this issue.

TOPICAL MODALITIES

Many topical treatments have been used as both monotherapy and adjuvant methods to treat NMSC (see **Box 2**). Advantages of topical regimens include excellent cosmesis with less risk of scarring, convenience, and ability to treat large areas. Potential disadvantages include cost of the agents and patient compliance, especially in patients requiring long treatment duration. One must also be aware that treatment with topical therapy could potentially cause skip lesions and subsequently lead to false-negative margin findings that theoretically reduces the efficacy of surgical excision and Mohs micrographic surgery. In addition, results may be delayed, and patients may become discouraged and discontinue the medication.

Imiquimod

Imiquimod 5% cream is an immunomodulating agent that is Food and Drug Administration (FDA)-approved for topical use in the treatment of AKs and superficial BCC in immunocompetent adults. Imiquimod 3.75% has recently been approved by the FDA and can be used daily on larger areas of skin, the balding scalp, or the full face. In contrast, imiquimod 5% is indicated for use on areas of skin that are 25 cm^2 or smaller. Imiquimod has been used effectively (with varying treatment regimens) in the treatment of AKs, superficial BCC, nodular BCC, and SCCIS (**Table 1**). Imiquimod works by stimulating both innate and cell-mediated immune responses and has antiviral, antitumoral, and immunoregulatory properties. Antitumoral mechanisms of action of imiquimod are listed in **Box 4**.

Imiquimod should be applied sparingly to focal areas when treating superficial BCC. A broader treatment area is recommended either on the scalp or face, but not both, when treating AKs. Imiquimod should be applied before bedtime and should be left on the skin for 6 to 10 hours. Imiquimod is generally well tolerated, and irritant reactions can be treated by temporary discontinuation of therapy and application of topical steroids. Therapy can be

Table 1
Treatment regimens for imiquimod 5%, 3.75%, and 2.5% cream

Tumor Type	Dosing	Treatment Duration	Results	References
AKs	5% cream qhs 2–3 times weekly	12–16 wk	50% complete and 75% partial clearance	Hadley et al[11]
	2.50% and 3.75% cream	2 wk on/off/on × 8 wk	Complete and partial clearance of 30.6% and 48.1% for imiquimod 2.5% and 35.6% and 59.4% for imiquimod 3.75%, respectively	Swanson et al[12]
Superficial BCC	5% cream qhs 3–7 times weekly	6–16 wk	50%–100%, >90% 5–7 times weekly 80% clearance at 5 years	Marks et al,[13] Geisse et al[14] Quirk et al[15]
Nodular BCC	5% cream qhs under occlusion 7d/wk	6–12 wk	70%–100% clearance, greatest efficacy at 12 wk	Huber et al,[16] Shumack et al[17]
SCCIS	5% cream qd-qod	6–16 wk	90%–100% clearance	Mackenzie-Wood et al[18]
SCC	5% cream 5–7 times per wk	12 wk	Limited follow-up	Martin-Garcia[19]

Abbreviations: qd, every day; qhs, every night before bedtime; qod, every other day.

resumed as necessary at a decreased frequency as indicated. Erythema involving the area of application is seen in most patients treated with imiquimod. Pruritus, burning sensation, stinging sensation, and tenderness are other common side effects. Other reported adverse events include hypopigmentation, fever, diarrhea, and fatigue.

AK

Imiquimod is FDA approved for the treatment of AKs involving the head and neck. Many treatment regimens have been used in treating AKs with varying degrees of success. A meta-analysis and systemic review evaluating efficacy and toxicity in the treatment of AKs concluded that imiquimod 5% cream 2 to 3 times weekly for 12 to 16 weeks resulted in complete clearing in 50% of patients (partial clearing of 75%) versus 5% of those treated with placebo. Toxicity was limited to irritant contact dermatitis and was well managed with temporary cessation of the drug.[11]

Superficial BCC

Imiquimod 5% cream is FDA approved for the treatment of superficial BCCs less than 2 cm in diameter on the neck, trunk, and extremities. Optimal dosing consists of nightly application 5 to 7 times a week for 6 to 16 weeks (depending

on the patient's clinical response). Cure rates have been shown to be greater than 90%.[13,14]

Nodular BCC

Treatment responses to imiquimod for nodular BCC are not as high as those seen in superficial BCC. In two phase 2 studies, the highest response rates achieved using imiquimod 5% cream twice daily for 12 weeks was around 75%.[17] Therefore, this modality should be limited to patients with small tumors in low-risk areas who cannot undergo surgery or receive radiation therapy or cryotherapy.

SCCIS

SCCIS, or Bowen disease, responds to treatment with imiquimod 5% cream. In an open-label study of 16 patients with SCCIS of the lower extremities, a 93% cure rate was attained using imiquimod 5% cream once daily for up to 16 weeks.[18]

SCC

Imiquimod is not recommended for the treatment of invasive SCC. In a case report and case series, Marin-Garcia[19] achieved optimal results with nightly applications 5 to 7 times weekly for 12 weeks. However, follow-up of these patients was limited. Therefore, imiquimod may be a viable

Box 4
Antitumoral mechanisms of action of imiquimod

Induced production of cytokines, including interferon (IFN)-α, tumor necrosis factor (TNF)-α, interleukin (IL)-1, IL-2, IL-6, IL-8, and IL-12, by human peripheral blood mononuclear cells

Stimulation of monocytes, macrophages, and toll-like receptor (TLR)-7- and TLR-8-bearing plasmacytoid dendritic cells, and epidermal Langerhans cells. Stimulation of TLRs induces the production of proinflammatory cytokines involved in the innate immune system

Production of IL-6, IL-8, and IFN-α by keratinocytes, leading to a T_H1-dominant response

Increase in type I IFN, improving the response to endogenous IFN-α, usually low in AKs

Suppression of type I IFN signaling proteins, which is an early event leading to SCC

Induction of FasR (CD95), a member of the TNF receptor family, involved in apoptosis

Induction of proapoptotic pathways associated with B-cell lymphoma/leukemia 2 (Bcl-2)–associated X (Bax) protein

Induction of caspases 3 and 9, which have been linked to stress signaling, mitochondrial death pathways, and apoptosis

Induction of E-selectin (a ligand for lymphocyte antigen expressed by skin-resident T cells that are responsible for immunosurveillance) on blood vessels of invasive SCCs, which is usually absent in SCCs

Reduction of T-regulatory cells, which express FOXP3, infiltrating SCCs. These T-regulatory cells cause impairment of effector T cells (responsible for immunosurveillance), surround the tumor, and prevent cells from reaching the tumor

treatment option in patients who refuse surgery or are not good surgical candidates.

5-Fluorouracil

5-Fluorouracil (5-FU) is a structural analogue of thymine that inhibits thymidylate synthetase, a critical enzyme in DNA synthesis. 5-FU prevents cellular proliferation, ultimately resulting in cell death. The effects are most pronounced in rapidly dividing cells. 5-FU has been used to treat various malignancies, including breast cancer, colorectal cancer, and tumors of the head and neck.[20] The use of 5-FU as a topical agent began after a case report describing resolution of AKs in a patient receiving systemic 5-FU.[21]

In 1963, a hydrophilic ointment of 20% 5-FU was initially used in the treatment of patients with diffuse AKs for 4 weeks.[22] Further studies testing multiple concentrations of 5-FU showed that the 5% ointment was comparable with the 20% ointment.[22] Since then, 5-FU has been used to treat multiple skin conditions, including extensive AKs, SCCIS, actinic cheilitis, porokeratosis, and verruca vulgaris.

The principal indication of 5-FU is for the treatment of AKs, with twice daily dosing for 1 month.[23] 5-FU is a practical alternative to treating large areas with extensive actinic damage on the face and neck without damaging normal skin. 5-FU has also been used successfully in the treatment of superficial BCC, actinic cheilitis, and Bowen disease,[24] especially when used in conjunction with other modalities such as ED&C.

The standard of care for the treatment of AKs has been with 5% 5-FU. More recently, 1.0% and 0.5% cream formulations have become available. One study showed the 0.5% formulation to be as efficacious as and better tolerated than the conventional 5% formulation.[25] The 0.5% formulation contains 5-FU in a patented porous microsphere delivery system that delivers a therapeutic dose of 5-FU while minimizing systemic absorption. 5-FU is commercially available as 1%, 2%, and 5% solutions and 0.5%, 1%, and 5% creams. The 1%, 2%, and 5% formulations should be applied twice daily, whereas the 0.5% formulation is to be used once daily. Treatment durations range from 2 to 6 weeks depending on the site treated and the patient's response and tolerability of the treatment. Patients should be instructed to avoid excessive application and to avoid sensitive areas such as the oral commissure, nasolabial creases, and eyes.

Topical 5-FU should be avoided in patients with known allergies to 5-FU and in patients who have known deficiency of dihydropyrimidine dehydrogenase (DPD), an enzyme critical in the metabolism of 5-FU.[26]

Erythema, irritation, burning sensation, pruritus, pain, hypopigmentation, and hyperpigmentation are the most common adverse effects. Symptoms are expected within the initial 5 to 10 days of treatment. Allergic contact dermatitis caused by 5-FU has also been reported.[27] An inflammatory reaction is expected, including crusting, edema, and oozing. Frequency of application or strength of 5-FU may be reduced in patients who experience severe reactions. Topical steroids may be used concomitantly and 1 to 2 weeks after treatment with topical 5-FU to reduce inflammation.[28]

Diclofenac

Diclofenac is a nonsteroidal antiinflammatory drug that is a potent inhibitor of inducible cyclooxygenase (COX) 2, resulting in a reduction of prostaglandin synthesis. COX is the rate-limiting enzyme in the synthesis of prostaglandins from arachidonic acid.[28] Increased production of prostaglandins may be associated with the development of NMSC.[29] Prostaglandin E2 plays a role in Bcl-2 gene expression, IL-6 production, and inhibition of apoptotic pathways. COX-2 has been shown to be overexpressed in a variety of different malignancies, including colon carcinoma, SCC of the esophagus, and skin cancers (AKs, melanoma, and NMSC). It is thought that by inhibiting COX-2, tumor growth can be slowed via inhibition of angiogenesis, apoptosis, and tumor invasion.[30] By the same principle, multiple UV-induced proinflammatory cytokines, such as IL-1, TNF-α, and transforming growth factor β also capable of inducing COX-2, may be inhibited by diclofenac. Hyaluronic acid 2.5% vehicle gel decreases the diffusion of diclofenac through the skin and subsequently increases the contact time with the epidermis, thereby increasing uptake of diclofenac by the atypical cells.[31] Topical diclofenac 3% gel has been used successfully in the treatment of AKs and is usually well tolerated. In one study, twice-daily application for 60 to 90 days was shown to decrease the number of AKs by 64%, and 33% of patients had complete clearance.[30]

Retinoids

All-trans retinoic acid (tretinoin) was the first topical retinoid studied and found to be beneficial in the treatment of AKs. Tretinoin has been shown to reduce the number of AKs on facial skin by up to 50% when used as monotherapy over a period of 6 months.[32] However, there was no significant improvement of lesions on the scalp and extremities.[32] Tretinoin may also be used in combination with 5-FU in the treatment of AKs.[32] Use of tretinoin leads to enhanced penetration of 5-FU and enhanced efficacy.

Tazarotene is a prodrug that is hydrolyzed in the tissue to form the active metabolite, tazaratenic acid. Tazarotenic acid has a high affinity for the retinoic acid receptor γ nuclear receptor in the epidermis. By binding to this receptor, cell proliferation and differentiation is regulated. A few small studies have shown tazarotene to be an effective treatment of NMSC. Peris and colleagues[33] achieved 53% clearance, 47% decreased size, and no tumor progression in a cohort of patients treated for BCC with 0.1% tazarotene gel once daily for 5 to 8 months.

Side effects include erythema, burning sensation, and pruritus. Tazarotene is a pregnancy category X medication and should be avoided in pregnant patients,[34–36] whereas tretinoin is a pregnancy category C medication. Caution must be taken in patients who continue to have significant sun exposure.

The use of systemic retinoids in high-risk patient populations has been shown to be effective in the chemoprevention of NMSC.[37,38] An in-depth discussion of systemic retinoids in organ transplant patients may be found in an article elsewhere in this issue.

Newer Topical Agents

Ingenol mebutate

Ingenol mebutate (IM) is an extract from the plant *Euphorbia peplus* (milkweed), which has been used for several years as a home remedy treatment of skin conditions, including AKs and skin cancers.[39] IM is thought to work by disrupting the plasma membrane, leading to mitochondrial swelling of dysplastic keratinocytes and subsequent cell death. IM also promotes healing and restoration of the normal clinical and histologic morphology.[39] Further generation of tumor-specific antibodies, along with proinflammatory cytokines and neutrophil infiltration, results in antibody-dependent cellular cytotoxicity that eliminates residual cells.[40] IM comes in formulations of 0.025% and 0.050%. Several controlled studies have shown IM to be efficacious in the treatment of AKs.[41,42] IM is generally well tolerated. Adverse effects include mild erythema, scaling, and crusting.

Resiquimod

Resiquimod is a TLR 7/8 agonist that has comparable stimulatory effects on monocytic cells, although it is 10- to 100-times more potent than imiquimod.[43–45] In addition, resiquimod induces IL-1 receptor antagonist, granulocyte/macrophage colony-stimulating factor, granulocyte colony-stimulating factor, macrophage inflammatory protein, macrophage inflammatory protein 1β, inflammatory protein 1α, and monocyte chemotactic protein.[45] One phase 2 study consisting of 132 patients showed an efficacy of 40.0% to 74.2% in the treatment of AKs when treating 4 to 8 lesions on the scalp with various concentrations of resiquimod 3 times weekly. There was no difference in efficacy among the various concentrations, but lower concentrations produced better tolerability.[46]

EMERGING NONSURGICAL MODALITIES
Chemical Peels

Chemical peeling is defined as the application of a topical agent to the skin, resulting in a variable degree of injury to the epidermis and dermis. The depth of penetration depends on the type and strength of the chemical. In general, superficial peels cause epidermal injury and sometimes extend into the superficial papillary dermis, medium-depth peels cause injury through the papillary dermis to the upper reticular dermis, and deep peels affect the midreticular dermis. Chemical peels have been shown to reduce AKs lesions by up to 75%. Chemical peels are effective in the treatment and prevention of AKs. Once-daily application of a medium-depth peel, such as Jessner solution (**Table 2**) followed by 35% trichloroacetic acid, was shown to be as safe and efficacious as twice-daily application of 5% 5-FU cream for 3 weeks.[47]

Chemical peels are a reasonable alternative in patients with poor compliance with diffuse actinic damage. Disadvantages include prolonged healing time and risk of secondary infection. The procedure is also considered elective and is unlikely to be covered by insurance.

Lasers

Laser ablation with either CO_2 or erbium:YAG has been shown to reduce the number of AKs by up to 94% in several studies.[48,49] Lasers induce coagulative necrosis, hyperthermia, and ablation leading to tumor destruction. Large areas can be treated with the potential for cosmetic rejuvenation. Laser ablation has also been shown to be effective in both the treatment and prevention of NMSCs.[50–52] However, laser treatment of SCC and BCC is limited by the need to keep treatment superficial secondary to risk of scarring. Treatment with laser also causes nonspecific thermal damage, making it difficult to elucidate the extent of tumor being treated.

Intralesional Therapy

Although intralesional therapy is not widely used, various agents have been used successfully in the treatment of primary cutaneous malignancies when delivered intralesionally. Intralesional therapy can be used to treat many lesions

Table 2 Jessner solution	
Resorcinol	14 g
Salicylic acid	14 g
85% lactic acid	14 g
95% ethanol (qs ad)	100 mL

Abbreviation: qs ad, a sufficient quantity to make.

simultaneously, provides good cosmesis, and can be done quickly with very little downtime. However, the effectiveness of this treatment modality is unknown, injections can be painful, medications are costly, and the patients require multiple treatment visits.

5-FU
The use of topical 5-FU for the treatment of AKs and NMSC is well established. 5-FU has also been shown to be efficacious in the treatment of BCC and SCC when delivered intralesionally. Treatment intervals are usually once weekly. Thorough and complete infiltration of the tumor is essential. If clinical necrosis of the tumor is not appreciated in 2 to 3 weeks, an alternative treatment should be considered.[53] A multicentered open-label study and a multicenter, randomized, open-label study demonstrated 100% eradication of BCCs when treated with 0.5 mL of 5-FU/epi gel 3 times weekly for 2 weeks.[54] Another study showed a cure rate of 96% of SCC treated once weekly for up to 6 weeks.[53] Although treatment with intralesional 5-FU shows promise, further study is needed.

Bleomycin
Bleomycin is named for a group of sulfur-containing glycopeptide cytotoxic antibiotics derived from *Streptomyces verticillus* and has been shown to have antiviral, antitumoral, and antibacterial effects.[55,56] Bleomycin affects the G_2 and S phases of rapidly dividing cells, leading to breakage of single-stranded DNA, inhibiting DNA repair by the inhibition of DNA ligase, causing apoptosis and subsequent epidermal necrosis. Although bleomycin is most commonly used to treat warts, treatment with intralesional bleomycin has also been described as an effective treatment of multiple BCCs.[57] Side effects include local pain, burning sensation, and potential tissue necrosis at the injection site. Raynaud phenomenon has been described after the treatment of lesions on the distal fingers and remains localized to the digits being treated.[58,59] Because of the pain associated with the injection of bleomycin, many clinicians anesthetize the area of treatment before injection.

IFN-α
IFN-α has been shown to be effective in treating BCC and SCC. The postulated mechanism is unclear, but it is thought to induce apoptosis of tumor cells via CD95 receptor-ligand interaction, inducing infiltration of cytotoxic lymphocytes.[60] Kim and coworkers[61] demonstrated complete clearance in a case series of patients treated with intralesional IFN-α for BCC and SCC with 1×10^6 to 2×10^6 IU 3 times weekly for 3 weeks.

There was no sign of recurrence at 33 months. Adverse events include fatigue, fever, myalgia, anorexia, nausea, vomiting, and headache.

PDT

PDT is a relatively new treatment that is FDA approved for the treatment of nonhypertrophic AKs of the head and scalp. PDT has also been used off-label in the treatment of various other dermatoses (Box 5) as well as NMSC (Table 3) and has become an emerging alternative for nonaggressive tumors in poor surgical candidates.

PDT involves the application of a topical photosensitizer that, when metabolized and activated by exposure to a light source, leads to destruction of neoplastic cells. Two hematoporphyrin derivatives, δ-aminolevulinic acid (ALA) and methyl aminolevulinate (MAL), have been used as topical photosensitizers. These two molecules are small enough to pass though the epidermis. ALA was developed in the United States, where MAL was primarily used in Europe until recently. MAL is approved in Europe for the treatment of AKs, BCC, and SCCIS. After topical application, the photosensitizer is preferentially taken up by the neoplastic, more metabolically active cells and converted to protoporphyrin IX. Protoporphyrin IX has absorption bands at 408, 510, 543, 583, and 633 nm; therefore, multiple light sources, including blue light, red light, intense pulsed light, and pulsed dye laser, has been used with success.

Box 5
PDT for NMSC

FDA approved

AKs (nonhypertrophic AKs of the head and scalp)

Commonly used in North America and Europe

SCCIS

BCC (superficial and nodular types)

Small case series, anecdotal reports, or investigational studies

Chemoprevention of NMSC

Cutaneous B-cell lymphoma

Cutaneous T-cell lymphoma

Keratoacanthoma

Actinic cheilitis

Extramammary Paget disease

Gorlin syndrome (basal cell nevus syndrome)

Protoporphyrin IX accumulates at levels of up to 10-fold greater than in normal tissue.[62] Incubation time for ALA is variable. Initial studies used an incubation time of 14 to 18 hours. However, more recent trials have shown similar efficacy with incubation of 1 to 2 hours.[63,64] The standard incubation time for MAL is 3 hours.

Blue light (corresponding to the 408-nm band) and red light (corresponding to the 633-nm band) are the most commonly used light sources for PDT. Blue light sources demonstrate better absorption but do not penetrate the skin as well as red light sources because of their shorter wavelength.[65] Therefore, blue light may be better for superficial lesions such as AKs, whereas treatment with red light may be reserved for lesions present deeper in the dermis.[9,19] When exposed to a light source, protoporphyrin IX is activated, leading to direct damage to the cell membranes, organelles, and surrounding vasculature, as well as subsequent activation of an inflammatory cascade leading to clearance of malignant cells.[63,66,67]

AKs

PDT has become a popular and effective treatment modality for AKs. PDT has been shown to be the preferred treatment by patients when compared with cryotherapy with regard to efficacy, cosmetic outcome, and skin discomfort.[68] With regard to tolerability, PDT seems to be superior to treatment with 5-FU.[69,70] PDT offers the advantage of excellent patient compliance requiring 1 to 2 office visits as opposed to applying a cream twice daily for several weeks. The disadvantage of PDT compare with other treatment modalities include the requirement for an office visit usually lasting a few hours, cost, discomfort during the procedure, and redness and photosensitivity after the procedure. In addition, PDT is less effective in the treatment of thick hyperkeratotic AKs. However, this shortcoming can be ameliorated with light curettage or dermabrasion before the procedure to remove the overlying scale. Residual lesions after PDT should be biopsied to rule out SCC.

The efficacy of PDT in the treatment of AKs has been well documented. Clearance rates of up to 91% have been reported with ALA-PDT, with 75% to 89% clearance at 12 weeks.[64] Clearance at 3 months with MAL-PDT has been shown to be around 90% using a regiment of 2 treatments 1 week apart.[71–73] The efficacy of ALA-PDT has been shown to be similar to or greater than that of cryotherapy.[71] The efficacy of ALA-PDT seems to be similar to that of 5-FU.[69,70] Regarding the long-term efficacy of ALA-PDT, a multicenter trial

Table 3
Treatment regimens for PDT

Tumor Type	Photosensitizer	Treatment Regimen	Results	References
AKs	ALA	1 treatment followed by a second treatment at 8 wk if necessary	91% clearance, with 75%–89% clearance at 12 wk	Piacquadio et al,[64] Tschen et al[74]
	MAL (3 h incubation)	2 treatments, 1 wk apart	89%–91%	Freeman et al,[71] Tarstedt et al,[72] Pariser et al[73]
	MAL (1 h incubation)	2 treatments; 1 wk apart	74 (thin lesions), 78% thick hyperkeratotic lesions	Braathen et al[9]
Superficial BCC	ALA	1 treatment	79%–99%	Morton et al,[10] Blume & Oseroff,[66] Clark et al,[82] Kennedy et al[83]
	MAL	1 treatment followed by a second treatment at 12 wk if necessary	97%	Braathen et al,[9] Basset-Seguin et al[84]
Nodular BCC	ALA	1–2 treatments	59%–92%	Caekelbergh et al[85]
	MAL	2 treatments, 1 wk apart	73%–91%	Soler et al,[86] Tope et al,[87] Foley et al[88]
SCCIS	ALA	1 treatment followed by a second treatment at 2 mo if necessary	75%–88% (100% clearance with 2 treatments)	Salim et al,[89] Morton et al[10]
	MAL	2 treatments, 1 wk apart	93% 73% at 3 mo, 53% at 2 y	Morton et al[10] Calzavara-Pinton et al[90]

Abbreviations: ALA, 5-aminolevulinic acid; MAL, methyl aminolevulinate.

demonstrated a recurrence rate of 19% for histologically proven AKs over a 12-month period.[74]

SCCIS

Several large randomized trials have shown both ALA-PDT and MAL-PDT to be effective in the treatment of SCCIS. A randomized controlled trial found MAL-PDT, with a 3-month clearance rate to be 93%, superior to both cryosurgery (86% clearance) and topical 5-FU (83% clearance). The recurrence rate at 1 year was 15% for the PDT-treated lesions, which was similar to that of lesions treated by 5-FU (17%) and cryotherapy (21%).[10] Cosmetic outcomes are better than 5-FU initially but equivalent at 1-year follow-up.[10] Regarding ALA-PDT, 2 treatments approximately 8 weeks apart seem to be the most effective regimen for complete clearance.[75] For thicker lesions, a longer wavelength (ie, MAL-PDT) may be more suitable.

MAL-PDT is approved for the treatment of SCCIS in Europe and is used as a first-line treatment in many cases. Long-term clearance rates with surgical excision still remain higher than nonsurgical interventions.[76] However, PDT may be a valuable treatment option for poor surgical candidates with larger lesions in a difficult anatomic location.[77–79]

SCC

Because of the invasive nature and risk of metastasis with SCC, PDT is not recommended.[9]

Superficial BCC

PDT is a viable and effective option for the treatment of superficial BCC, especially in instances in which surgical treatment carries a high risk of complication or result in an unsatisfactory cosmetic outcome.[9] The optimal treatment protocol is uncertain. Most protocols use MAL-PDT and consist of 1 or 2 treatment sessions 1 week apart, with retreatment at 2 to 3 months if necessary. Light curettage or other physical debridement is done before treatment. Clearance rates are similar to those of other nonsurgical modalities.

Nodular BCC

MAL-PDT is approved in Europe for the treatment of nodular BCC. Treatment consists of debulking the tumor, followed by 2 treatments 7 days apart with retreatment at 3 months if warranted. ALA-PDT is not recommended for the treatment of nodular BCC at this time.[9]

Oral Capecitabine

Capecitabine is an oral fluoropyrimidine carbamate that is converted predominantly in tumor cells to 5-FU by a thymidine phosphorylase (tumor-associated angiogenic factor, dThdPase). 5-FU is catabolized by DPD into an inactive metabolite. The susceptibility of tumor cells to 5-vFU therapy depends on the ratio of activity of DPD and dThdPase. Capecitabine is approved for the treatment of colorectal carcinoma and metastatic breast cancer.

Wollina and colleagues[80] reported 4 patients with advanced SCC of the skin who were treated with oral capecitabine and IFN subcutaneously, resulting in complete remission in 2 patients and partial response in the other 2. IFN acts synergistically by causing a forced accumulation of 5-FU in tumor cells as a result of stimulation of dThdPase. Cartei and colleagues[81] reported 14 patients with cutaneous SCC treated with oral capecitabine, resulting in 2 partial remissions and 3 minimal remissions. Further evaluation and validation by prospective trials is warranted.

SUMMARY

Although surgical modalities remain the mainstay of treatment of NMSC, many nonsurgical options have emerged as viable alternatives in patients who are poor surgical candidates or have diffuse disease in difficult locations. The dermatologic surgeon should be knowledgeable and have a thorough understanding of all treatment options to assist the patient in making the most informed decision possible, ultimately leading to an optimal outcome.

REFERENCES

1. Werlinger Kd, Upton G, Moore Ay. Recurrence rates of primary nonmelanoma skin cancers treated by surgical excision compared to electrodessication-curettage in a private dermatological practice. Dermatol Surg 2002;28(12):1138–42 [discussion: 1142].
2. Silverman MK, Kopf AW, Gladstein AH, et al. Recurrence rates of treated basal cell carcinomas. Part 4: x-ray therapy. J Dermatol Surg Oncol 1992;18(7):549–54.
3. Sheridan AT, Dawber RP. Curettage, electrosurgery and skin cancer. Australas J Dermatol 2000;41(1):19–30.
4. Ahmed I, Berth-Jones J, Charles-Holmes S, et al. Comparison of cryotherapy with curettage in the treatment of Bowen's disease: a prospective study. Br J Dermatol 2000;143(4):759–66.
5. Wang I, Bendsoe N, Klinteberg CA, et al. Photodynamic therapy vs. cryosurgery of basal cell carcinomas: results of a phase III clinical trial. Br J Dermatol 2001;144(4):832–40.
6. Bath-Hextall FJ, Perkins W, Bong J, et al. Interventions for basal cell carcinoma of the skin. Cochrane Database Syst Rev 2007;1:CD003412.
7. Hall VL, Leppard BJ, Mcgill J, et al. Treatment of basal-cell carcinoma: comparison of radiotherapy and cryotherapy. Clin Radiol 1986;37(1):33–4.
8. Thissen MR, Nieman FH, Ideler AH, et al. Cosmetic results of cryosurgery versus surgical excision for primary uncomplicated basal cell carcinomas of the head and neck. Dermatol Surg 2000;26(8):759–64.
9. Braathen LR, Szeimies RM, Basset-Seguin N, et al. Guidelines on the use of photodynamic therapy for nonmelanoma skin cancer: an international consensus. International Society for Photodynamic Therapy in Dermatology, 2005. J Am Acad Dermatol 2007;56(1):125–43.
10. Morton C, Horn M, Leman J, et al. Comparison of topical methyl aminolevulinate photodynamic therapy with cryotherapy or fluorouracil for treatment of squamous cell carcinoma in situ: results of a multicenter randomized trial. Arch Dermatol 2006;142(6):729–35.
11. Hadley G, Derry S, Moore RA. Imiquimod for actinic keratosis: systematic review and meta-analysis. J Invest Dermatol 2006;126(6):1251–5.
12. Swanson N, Abramovits W, Berman B, et al. Imiquimod 2.5% and 3.75% for the treatment of actinic keratoses: results of two placebo-controlled studies of daily application to the face and balding scalp for two 2-week cycles. J Am Acad Dermatol 2010;62(4):582–90.
13. Marks R, Gebauer K, Shumack S, et al. Imiquimod 5% cream in the treatment of superficial basal cell carcinoma: results of a multicenter 6-week dose-response trial. J Am Acad Dermatol 2001;44(5):807–13.
14. Geisse JK, Rich P, Pandya A, et al. Imiquimod 5% cream for the treatment of superficial basal cell carcinoma: a double-blind, randomized, vehicle-controlled study. J Am Acad Dermatol 2002;47(3):390–8.

15. Quirk C, Gebauer K, De'Ambrosis B, et al. Sustained clearance of superficial basal cell carcinomas treated with imiquimod cream 5%: results of a prospective 5-year study. Cutis 2010;85(6):318–24.

16. Huber A, Huber JD, Skinner RB Jr, et al. Topical imiquimod treatment for nodular basal cell carcinomas: an open-label series. Dermatol Surg 2004;30(3):429–30.

17. Shumack S, Robinson J, Kossard S, et al. Efficacy of topical 5% imiquimod cream for the treatment of nodular basal cell carcinoma: comparison of dosing regimens. Arch Dermatol 2002;138(9):1165–71.

18. Mackenzie-Wood A, Kossard S, De Launey J, et al. Imiquimod 5% cream in the treatment of Bowen's disease. J Am Acad Dermatol 2001;44(3):462–70.

19. Martin-Garcia RF. Imiquimod: an effective alternative for the treatment of invasive cutaneous squamous cell carcinoma. Dermatol Surg 2005;31(3):371–4.

20. Longley DB, Harkin DP, Johnston PG. 5-Fluorouracil: mechanisms of action and clinical strategies. Nat Rev Cancer 2003;3(5):330–8.

21. Falkson G, Schulz EJ. Skin changes in patients treated with 5-fluorouracil. Br J Dermatol 1962;74:229–36.

22. Dillaha CJ, Jansen GT, Honeycutt WM, et al. Selective cytotoxic effect of topical 5-fluorouracil. Arch Dermatol 1963;88:247–56.

23. Drake LA, Ceilley RI, Cornelison RL, et al. Guidelines of care for actinic keratoses. Committee on Guidelines of Care. J Am Acad Dermatol 1995;32(1):95–8.

24. Bargman H, Hochman J. Topical treatment of Bowen's disease with 5-fluorouracil. J Cutan Med Surg 2003;7(2):101–5.

25. Loven K, Stein L, Furst K, et al. Evaluation of the efficacy and tolerability of 0.5% fluorouracil cream and 5% fluorouracil cream applied to each side of the face in patients with actinic keratosis. Clin Ther 2002;24(6):990–1000.

26. Johnson MR, Hageboutros A, Wang K, et al. Life-threatening toxicity in a dihydropyrimidine dehydrogenase-deficient patient after treatment with topical 5-fluorouracil. Clin Cancer Res 1999;5(8):2006–11.

27. Goette DK, Odom RB, Arrott JW, et al. Treatment of keratoacanthoma with topical application of fluorouracil. Arch Dermatol 1982;118(5):309–11.

28. Peters DC, Foster RH. Diclofenac/hyaluronic acid. Drugs Aging 1999;14(4):313–9 [discussion: 320–1].

29. Marks F, Furstenberger G, Muller-Decker K. Metabolic targets of cancer chemoprevention: interruption of tumor development by inhibitors of arachidonic acid metabolism. Recent Results Cancer Res 1999;151:45–67.

30. Masferrer JL, Leahy KM, Koki AT, et al. Antiangiogenic and antitumor activities of cyclooxygenase-2 inhibitors. Cancer Res 2000;60(5):1306–11.

31. Berman B, Villa AM, Ramirez CC. Mechanisms of action of new treatment modalities for actinic keratosis. J Drugs Dermatol 2006;5(2):167–73.

32. Tutrone WD, Saini R, Caglar S, et al. Topical therapy for actinic keratoses, II: diclofenac, colchicine, and retinoids. Cutis 2003;71(5):373–9.

33. Peris K, Fargnoli MC, Chimenti S. Preliminary observations on the use of topical tazarotene to treat basal-cell carcinoma. N Engl J Med 1999;341(23):1767–8.

34. Weinstein GD, Koo JY, Krueger GG, et al. Tazarotene cream in the treatment of psoriasis: two multicenter, double-blind, randomized, vehicle-controlled studies of the safety and efficacy of tazarotene creams 0.05% and 0.1% applied once daily for 12 weeks. J Am Acad Dermatol 2003;48(5):760–7.

35. Marks R. Pharmacokinetics and safety review of tazarotene. J Am Acad Dermatol 1998;39(4 Pt 2):S134–8.

36. Weinstein GD, Krueger GG, Lowe NJ, et al. Tazarotene gel, a new retinoid, for topical therapy of psoriasis: vehicle-controlled study of safety, efficacy, and duration of therapeutic effect. J Am Acad Dermatol 1997;37(1):85–92.

37. De Graaf YG, Euvrard S, Bouwes Bavinck JN. Systemic and topical retinoids in the management of skin cancer in organ transplant recipients. Dermatol Surg 2004;30(4 Pt 2):656–61.

38. Chakrabarty A, Geisse JK. Medical therapies for non-melanoma skin cancer. Clin Dermatol 2004;22(3):183–8.

39. Ogbourne SM, Suhrbier A, Jones B, et al. Antitumor activity of 3-ingenyl angelate: plasma membrane and mitochondrial disruption and necrotic cell death. Cancer Res 2004;64(8):2833–9.

40. Challacombe JM, Suhrbier A, Parsons PG, et al. Neutrophils are a key component of the antitumor efficacy of topical chemotherapy with ingenol-3-angelate. J Immunol 2006;177(11):8123–32.

41. Siller G, Gebauer K, Welburn P, et al. Pep005 (ingenol mebutate) gel, a novel agent for the treatment of actinic keratosis: results of a randomized, double-blind, vehicle-controlled, multicentre, phase IIa study. Australas J Dermatol 2009;50(1):16–22.

42. Anderson L, Schmieder GJ, Werschler WP, et al. Randomized, double-blind, double-dummy, vehicle-controlled study of ingenol mebutate gel 0.025% and 0.05% for actinic keratosis. J Am Acad Dermatol 2009;60(6):934–43.

43. Tomai MA, Gibson SJ, Imbertson LM, et al. Immunomodulating and antiviral activities of the imidazoquinoline S-28463. Antiviral Res 1995;28(3):253–64.

44. Testerman TL, Gerster JF, Imbertson LM, et al. Cytokine induction by the immunomodulators imiquimod and S-27609. J Leukoc Biol 1995;58(3):365–72.

45. Jones T. Resiquimod 3M. Curr Opin Investig Drugs 2003;4(2):214–8.

46. Szeimies RM, Bichel J, Ortonne JP, et al. A phase II dose-ranging study of topical resiquimod to treat actinic keratosis. Br J Dermatol 2008;159(1):205–10.

47. Lawrence N, Cox SE, Cockerell CJ, et al. A comparison of the efficacy and safety of Jessner's solution and 35% trichloroacetic acid vs 5% fluorouracil in the treatment of widespread facial actinic keratoses. Arch Dermatol 1995;131(2):176–81.

48. Jiang SB, Levine VJ, Nehal KS, et al. Er:YAG laser for the treatment of actinic keratoses. Dermatol Surg 2000;26(5):437–40.

49. Iyer S, Friedli A, Bowes L, et al. Full face laser resurfacing: therapy and prophylaxis for actinic keratoses and non-melanoma skin cancer. Lasers Surg Med 2004;34(2):114–9.

50. Humphreys TR, Malhotra R, Scharf MJ, et al. Treatment of superficial basal cell carcinoma and squamous cell carcinoma in situ with a high-energy pulsed carbon dioxide laser. Arch Dermatol 1998; 134(10):1247–52.

51. Hantash BM, Stewart DB, Cooper ZA, et al. Facial resurfacing for nonmelanoma skin cancer prophylaxis. Arch Dermatol 2006;142(8):976–82.

52. Iyer S, Bowes L, Kricorian G, et al. Treatment of basal cell carcinoma with the pulsed carbon dioxide laser: a retrospective analysis. Dermatol Surg 2004; 30(9):1214–8.

53. Morse LG, Kendrick C, Hooper D, et al. Treatment of squamous cell carcinoma with intralesional 5-fluorouracil. Dermatol Surg 2003;29(11):1150–3 [discussion: 1153].

54. Miller BH, Shavin JS, Cognetta A, et al. Nonsurgical treatment of basal cell carcinomas with intralesional 5-fluorouracil/epinephrine injectable gel. J Am Acad Dermatol 1997;36(1):72–7.

55. James MP, Collier PM, Aherne W, et al. Histologic, pharmacologic, and immunocytochemical effects of injection of bleomycin into viral warts. J Am Acad Dermatol 1993;28(6):933–7.

56. Munkvad M, Genner J, Staberg B, et al. Locally injected bleomycin in the treatment of warts. Dermatologica 1983;167(2):86–9.

57. Gyurova MS, Stancheva MZ, Arnaudova MN, et al. Intralesional bleomycin as alternative therapy in the treatment of multiple basal cell carcinomas. Dermatol Online J 2006;12(3):25.

58. Amer M, Diab N, Ramadan A, et al. Therapeutic evaluation for intralesional injection of bleomycin sulfate in 143 resistant warts. J Am Acad Dermatol 1988;18(6):1313–6.

59. Shumer SM, O'keefe EJ. Bleomycin in the treatment of recalcitrant warts. J Am Acad Dermatol 1983;9(1): 91–6.

60. Buechner SA, Wernli M, Harr T, et al. Regression of basal cell carcinoma by intralesional interferon-alpha treatment is mediated by Cd95 (Apo-1/Fas)-Cd95 ligand-induced suicide. J Clin Invest 1997; 100(11):2691–6.

61. Kim KH, Yavel RM, Gross VL, et al. Intralesional interferon alpha-2b in the treatment of basal cell carcinoma and squamous cell carcinoma: revisited. Dermatol Surg 2004;30(1):116–20.

62. Angell-Petersen E, Sorensen R, Warloe T, et al. Porphyrin formation in actinic keratosis and basal cell carcinoma after topical application of methyl 5-aminolevulinate. J Invest Dermatol 2006;126(2):265–71.

63. Touma D, Yaar M, Whitehead S, et al. A trial of short incubation, broad-area photodynamic therapy for facial actinic keratoses and diffuse photodamage. Arch Dermatol 2004;140(1):33–40.

64. Piacquadio DJ, Chen DM, Farber HF, et al. Photodynamic therapy with aminolevulinic acid topical solution and visible blue light in the treatment of multiple actinic keratoses of the face and scalp: investigator-blinded, phase 3, multicenter trials. Arch Dermatol 2004;140(1):41–6.

65. Garcia-Zuazaga J, Cooper KD, Baron Ed. Photodynamic therapy in dermatology: current concepts in the treatment of skin cancer. Expert Rev Anticancer Ther 2005;5(5):791–800.

66. Blume JE, Oseroff AR. Aminolevulinic acid photodynamic therapy for skin cancers. Dermatol Clin 2007; 25(1):5–14.

67. Kalisiak MS, Rao J. Photodynamic therapy for actinic keratoses. Dermatol Clin 2007;25(1):15–23.

68. Morton C, Campbell S, Gupta G, et al. Intraindividual, right-left comparison of topical methyl aminolaevulinate-photodynamic therapy and cryotherapy in subjects with actinic keratoses: a multicentre, randomized controlled study. Br J Dermatol 2006;155(5):1029–36.

69. Smith S, Piacquadio D, Morhenn V, et al. Short incubation PDT versus 5-FU in treating actinic keratoses. J Drugs Dermatol 2003;2(6):629–35.

70. Kurwa HA, Yong-Gee SA, Seed PT, et al. A randomized paired comparison of photodynamic therapy and topical 5-fluorouracil in the treatment of actinic keratoses. J Am Acad Dermatol 1999; 41(3 Pt 1):414–8.

71. Freeman M, Vinciullo C, Francis D, et al. A comparison of photodynamic therapy using topical methyl aminolevulinate (Metvix) with single cycle cryotherapy in patients with actinic keratosis: a prospective, randomized study. J Dermatolog Treat 2003;14(2):99–106.

72. Tarstedt M, Rosdahl I, Berne B, et al. A randomized multicenter study to compare two treatment regimens of topical methyl aminolevulinate (Metvix)-PDT in actinic keratosis of the face and scalp. Acta Derm Venereol 2005;85(5):424–8.

73. Pariser DM, Lowe NJ, Stewart DM, et al. Photodynamic therapy with topical methyl aminolevulinate for actinic keratosis: results of a prospective randomized multicenter trial. J Am Acad Dermatol 2003;48(2):227–32.

74. Tschen EH, Wong DS, Pariser DM, et al. Photodynamic therapy using aminolaevulinic acid for patients with

nonhyperkeratotic actinic keratoses of the face and scalp: phase iv multicentre clinical trial with 12-month follow up. Br J Dermatol 2006;155(6):1262–9.

75. Morton CA, Whitehurst C, Moseley H, et al. Comparison of photodynamic therapy with cryotherapy in the treatment of Bowen's disease. Br J Dermatol 1996;135(5):766–71.

76. Thestrup-Pedersen K, Ravnborg L, Reymann F. Morbus Bowen. A description of the disease in 617 patients. Acta Derm Venereol 1988;68(3):236–9.

77. Ball SB, Dawber RP. Treatment of cutaneous Bowen's disease with particular emphasis on the problem of lower leg lesions. Australas J Dermatol 1998;39(2):63–8 [quiz: 69–70].

78. Morton CA. Methyl aminolevulinate: actinic keratoses and Bowen's disease. Dermatol Clin 2007; 25(1):81–7.

79. Morton CA, Whitehurst C, Mccoll JH, et al. Photodynamic therapy for large or multiple patches of Bowen disease and basal cell carcinoma. Arch Dermatol 2001;137(3):319–24.

80. Wollina U, Hansel G, Koch A, et al. Oral capecitabine plus subcutaneous interferon alpha in advanced squamous cell carcinoma of the skin. J Cancer Res Clin Oncol 2005;131:300–4.

81. Cartei G, Cartei F, Interlandi G, et al. Oral 5-fluorouracil in squamous cell carcinoma of the skin in the aged. Am J Clin Oncol 2000;23:181–4.

82. Clark C, Bryden A, Dawe R, et al. Topical 5-aminolaevulinic acid photodynamic therapy for cutaneous lesions: outcome and comparison of light sources. Photodermatol Photoimmunol Photomed 2003; 19(3):134–41.

83. Kennedy JC, Pottier RH, Pross DC. Photodynamic therapy with endogenous protoporphyrin IX: basic principles and present clinical experience. J Photochem Photobiol B 1990;6(1–2):143–8.

84. Basset-Seguin N, Ibbotson SH, Emtestam L, et al. Topical methyl aminolaevulinate photodynamic therapy versus cryotherapy for superficial basal cell carcinoma: a 5 year randomized trial. Eur J Dermatol 2008;18(5):547–53.

85. Caekelbergh K, Nikkels AF, Leroy B, et al. Photodynamic therapy using methyl aminolevulinate in the management of primary superficial basal cell carcinoma: clinical and health economic outcomes. J Drugs Dermatol 2009;8(11):992–6.

86. Soler AM, Warloe T, Berner A, et al. A follow-up study of recurrence and cosmesis in completely responding superficial and nodular basal cell carcinomas treated with methyl 5-aminolaevulinate-based photodynamic therapy alone and with prior curettage. Br J Dermatol 2001;145(3):467–71.

87. Tope WD, Menter A, El-Azhary RA, et al. Comparison of topical methyl aminolevulinate photodynamic therapy versus placebo photodynamic therapy in nodular BCC. J Eur Acad Dermatol Venereol 2004; 18(Suppl 2):413–4.

88. Foley P, Freeman M, Menter A, et al. Photodynamic therapy with methyl aminolevulinate for primary nodular basal cell carcinoma: results of two randomized studies. Int J Dermatol 2009;48(11):1236–45.

89. Salim A, Leman JA, McColl JH, et al. Randomized comparison of photodynamic therapy with topical 5-fluorouracil in Bowen's disease. Br J Dermatol 2003;148(3):539–43.

90. Calzavara-Pinton PG, Venturini M, Sala R, et al. Methylaminolaevulinate-based photodynamic therapy of Bowen's disease and squamous cell carcinoma. Br J Dermatol 2008;159(1):137–44.

Special Considerations for Mohs Micrographic Surgery on the Eyelids, Lips, Genitalia, and Nail Unit

Kyle L. Horner, MD, MS, Christopher C. Gasbarre, DO*

KEYWORDS

• Mohs • Eyelid • Lip • Genitalia • Nail

The American Academy of Dermatology's *Guidelines of Care for Mohs Micrographic Surgery* were developed to promote the continued delivery of quality care to our patients by using the Mohs technique for certain tumors and on specific anatomic sites where complete removal of the tumor with maximal normal tissue preservation and the lowest recurrence risk is needed. The need to maximize normal tissue preservation on the eyelids, lips, genitalia, and nail unit apparatus is of the utmost importance for obvious reasons, including the need to maintain free margins, functional competence, and aesthetic values. Basal cell carcinomas (BCCs) may have a potentially higher risk of recurrence with other types of treatment modalities in the periorbital and perioral areas. Likewise, squamous cell carcinomas (SCCs) of the periorbital skin/canthus, genitalia, lip, and nail bed/matrix have a higher risk of local recurrence. Less common tumors that favor these areas, such as verrucous carcinoma, sebaceous carcinoma, microcystic adnexal carcinoma (MAC), extramammary Paget disease, and erythroplasia of Queyrat, may also be successfully treated with Mohs micrographic surgery (MMS).[1]

When the choice is made to proceed with MMS for tumors at these sites, there are other considerations that the prudent dermatologic surgeon must take into account to have optimal outcomes.

The unique anatomy, free margins, and specially adapted form and function at these sites must be appreciated to remove the tumor and minimize collateral damage and thus lessen any potential side effects for the patient. Often, specialized instruments may be needed to work on these locations. These sites may contain transitions between thicker, hair-bearing skin and thin glabrous skin, with more laxity, which can sometimes challenge the inexperienced surgeon to remove the layers without damage or scalpel chatter, and at an optimally consistent level. Because of the lower prevalence of skin cancers at these sites (ie, MMS may not be performed so frequently in these anatomic locations), the occurrence of rare tumors, and given the unique histology of mucosal skin and nail matrix, the pathology on frozen sections, can be more difficult to interpret. Transitions from acral skin to nail matrix, mucosal eyelid to tarsal plate to cutaneous eyelid skin, or cutaneous lip to mucosal lip can frequently require more care when positioning, embedding, and sectioning tissue specimens, so experienced Mohs histotechnicians should be used whenever possible. Because of the superficiality of skeletal muscle and generally excellent vascular supply to these areas, bleeding is always a concern when performing surgery at these sites. In particular, electrocautery/coagulation for hemostasis must be used carefully and judiciously near

The authors have nothing to disclose.
Dermatologic Surgery and Cutaneous Oncology, Cleveland Clinic Foundation, 9500 Euclid Avenue, A-61, Cleveland, OH 44195, USA
* Corresponding author.
E-mail address: gasbarc@ccf.org

Dermatol Clin 29 (2011) 311–317
doi:10.1016/j.det.2011.01.005

the cornea and nail matrix to prevent accidental scarring to the eye or permanent undue dystrophy of the future nail plate.

The remainder of this discussion details site-specific tumors amenable to MMS and also briefly mentions pertinent anatomy, site-specific instruments, potential adverse outcomes, and repair options for these locations. Many books and journal articles cover these subjects in more depth.[2–10]

EYELIDS/PERIORBITAL

The eyelids are composed of cutaneous skin (<1 mm thick), orbicularis oculi muscle, the tarsal plate, and the conjunctiva.[6] At the eyelid margin the skin tightly adheres to the tarsal plate. In the vertical dimension the inferior tarsal plate is 3 to 5 mm tall and the superior tarsal plate is 10 to 12 mm high.[11] The tarsal plates connect to the bony orbital rim by the medial and lateral canthal ligaments. These ligaments can be cut intentionally for more laxity if needed (eg, for a large wedge repair), or sutured to different areas of the orbital rim to perform a canthopexy. The lacrimal gland with its canaliculi sits in the superior and lateral area of the upper eyelid, and the lacrimal caruncle, canaliculi, and sac are located in the medial/inferior canthus area.[2] If these features are inadvertently damaged during surgery they can cause dry or watery eyes, respectively.

Specialized tools used for MMS on the eyelids include, but are not limited to, corneal shields (we favor plastic shields over the metal ones used for laser to eliminate the risk of inadvertent damage to the cornea and sclera during electrocoagulation), chalazion clamps, small curved iris scissors, Castroviejo scissors and needle holder, Bishop-Harmon forceps, Stevens tenotomy or gradle scissors, micro/beaver blades, 15-c scalpel blades, and micro-tipped/fine-tipped, Teflon-coated, electrosurgery tips.

Approximately 5% to 10% of skin cancers occur in the periocular region (Table 1).[12] Risk factors for periocular neoplasms include advancing age, fair skin, family history, and chronic sun exposure.[13] The most common malignancies are BCC (90%), sebaceous carcinoma (5%), SCC (4%), followed by malignant melanoma (1%), lymphoma, Kaposi sarcoma, MAC, and rarely Merkel cell carcinoma (Box 1).[13–17] BCCs (~70% of the time), SCCs (~68%), and melanoma (~57%) occur more commonly on the lower lid.[18–20] On the other hand, sebaceous carcinoma occurs on the upper eyelid 63% of the time because the upper eyelid has more sebaceous glands than the lower lid.[15] Most BCCs and SCCs involve the lower eyelid, followed by the medial canthus or upper eyelid and

then lateral canthus.[13,20] Eyelid BCCs, SCCs, sebaceous carcinoma, and Merkel cell carcinoma have all been treated with traditional frozen section MMS, and malignant melanoma has been treated with modified slow Mohs with paraffin-embedded tissue, all with lower recurrence rates versus surgical excision (Table 2).[14,18,21,22]

Adverse outcomes that may occur whenever surgery is attempted on the eyelids include the normal complications seen in any skin surgery repair such as scarring, dehiscence, flap failure

Table 1 Percentage of skin cancers by anatomic site	
Periorbital/eyelids	5–10
Lips	3–4
Penis	0.5 (of all cancers)
Vulva	1 (of all cancers in women)
Nail unit	~0.3

Data from Refs.[12,26,31,32]

Box 1
Tumors amenable to MMS by anatomic site

Periocular/eyelids

BCC

SCC

Sebaceous carcinoma

Melanoma in situ

MAC

Merkel cell carcinoma

Lips

BCC

SCC

SCC in situ

MAC

Genitalia

SCC

BCC

Extramammary Paget disease

Dermatofibrosarcoma protuberans

Granular cell tumor

Nail unit

SCC

Keratoacanthoma

Melanoma in situ

or graft necrosis, hematoma, and infection. Site-specific complications may include ectropion, trichiasis, lagophthalmos, ptosis, keratoconjunctivitis, sicca, watery eye, webbing, entropion, and orbital hemorrhage.[13,23]

Repair options for Mohs defects on the eyelids or periocular skin include, but are not limited to, secondary intention healing, direct closure, grafting, pentagonal excision with direct closure, lateral canthotomy and inferior cantholysis with direct closure, Tenzel semicircular advancement flap, Mustardé laterally based cheek rotation flap, Hughes tarsoconjunctival flap, hinge flap with or without cheek advancement flap, Cutler-Beard bridge flap, glabellar flap, forehead flap, and the spiral flap.[6,24]

It is important to consult or refer to oculoplastic colleagues when a repair is beyond the skill or expertise of the Mohs surgeon. If the Mohs surgeon is comfortable performing the repair, it is important to pay close attention to suturing technique, placing any sutures or knots on the cutaneous side of the eyelid, including throwing the deep sutures with the knots facing outward and away from the cornea so as to not cause abrasion and resultant scar. This technique is counter to the typical dermal buried suture technique. Here, suture is passed through the wound edge superficial to deep and deep to superficial so that the knot is more superficial and not buried toward the cornea. It is also important to close the muscle layer and cutaneous layers, paying attention to tarsal plate alignment. The mucosal side can be closed via a buried or subcuticular suture; however, if the muscle and cutaneous eyelid are well approximated, the mucosal eyelid often heals nicely by secondary intent. If necessary, a Frost suture (a horizontal mattress through the lower lid taped to the superior brow) may be used to reduce downward traction and possible cicatricial ectropion.[25] Proper eye patches when needed and good postoperative wound care instructions for the patient can help put the patient at ease and alleviate their fear before leaving the office.

LIPS

The lips encompass the cutaneous upper and lower lips, the white roll (where the cutaneous lip joins the vermillion), the vermillion, the red line (where the vermillion joins the mucosal lip), and the mucosa. The orbicularis oris muscle is contained within the lips and the inferior labial artery lies just posterior and inferior to the red line on the mucosal side of the lower lip. Likewise the superior labial artery is superior and posterior to the red line on the mucosal side of the upper lip. Both of these arteries run between the orbicularis

Table 2
Recurrence rates by site: MMS Versus WLE

Site	Tumor	MMS (%)	Median or Mean Follow-up (Years)	WLE (%)	Median or Mean Follow-up (Years)	References
Periorbital	SCC	0–3.6	2.75–5	6+	2.6–4	13,18,45
Periorbital	BCC	0–2	5	5–26	2.6–4	13,21,23,46,47
Periorbital	Melanoma in situ	0–5	2–5	21–25	2–5	17
Periorbital	Sebaceous carcinoma	11–12	3.1	9–36	5	17,22,48
Periorbital	MAC	5–12	5	40–60	Variable	17
Lip	SCC	0–8	5	10+	Variable	27–29
Lip	BCC	0–3	3–5	12.5	2.6	28,49
Genitalia	Extramammary Paget disease	16–23	3.25–5	31–61	Variable	37
Penis	SCC	5.9–32	Variable	3–30	Variable	31,39
Vulva	SCC	27	Variable	38	2.6	36,50
Nail unit	SCC	4–8	5	5 (WLE) 56 (LSE)	<3	40,51
Nail unit	Melanoma	21	7.7	0–11 (with amputation)	Variable	44

Abbreviation: LSE, limited surgical excision.

oris muscle and the mucosal lining of the inner lip.[8] Direct pressure by an able-bodied assistant on both sides of the proposed surgical field achieves excellent hemostasis with minimal discomfort to the patient. Alternatively a large chalazion or similar clamp(s) can be applied to achieve hemostasis. Precise realignment of the white roll, vermillion, and red line are necessary for an optimal cosmetic outcome because even the layperson's eye is adept at recognizing uneven lines on the lips.

The lip does not normally require specialized instrumentation for Mohs; however, we have used a dental roll or tightly rolled gauze behind the lip (between the mucosal lip and teeth/gums) to evert the lip and serve as a more rigid backing support, so precise cuts can be delivered with the scalpel. This strategy also serves to catch any blood that may go into the patient's mouth, with potentially off-putting tastes or sensation. It is important to use a soft suture such as fast gut or silk on the vermillion or mucosal lip, so as to decrease the discomfort of a rigid suture end irritating surrounding tissue postoperatively.

Lip carcinomas account for only about 0.6% of all cancers (3%–4% of all skin cancers), with women affected by mostly upper lip tumors (75%) and men affected by mostly lower lip tumors (74%) (see **Table 1**).[26,27] On the upper lip, BCCs are the most common, followed by SCCs, SCC in situ, and MAC, whereas on the lower lip, SCC is more common followed by BCC and SCC in situ (see **Box 1**).[27,28] The nodal metastatic rate for lip SCC can be as high as 13.7% to 20%, and the 5-year survival with metastases to the lymph nodes is 50% or less in most studies.[27,29] MMS recurrence rates for both SCCs and BCCs treated on the lips are lower than with wide local excision (WLE) (see **Table 2**).

Repair options for partial thickness defects on the lips may include secondary intention healing, mucosal advancement flaps, surgical vermilionectomy, linear closure, and V to Y and A to T flaps. For deeper defects into or through the orbicularis oris muscle or for full-thickness defects, wedge resections and cross-lip (eg, Abbe) flaps can be used.[30]

Functional complications occurring from lip surgery can include pain, bleeding, difficulty eating, long-lasting dysesthesias, or dysphonia.[30] In men, the coarse beard terminal hairs can be inadvertently brought closer to the vermillion lip during reconstruction, causing irritation to the opposing lip.[3] Aesthetically, asymmetry or imprecise alignment of the white roll/vermillion can be seen readily by even the layperson, so care must be taken to reapproximate this junction carefully.

Marking the white line with a surgical marker before anesthesia or scoring it superficially with a scalpel after anesthesia (which does not scar and does not rub off) are effective ways to denote this critical aesthetic line, making the reapproximation easier during the reconstructive phase. Also, mucosal advancement flaps can cause mismatch in color and feminization of the lip in men.[30]

GENITALIA

The female external genitalia consist of the mons pubis, prepuce of the clitoris, glans of the clitoris, external urethral orifice, Skene duct openings, vestibule of the vagina, Bartholin gland duct openings, labia minora, labia majora, and the perineal raphe. The male external genitalia encompass the penile shaft, neck and corona of the glans, opening of the Tyson glands, the foreskin (if uncircumcised), the glans, the external urethral orifice, the scrotum, and the perineal raphe. On the dorsal side of the penile shaft lie the superficial dorsal vein, the lateral superficial veins, the deep dorsal vein, and the dorsal arteries and nerves.[2,10,31]

For the Mohs surgeon, few special instruments are needed for genital surgery. Because of the delicate nature of the skin in some areas, a sharp pair of curved iris scissors or Castroviejo scissors may be used to remove the layers. Urethral sounds or catheters may be introduced into the urethra for some protection and stabilization if necessary. Copious antiseptics and postoperative antibiotics should be used in these areas because they are more prone to surgical postoperative infections. Lidocaine with epinephrine has been used on the penis without side effects or complications and helps with hemostasis, which can be difficult secondary to its vascular nature.

In the United States, the incidence of penile cancer is approximately 0.5% of all cancers, but in underdeveloped countries it can be as high as 20%.[31] Vulvar cancers account for 1% of all malignancies in women (see **Table 1**).[32] For both men and women, SCC accounts for most genital cancers (>95%) with BCCs, extramammary Paget disease, melanoma, verrucous carcinoma, dermatofibrosarcoma protuberans, and granular cell tumor accounting for some (see **Box 1**).[33–35] Risk factors include phimosis, chronic inflammatory conditions, ultraviolet A phototherapy, and especially human papillomavirus (HPV).[35] SCC of the penis can have high recurrence rates with any penile-preserving surgery including Mohs (as high as 50%).[34] Likewise, vulvar SCC has a 23% chance of recurrence.[36] For large tumors, referral to a urological or gynecologic surgeon for other options such as nontissue-sparing surgery and sentinel lymph node biopsy is prudent. MMS (especially with multiple preoperative scouting biopsies) is becoming the surgery of choice for extramammary Paget disease, with overall lower recurrence rates (16%–23% vs 31%–61% for standard excision) (see **Table 2**).[37,38]

A multidisciplinary approach should be taken for genital cancers and may involve urologists, gynecologists, oncologists, radiation oncologists, plastic surgeons, dermatologic surgeons, dermatologists, and dermatopathologists.[33] Repair options for genital surgery include secondary intention healing, primary closures, split or full-thickness skin graft, and fasciocutaneous or myocutaneous flaps.[30,33]

Complications of genital surgery include but are not limited to infection, pain, urethral meatal strictures, deformity, phimosis, decreased libido, and decreased sexual satisfaction.[35,39]

NAIL UNIT

The nail unit consists of the proximal nail fold (consisting of the eponychium and cuticle), the lateral nail folds, distal hyponychium, proximal matrix, proximal nail fold, distal matrix, and the nail plate itself.[9] The extensor tendon of the phalanx inserts at the base of the proximal matrix approximately 2 to 3 mm distal to the distal interphalangeal joint or 12 mm proximal to the cuticle.[9] It is important to know these landmarks to maintain function and to limit the damage to the proximal matrix, which can cause visible nail destruction.

Several nail-specific instruments are helpful when conducting surgery of the nail unit. These instruments include a tourniquet (a Penrose drain works well, but one can put a sterile glove on the patient's hand, cut off the tip of the operative finger, and roll it back proximally, which also makes an adequate tourniquet as well as sterile field), freer septum elevator, platypus nail puller, nail nipper, and English anvil nail splitter. Anesthesia is generally obtained by proximal digital block with supplemental wing block or distal digital blocks with 1% or 2% lidocaine with or without epinephrine, although the use of epinephrine has a small chance of unexpected localized ischemia.[9] A preoperative radiograph of the digit and hand should be strongly considered for anything more than in situ disease to rule out bone involvement.[40]

Tumors of the nail unit are rare, with SCC (most commonly on the thumb) being the most common, followed by melanoma, BCC, keratoacanthomas, and Kaposi sarcoma (see **Table 1**, **Box 1**).[9,40] Risk factors for subungual SCCs include HPV,

trauma, chronic inflammation, and radiation exposure.[41] Although a delay in treatment is common with subungual SCCs, the metastatic rate is low compared with other anatomic sites.[42] Only several hundred reported cases of SCC and approximately 23 cases of BCC of the nail unit have been reported in the literature.[41,43] Nail apparatus melanoma is one of the rarest forms of melanoma, with an incidence of less than 4% of all melanomas. It has a poor survival rate and is difficult to detect because 15% to 65% of the time it is amelanotic.[44] Although not the standard of care, if MMS is used for nail apparatus melanoma, immunohistochemistry should be considered to enhance the accuracy of the histologic evaluation (see **Table 2**).[44] For larger tumors, or those invading bone, the Mohs surgeon should consider a consultation with a hand surgeon to discuss a combined case, WLE, or amputation as indicated.

Secondary intention healing may be the most common closure after MMS of the nail unit, but skin grafts and primary closures have also been used successfully.[42,43]

Complications include permanent nail dystrophy, partial or complete nail loss, nail spicules, long-lasting pain/redness/swelling, stiffness of the interphalangeal joints, and reduced active movement of the distal interphalangeal joint.[42]

SUMMARY

MMS on the eyelids, lips, genitalia and the nail unit is uncommon, and there are unique challenges to these anatomic sites. As long as the Mohs surgeon understands the anatomy, is facile with the specialized instruments, is experienced and comfortable with the histology of the more uncommon malignant neoplasms encountered, is adept at some standard repair options, and appreciates the potentially severe adverse outcomes if the repair does not go as expected, they can help patients by performing a tissue-sparing (and sometimes amputation-sparing) procedure with the highest cure rates available. Comparing data between MMS and WLEs is difficult, because high-quality trials comparing the methods are lacking and there is no standard way to report the data (eg, follow-up periods are variable). Site-specific data are even more difficult to come by, but **Table 2** is an earnest and honest attempt to summarize the available evidence. MMS should be considered the treatment of choice on most malignant neoplasms of the eyelids and lips. There is little doubt that MMS can preserve tissue and possibly avoid digital amputation or penectomy in certain situations, but genitalia-specific and nail apparatus–specific tumors must be taken on a case by case basis and approached with the best interest of the patient in mind. Relying on our surgical colleagues to comanage a difficult case should be embraced as well, if it benefits the patient.

REFERENCES

1. Drake LA, Dinehart SM, Goltz RW, et al. Guidelines of care for Mohs micrographic surgery. American Academy of Dermatology. J Am Acad Dermatol 1985;33:271–8.
2. Netter Frank H. Atlas of human anatomy. 4th edition. Philadelphia: Saunders Elsevier; 2006.
3. Baker Shan R. Local flaps in facial reconstruction. 2nd edition. Philadelphia: Mosby; 2007.
4. Vidimos AT, Ammirati CT, Poblete-Lopez C. Requisites in dermatology: dermatologic surgery. Philadelphia: Saunders Elsevier; 2009.
5. Robinson JK, Hanke CW, Sengelmann RD, et al. Surgery of the skin: procedural dermatology. Philadelphia: Elsevier Mosby; 2005.
6. Ahmad J, Mathes DW, Itani KM. Reconstruction of the eyelids after Mohs surgery. Semin Plast Surg 2008;22:306–18.
7. Schessler MJ, McClellan WT. Lower eyelid reconstruction following Mohs surgery. W V Med J 2009; 105:19–23.
8. Gloster HM Jr. Second intention healing for intermediate and large postsurgical defects of the lip. J Am Acad Dermatol 2007;57:832–5.
9. Clark RE, Madani S, Bettencourt MS. Nail surgery. Dermatol Clin 1998;16:145–65.
10. Schlosser BJ, Mirowski GW. Approach to the patient with vulvovaginal complaints. Dermatol Ther 2010; 23:438–48.
11. Wesley RE, McCord CD Jr, Jones NA. Height of the tarsus of the lower eyelid. Am J Ophthalmol 1980;90: 102–5.
12. Kroll DM. Management and reconstruction of periocular malignancies. Facial Plast Surg 2007;23:181–9.
13. Nemet AY, Deckel Y, Martin PA, et al. Management of periocular basal and squamous cell carcinoma: a case series of 485 cases. Am J Ophthalmol 2006;142:293–7.
14. Pathai S, Barlow R, Williams G, et al. Mohs' micrographic surgery for Merkel cell carcinomas of the eyelid. Orbit 2005;24:273–5.
15. Shields JA, Demirci H, Marr BP, et al. Sebaceous carcinoma of the ocular region: a review. Surv Ophthalmol 2005;50:103–22.
16. Leibovitch I, Huilgol SC, Richards S, et al. Periocular microcystic adnexal carcinoma: management and outcome with Mohs' micrographic surgery. Ophthalmologica 2006;220:109–13.
17. Moul DK, Chern PL, Shumaker PR, et al. Mohs micrographic surgery for eyelid and periorbital skin cancer. Int Ophthalmol Clin 2009;49:111–27.
18. Malhotra R, Huigol SC, Huynh NT, et al. The Australian Mohs database: periocular squamous cell carcinoma. Ophthalmology 2004;111:617–23.
19. Then SY, Malhotra R, Barlow R, et al. Early cure rates with narrow-margin slow-Mohs surgery for periocular malignant melanoma. Dermatol Surg 2009;35: 17–23.
20. Levin F, Khalil M, McCormick A, et al. Excision of periocular basal cell carcinoma with stereoscopic microdissection of surgical margins for frozen-section control. Arch Ophthalmol 2009;127:1011–5.
21. Malhotra R, Huilgol SC, Huynh NT, et al. The Australian Mohs database, part II: periocular basal cell carcinoma outcome at 5-year follow-up. Ophthalmology 2004;111:631–6.
22. Spencer JM, Nossa R, Tse DT, et al. Sebaceous carcinoma of the eyelid treated with Mohs micrographic surgery. J Am Acad Dermatol 2001;44: 1004–9.
23. Hamada S, Kersey T, Thaller VT. Eyelid basal cell carcinoma: non-Mohs excision, repair, and outcome. Br J Ophthalmol 2005;89:992–4.
24. Lin H, Li W. Use of the spiral flap for closure of small defects of the lower eyelid. Ann Plast Surg 2009;63: 514–6.
25. Frost A. Supporting suture in ptosis operations. Am J Opthalmol 1934;17:633.
26. Griffiths RW, Suvarna SK, Stone J. Basal cell carcinoma histological clearance margins: an analysis of 1539 conventionally excised tumours. Wider still and deeper? J Plast Reconstr Aesthetic Surg 2007;60:41–7.
27. Holmkvist KA, Roenigk RK. Squamous cell carcinoma of the lip treated with Mohs micrographic surgery: outcome at 5 years. J Am Acad Dermatol 1998;38:960–6.
28. Leibovitch I, Huilgol SC, Selva D, et al. Cutaneous lip tumours treated with Mohs micrographic surgery: clinical features and surgical outcome. Br J Dermatol 2005;153:1147–52.
29. Rowe DE, Carroll RJ, Day CL. Prognostic factors for local recurrence, metastasis, and survival rates in squamous cell carcinoma of the skin, ear, and lip. J Am Acad Dermatol 1992;26:976–90.
30. Leonard AL, Hanke CW. Second intention healing for intermediate and large postsurgical defects of the lip. J Am Acad Dermatol 2007;57:832–5.
31. Haseebuddin M, Brandes SB. The prepuce: preservation and reconstruction. Curr Opin Urol 2008;18: 575–82.
32. Hacker NF. Vulvar cancer. 4th edition. Philadelphia: Lippincott Williams & Wilkins; 2005.
33. Moodley M, Moodley J. Dermatofibrosarcoma protuberans of the vulva: a case report and review of the literature. Gynecol Oncol 2000;78:74–5.
34. Wells MD, Taylor RS. Mohs micrographic surgery for penoscrotal malignancy. Urol Clin North Am 2010;37:403–9.

35. Pizzocaro G, Algaba F, Horenblas S, et al. EAU penile cancer guidelines 2009. Eur Urol 2010;57: 1002–12.

36. Groenen SM, Timmers PJ, Burger CW. Recurrence rate in vulvar carcinoma in relation to pathological margin distance. Int J Gynecol Cancer 2010;20:869–73.

37. Appert DL, Otley CC, Phillips PK, et al. Role of multiple scouting biopsies before Mohs micrographic surgery for extramammary Paget's disease. Dermatol Surg 2005;31:1417–22.

38. Lee KY, Roh MR, Chung WG, et al. Comparison of Mohs micrographic surgery and wide excision for extramammary Paget's disease: Korean experience. Dermatol Surg 2009;35:34–40.

39. Antunes AA, Dall'Oglio MF, Srougi M. Organ-sparing treatment for penile cancer. Nat Clin Pract Urol 2007;4:596–604.

40. Goldminz D, Bennett RG. Mohs micrographic surgery of the nail unit. J Dermatol Surg Oncol 1992;18:721–6.

41. Kelly KJ, Kalani AD, Storrs S, et al. Subungual squamous cell carcinoma of the toe: working toward a standardized therapeutic approach. J Surg Educ 2008;65:297–301.

42. de Berker DA, Dahl MG, Malcolm AJ, et al. Micrographic surgery for subungual squamous cell carcinoma. Br J Plast Surg 1996;49:414–9.

43. Forman SB, Ferringer TC, Garrett AB. Basal cell carcinoma of the nail unit. J Am Acad Dermatol 2007;56:811–4.

44. Brodland DG. The treatment of nail apparatus melanoma with Mohs micrographic surgery. Dermatol Surg 2001;27:269–73.

45. Thosani MK, Schneck G, Jones EC. Periocular squamous cell carcinoma. Dermatol Surg 2008; 34:585–99.

46. Hauben DJ, Zirkin H, Mahler D, et al. The biologic behavior of basal cell carcinoma: analysis of recurrence in excised basal cell carcinoma: part II. Plast Reconstr Surg 1982;69:110–6.

47. Morris DS, Elzaridi E, Clarke L, et al. Periocular basal cell carcinoma: 5-year outcome following slow Mohs surgery with formalin-fixed paraffin-embedded sections and delayed closure. Br J Ophthalmol 2009;93:474–6.

48. Snow SN, Larson PO, Lucarelli MJ, et al. Sebaceous carcinoma of the eyelids treated by Mohs micrographic surgery: report of nine cases with review of the literature. Dermatol Surg 2002;28:623–31.

49. Huynh NT, Veness MJ. Basal cell carcinoma of the lip treated with radiotherapy. Australas J Dermatol 2002;43:15–9.

50. Dudley C, Kircik LH, Bullen R, et al. Vulvar squamous cell carcinoma metastatic to the skin. Dermatol Surg 1998;24:889–92.

51. Dalle S, Depape L, Phan A, et al. Squamous cell carcinoma of the nail apparatus: clinicopathological study of 35 cases. Br J Dermatol 2007;156: 871–4.

Multidisciplinary Approach to Large Cutaneous Tumors of the Head and Neck

Peter C. Revenaugh, MD[a], Rahul Seth, MD[a],
Jennifer Lucas, MD[b], Michael A. Fritz, MD[a],*

KEYWORDS

- Mohs micrographic surgery
- Head and neck cutaneous malignancy
- Basal cell carcinoma • Squamous cell carcinoma
- Head and neck cutaneous malignancy
- Head and neck reconstruction

Nonmelanoma skin cancers are the most common malignancies in the United States and most frequently occur in areas of direct sun exposure, such as the head and neck regions. Tumors in so-called high-risk areas as well as recurrent tumors have been successfully approached using Mohs micrographic surgery (MMS) with established advantages over other methods of resection and margin control.[1,2] However, large tumors, aggressive pathology, and involvement of multiple aesthetic units or critical structures can complicate excision under local anesthesia and warrant extensive reconstruction.

As a result, extensive or massive cutaneous tumors of the head and neck are traditionally approached in the operating suite under general anesthesia where excision with predetermined margins is easily accomplished and reconstructive capabilities are readily available. In such instances, MMS is rarely used and frozen-section analysis is commonly employed to ensure marginal clearance, albeit with known compromise of accuracy

and consequently inferior tumor control.[1,3] Given these limitations, periods of observation for recurrence have been advocated prior to definitive reconstruction of defects, resulting in additional patient morbidity and psychosocial compromise.

The seemingly obvious need for optimal margin clearance when managing complex, massive, or multiple cutaneous malignancies necessitates a shift in current resection paradigms. As a result, the authors have begun a unique and now routine collaborative approach to large tumors, which concurrently employs multiple subspecialties to ensure both optimal oncologic management and appropriate aesthetic and functional reconstruction. Currently at the authors' institution, dermatologic surgeons, facial plastic surgeons, head and neck surgeons, and additional subspecialties manage tumors in a single operative setting. This method of intraoperative Mohs micrographic surgery (IMMS) provides efficient and reliable extirpation of large tumors and allows for immediate reconstruction of complex defects.

Disclosures: The authors have nothing to disclose.
[a] Department of Otolaryngology–Head and Neck Surgery, Head and Neck Institute, Cleveland Clinic, 9500 Euclid Avenue, Desk A71, Cleveland, OH 44195, USA
[b] Department of Dermatology, Dermatology and Plastic Surgery Institute, Cleveland Clinic, 9500 Euclid Avenue, Desk A61, Cleveland, OH 44195, USA
* Corresponding author.
E-mail address: fritzm1@ccf.org

Dermatol Clin 29 (2011) 319–324
doi:10.1016/j.det.2011.02.001
0733-8635/11/$ – see front matter © 2011 Elsevier Inc. All rights reserved.

ROLE OF MOHS MICROGRAPHIC SURGERY IN LARGE TUMORS

Mohs micrographic surgery is advantageous in the treatment of head and neck cutaneous malignancies for its ability to effectively evaluate the tumor margins while simultaneously preserving tissue. Marginal control is paramount in reducing the potential for metastatic disease, recurrence, and increasing overall and disease-free survival.[4–6] Several methods of treatment have been employed for head and neck cutaneous malignancies, including conventional excision, MMS, cryosurgery, and electrodessication and curettage. Only conventional excision and MMS are recommended, as the other methods cited result in operator-dependent outcomes and difficulty yielding histological evidence of adequate margins.[7] Conventional excision with adequate gross margins is commonly employed by nondermatologists for large or recurrent basal cell carcinomas (BCC) and squamous cell carcinomas (SCC). Current recommendations cite 4-5 mm surgical margins for well-defined small basal and squamous cell carcinomas and 4-15 mm margins for large BCC or SCC to achieve clearance in approximately 95% of tumors.[8,9] Intraoperative frozen-section analysis is often employed to confirm negative margins during conventional resection of large tumors in the operating suite. However, frozen-section analysis can be dependent upon artifact, proper orientation, sectioning method, and completeness of section.[10] Frozen-section analysis in the setting of recurrent facial cutaneous BCC reports a 72% rate of accuracy[3]; whereas, MMS reports 5-year cure rates of up to 98.9% for both primary and recurrent BCC and SCC.

MMS has been established as the gold standard for excision of higher-risk cutaneous malignancies, including large cutaneous tumors (>2 cm in diameter). Regardless of size, high-risk clinical features also include tumors that are recurrent, located in areas with high risk of recurrence[6] (midface, ear, and lip), and have ill-defined boundaries or aggressive pathology.[11] In such cases, the improved cure rate over conventional excision is most certainly attributable to the ability of MMS to assess 100% of the excised tumor margin as opposed to the estimated 1% of margin directly evaluated with traditional surgical excision and paraffin-section margin assessment. Optimal management of large (>5 cm), so-called giant BCC and large SCC is not well established.[6,12,13] Recent data indicates that Mohs excision of large BCC and SCC could be advantageous for definitive tumor control, but is not without challenges and potential limitations.

CHALLENGES IN MANAGEMENT OF LARGE TUMORS

Large cutaneous tumors of the head and neck provide unique challenges not only for Mohs clearance and adequate extirpation but also for functional and aesthetic reconstruction. Often, large tumors require increased operative time and multiple sections, which may be difficult to accomplish in an office-based setting. Longer operative times and the potential need for more extensive resection may also hinder the ability of patients to tolerate excision under local anesthesia. Necessity for deeper resection or resection involving critical structures, including bone, deep tissues, eyelid, orbit, or nasal mucosa, may also obviate office-based excision. Tumors with nodal metastasis, parotid extension, bone invasion, or intracranial extension along nerve branches may not be cleared with office-based MMS. Also, if several aesthetic subunits are involved, the resultant wound may require more complex reconstructive techniques than are available in an office-based setting and may require general anesthesia to accomplish them. Finally, resection of large tumors requiring delayed reconstruction with or without general anesthesia, or multiple-staged formalin-fixed tissue Mohs resections (so-called slow Mohs) are disadvantageous because of the inconvenience to patients, aesthetic concerns with a large wound, and potential risk for secondary infection or wound contracture.[14] Despite these limitations of office-based MMS in the setting of large tumors, the collaborative approach of IMMS, which the authors advocate, offers the advantages of total marginal assessment and clearance of large and complicated tumors coupled with the ability to immediately and efficiently reconstruct the resultant defect. Therefore, extensive tumors with or without deep invasion, those involving critical structures or multiple aesthetic subunits are ideal types to approach with a multidisciplinary technique. In properly selected patients, this approach can minimize the number of procedures, operative time, and potential morbidity for patients.

MULTIDISCIPLINARY TECHNIQUE
Preoperative

Successful multidisciplinary management of large cutaneous tumors via IMMS begins with proper preoperative planning. The dermatologic surgeon, head and neck surgeon, or facial plastic surgeon initially evaluates patients depending upon the referral source or patient preference and cross-referral for evaluation and management is then accomplished between these specialists. A discussion regarding management then ensues, ideally at a multidisciplinary tumor board involving surgeons, medical oncologists, and radiation oncologists.

Further evaluation by appropriate collaborative services and pertinent imaging should be obtained. Ophthalmology and oculoplastic surgery are consulted for assessment of ocular function and ability to salvage the orbit and periorbital structures in cases with orbital and periorbital involvement. When indicated, neurosurgeons assist in reviewing imaging with emphasis on margins and feasibility of resection for tumors that may have intracranial extension. Head and neck pathology specialists and dermatopathologists can be consulted to elucidate histologic features of the tumor. Radiation oncologists and medical oncologists are additionally involved in consideration of alternative or adjunctive therapies.

Aside from face-to-face discussions between members of the extirpative and Mohs surgical teams, a multidisciplinary reconstructive conference provides an ideal forum for management of particularly difficult cases. Here surgeons convene to discuss comprehensive management recommendations based on likely resection margins and reconstructive options.

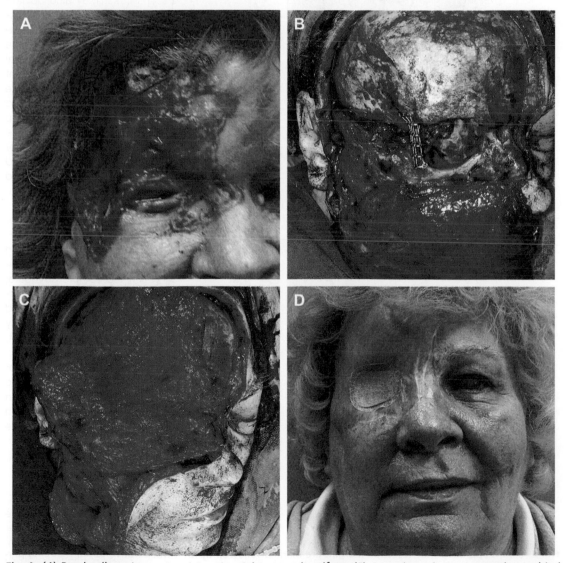

Fig. 1. (*A*) Basal cell carcinoma involving the right upper hemiface. (*B*) Extensive soft-tissue resection, orbital exenteration, subtotal rhinectomy, and partial maxillectomy was required to clear margins. (*C, D*) Reconstruction involved a free latissimus myogenous flap, split-thickness skin graft, and cervicofacial advancement flap with good postoperative contour and ability to accept orbital prosthesis.

Again, coordination between the ablative and Mohs surgical teams is paramount in scheduling and conducting a successful operation. Generally, block operating room time is coordinated with Mohs reading times, and patient volumes on these days are tightly controlled to ensure rapid efficient extirpation and margin clearance. The case then proceeds with head and neck oncologic surgeons

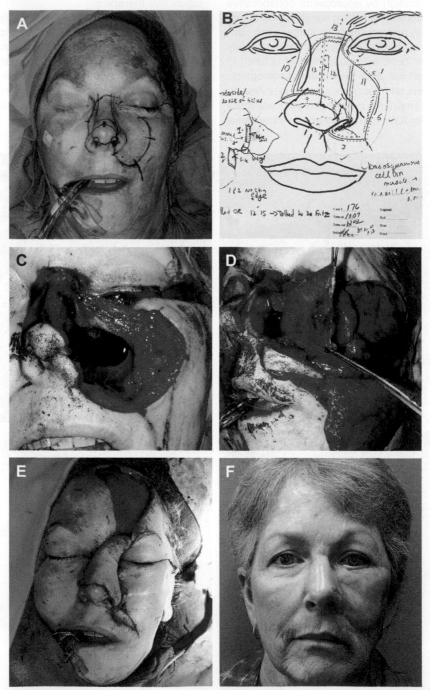

Fig. 2. (*A*) Preoperative wide resection margins are marked followed by (*B*) intraoperative tumor mapping performed by the Mohs surgeon. (*C*) Resection defect following subtotal rhinectomy, left medial maxillectomy, and left infraorbital nerve excision. (*D*) Anterolateral thigh fascia/fat flap reconstructed the nasal lining and cheek contour. (*E*) Cervicofacial, paramedian, and nasolabial island flaps provided cutaneous coverage. (*F*) Optimized cosmetic and functional reconstruction without recurrence is maintained at 2 years after surgery.

and facial plastic surgeons conducting the ablation in direct communication with Mohs teams and appropriate consulting services on a stand-by basis.

Intraoperative

Once general anesthesia has been induced and patients are properly positioned, the Mohs and extirpative surgeons demarcate initial resection margins, which are agreed upon by consensus. In contrast to the typical tissue-sparing approach employed in the Mohs suite, resection is more aggressive to ensure rapid margin clearance, ideally within the first 1 or 2 layers, the so-called wide-margin Mohs. Aesthetic subunits whose removal will not affect reconstructive results are often included in their entirety if there is potential tumor involvement. The specimen and resection bed are clearly marked and a detailed tumor map is created to ensure correct orientation while the resection proceeds. Appropriate orientation is again confirmed upon removal of the specimen.

The Mohs surgeons then take the specimen from the operating suite to the Mohs histology lab for processing and margin reading. The specimen is similarly mapped and marked in the standard Mohs fashion. Accommodations by the Mohs team allow for rapid reads of large tumors, which in the authors' experience, can be completed within 1 to 3 hours. Margins of particular concern are often identified and read as a high priority in order to expedite final clearance. Any areas in need of re-resection are clearly marked on the map and the Mohs surgeon returns to the operating suite for direct discussion and marking with the resecting surgeon.

While margins are being read, adjunctive procedures that do not alter the resection margins are pursued, thereby reducing potential time with patients under general anesthesia. These procedures comprise further oncologic and reconstructive procedures, including parotidectomy, maxillectomy or neck dissections. Reconstructive efforts, such as raising local, regional, or free tissue flaps and obtaining needed bone or cartilage grafts, are also commenced provided their shape and size are not dependent upon final margins and harvest does not alter the original resection bed.

Serial resection of additional layers with immediate Mohs interpretation is performed until negative margins are achieved. Full reconstruction is then performed once tumor clearance is verified. Patients are typically admitted postoperatively to the reconstructive service for monitoring based upon their particular level of care needs.

Case 1

A 71-year-old woman who presented with a large, neglected BCC involving the right hemiface, including extensive periorbital involvement (**Fig. 1**). She underwent an extensive soft-tissue resection, orbital exenteration, subtotal rhinectomy, and partial maxillectomy. Two layers were necessary to clear the tumor using IMMS. The first layer was 75% positive and a further 1-cm circumferential excision was required to obtain clear margins. Reconstruction was initiated during margin assessment and completed after final read. This reconstruction included a free latissimus myogenous flap with split-thickness skin graft and cervicofacial advancement flap.

Case 2

A 59-year-old woman with a multiple recurrent BCC that initially involved the left nasofacial sulcus. The patient suffered extensive recurrence after multiple excisions and radiation therapy. The affected area included the left nasofacial sulcus, nasal ala, dorsum, cheek, and lateral nasal wall mucosal surface (**Fig. 2**). IMMS was performed, including a subtotal rhinectomy, left medial maxillectomy, and left infraorbital nerve excision. A single layer was required to obtain negative peripheral margins. Concurrent with margin assessment, a free anterolateral thigh fat/fascial flap was harvested and a paramedian forehead and cervicofacial flap was elevated. After negative margins were confirmed, reconstruction was performed.

SUMMARY

IMMS is well suited for large cutaneous tumors, particularly recurrent or persistent after-resection tumors, or those in sites where extirpation and reconstruction may be extensive and complex. In these cases, a multidisciplinary approach may best serve patients by limiting procedures while assuring the most complete resection.

Ideally, a multidisciplinary approach to large tumors would provide: (1) accurate and efficient total marginal evaluation to ensure complete extirpation; (2) a tissue-sparing resection preserving cosmetically and functionally important areas of the face; (3) ability to perform immediate complex reconstruction if necessary; and (4) reduced operative time, limited additional procedures, and the least potential morbidity to patients.

Several investigators have advocated a multidisciplinary approach to cutaneous tumors involving

Mohs surgeons and head and neck surgeons, yet there is a paucity of literature describing successful paradigms.[13] The intraoperative multidisciplinary use of MMS for large cutaneous neoplasms was first described by Levine and colleagues[15] in 1979. Several small case series followed in the early 1980s but further studies were limited.[16,17] Recently, Ducic and colleagues[18] described their technique where preoperative Mohs creates a "ring of Mohs" clearing the cutaneous margins prior to definitive resection. Of course, this technique does not fully evaluate the deep margin intraoperatively but can be used for tumors where the cutaneous margin does not involve critical structures. The authors' implementation of IMMS provides a multidisciplinary approach to simultaneous rapid Mohs resection and same-setting reconstruction of large cutaneous tumors.

IMMS is a unique collaboration of multiple surgical subspecialties with the goal of providing tumor extirpation with assurance of complete margin clearance at the same setting as reconstruction. With dedicated efforts and resources, the Mohs surgeon can efficiently evaluate the initial large resection's margins and direct further resection as needed to completely clear the tumor. During margin assessment, the facial plastic/head and neck surgeon is able to perform additional extirpative or reconstructive efforts required by the defect. Therefore, an efficient system has been created allowing greater ability to obtain tumor-free margins and afford simultaneous reconstruction to restore form and function for even the most complex large cutaneous neoplasms.

REFERENCES

1. Rowe DE, Carroll RJ, Day CL Jr. Prognostic factors for local recurrence, metastasis, and survival rates in squamous cell carcinoma of the skin, ear, and lip. Implications for treatment modality selection. J Am Acad Dermatol 1992;26(6):976–90.
2. Cumberland L, Dana A, Liegeois N. Mohs micrographic surgery for the management of nonmelanoma skin cancers. Facial Plast Surg Clin North Am 2009;17(3):325–35.
3. Manstein ME, Manstein CH, Smith R. How accurate is frozen section for skin cancers? Ann Plast Surg 2003;50(6):607–9.
4. Mourouzis C, Boynton A, Grant J, et al. Cutaneous head and neck SCCs and risk of nodal metastasis - UK experience. J Craniomaxillofac Surg 2009;37(8):443–7.
5. Cherpelis BS, Marcusen C, Lang PG. Prognostic factors for metastasis in squamous cell carcinoma of the skin. Dermatol Surg 2002;28(3):268–73.
6. Brantsch KD, Meisner C, Schonfisch B, et al. Analysis of risk factors determining prognosis of cutaneous squamous-cell carcinoma: a prospective study. Lancet Oncol 2008;9(8):713–20.
7. Motley R, Kersey P, Lawrence C. Multiprofessional guidelines for the management of the patient with primary cutaneous squamous cell carcinoma. Br J Plast Surg 2003;56(2):85–91.
8. Wolf DJ, Zitelli JA. Surgical margins for basal cell carcinoma. Arch Dermatol 1987;123(3):340–4.
9. Brodland DG, Zitelli JA. Surgical margins for excision of primary cutaneous squamous cell carcinoma. J Am Acad Dermatol 1992;27(2 Pt 1):241–8.
10. Smith-Zagone MJ, Schwartz MR. Frozen section of skin specimens. Arch Pathol Lab Med 2005;129(12):1536–43.
11. Neville JA, Welch E, Leffell DJ. Management of nonmelanoma skin cancer in 2007. Nat Clin Pract Oncol 2007;4(8):462–9.
12. Lackey PL, Sargent LA, Wong L, et al. Giant basal cell carcinoma surgical management and reconstructive challenges. Ann Plast Surg 2007;58(3):250–4.
13. Jennings L, Schmults CD. Management of high-risk cutaneous squamous cell carcinoma. J Clin Aesthet Dermatol 2010;3(4):39–48.
14. Lawrence CM, Haniffa M, Dahl MG. Formalin-fixed tissue Mohs surgery (slow Mohs) for basal cell carcinoma: 5-year follow-up data. Br J Dermatol 2009;160(3):573–80.
15. Levine H, Bailin P, Wood B, et al. Tissue conservation in treatment of cutaneous neoplasms of the head and neck. Combined use of Mohs' chemosurgical and conventional surgical techniques. Arch Otolaryngol 1979;105(3):140–4.
16. Baker SR, Swanson NA. Complete microscopic controlled surgery for head and neck cancer. Head Neck Surg 1984;6(5):914–20.
17. Baker SR, Swanson NA, Grekin RC. An interdisciplinary approach to the management of basal cell carcinoma of the head and neck. J Dermatol Surg Oncol 1987;13(10):1095–106.
18. Ducic Y, Marra DE, Kennard C. Initial Mohs surgery followed by planned surgical resection of massive cutaneous carcinomas of the head and neck. Laryngoscope 2009;119(4):774–7.

Prosthetic Rehabilitation

Michael Huband, DDS

KEYWORDS

- Maxillofacial prosthetics • Maxillofacial prosthodontist
- Facial prostheses • Prosthetic • Craniofacial implants

Most patients requiring prosthetic facial rehabilitation have undergone ablative surgery for head and neck cancers.[1] These patients are often best treated by a multidisciplinary approach involving the surgeons performing ablative and reconstructive surgery and the maxillofacial prosthodontist. Presurgical and postsurgical planning should be coordinated by the responsible specialist before proceeding with the surgery. This coordination facilitates a more concerted effort between the various disciplines so that eradication of the disease and postsurgical outcome emerge favorably.[1–4] Prosthodontics is one of the 9 dental specialties recognized by the American Dental Association. Maxillofacial prosthetics is a subspecialty of prosthodontics dedicated to prosthetic correction and management of maxillofacial defects acquired from tumor ablative surgery, trauma, congenital defects, or alterations of growth and development. The number of practitioners who actively practice this subspecialty is very low; therefore, accessibility may be an issue. Resources available through the American Academy of Maxillofacial Prosthetics and the International Society for Maxillofacial Rehabilitation may be helpful in locating a maxillofacial prosthodontist.[4] Ideally, patients should be referred to the maxillofacial prosthodontist early in the treatment process. This early referral allows time for proper evaluation and consultation in which treatment options and the prosthetic rehabilitation process can be discussed with the patient and family.[1] Other valuable information, such as preoperative photographs and models, may be gathered early in the treatment process.

SURGICAL AND PROSTHETIC RECONSTRUCTION OPTIONS

Head and neck defects caused by ablative cancer surgery, trauma, and congenital malformation result in many functional and psychological difficulties for patients and those around them.[5] Surgical reconstruction techniques, prosthetic rehabilitation, or a combination of both to correct facial disfigurement may improve function, self-confidence, and psychological well-being of the patient.[5,6] The site, size, and cause of the defect, in conjunction with the patient's age, health, and desires, are used to determine the method of surgical reconstruction and prosthetic rehabilitation. In some cases, prosthetic rehabilitation may be preferred because of the complexity of the reconstructive surgery, anticipated complications from radiation therapy, and the value placed on aesthetics.[7,8] Surgical reconstruction with flaps taken from sun-exposed skin may result in a mismatch of shape, color, and texture. In these situations, a prosthesis may be the best choice to create symmetry and to blend with the tone and texture of the skin adjacent to the defect.[4] One of the greatest advantages of a prosthesis over surgical reconstruction is the ability to perform periodic surveillance of the surgical site. By using a prosthesis, it is possible to directly visualize recurrent areas that may be apparent from

The author has nothing to disclose.
Maxillofacial Prosthetics, Section of Dentistry, Head and Neck Institute, Cleveland Clinic, 9500 Euclid Avenue/A71, Cleveland, Ohio 44195, USA
E-mail address: Hubandm@ccf.org

Dermatol Clin 29 (2011) 325–330
doi:10.1016/j.det.2011.01.006

the perioperative period to the third year of follow-up. With surgical reconstruction, the ability to perform surveillance is markedly reduced.[4]

FABRICATION OF FACIAL PROSTHESES

Facial prostheses are used to replace, cover, and change the appearance of disfigured or missing anatomic structures. In addition, these prostheses may function to support devices such as eyeglasses, warm the incoming air, close an opening, and protect the underlying fragile tissues.[9] Prostheses also play an important role in restoring body image and assisting the reintegration of the patient with the society. However, prostheses have limitations and realistically cannot perfectly restore aesthetics and function. A well-made prosthesis is intended to pass "the grocery store or shopping mall test," that is, it will allow a person to walk through a public place without attracting attention. It is important for patients and those around them to have realistic expectations. Pictures available on the Internet may have been touched-up or may represent an unusually exceptional outcome. Dramatic results can be achieved in a Hollywood movie in which prostheses and hours of applying makeup are used to create special effects. However, this is not practical for patients in whom the prosthesis requires daily removal, cleaning, and skin care.

Facial prostheses are custom fabricated and most often made of silicone elastomers because of the material's clinical inertness, strength, durability, and ease of manipulation.[10] Creating a prosthesis is a labor-intensive process requiring many hours of work. The number of appointments vary with the complexity of the defect and the patient's expectations. The process involves the following steps: (1) making an impression of the affected area, (2) creating a cast or model of the affected area, (3) sculpting a prosthesis out of wax or clay (**Fig. 1**), (4) creating a mold of the sculpted form,

(5) casting the mold in a base material intrinsically colored to match the patient's overall skin tone (**Fig. 2**), and (6) extrinsic coloring and characterization to enhance details and create a prosthesis that matches the adjacent skin (**Figs. 3** and **4**).[9]

Many patients find the impression appointment the most stressful because the impression is made during the early phase of the doctor-patient relationship. In addition, the tissues may still be sensitive from surgery or radiation therapy. Often, the impression covers the eyes or nose and may lead to a claustrophobic feeling for the patient. This problem is best managed by the maxillofacial prosthodontist building a positive and trusted relationship with the patient, explaining the procedure in advance, reassuring the patient that the impression materials are safe, talking to the patient through the process, and allowing adequate time for healing and tissue remodeling before impression making. Adequate healing is important not only for patient comfort but also for ensuring that the impression made in the first step is accurate.[9] An accurate cast of the defect is required to produce a well-fitting prosthesis. In general, prosthesis fabrication begins 6 to 8 weeks after surgery or the completion of radiation therapy. This period is a guideline, and the actual determination of adequate healing is made clinically.

Matching the tone and characteristics of the skin adjacent to the defect can be demanding and complicated by the patient's exposure to sunlight or a dermatologic condition. Therefore, the patient's usual complexion should be considered. If the patient has a recent tan, sunburn, or rash, the mix of the base shade and extrinsic coloring should be delayed until these conditions are resolved. Patients should also be encouraged to use a sunblock to avoid these problems and to reduce the risk of premature aging and skin cancer. For patients who have an unusually wide variation in skin tone, such as a summer

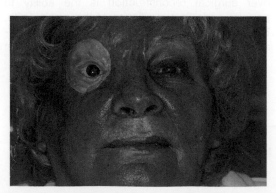

Fig. 1. Wax sculpture evaluated on the patient.

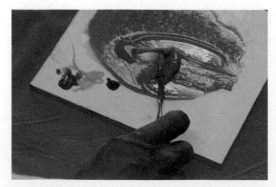

Fig. 2. Custom intrinsic coloring to match skin tone.

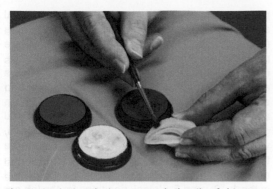

Fig. 3. Extrinsic coloring to match details of skin tone.

complexion and a winter complexion, multiple prostheses in differing colors may be fabricated for seasonal use.

RETENTION OF FACIAL PROSTHESES

Facial prostheses may be retained with a double-sided tape, portions of the prosthesis engaging anatomic undercuts in the defect, medical grade adhesive, osseointegrated implants, or a combination of these.[11–13] Adhesives are in wide use and may need to be reapplied during the day because retention is reduced by humidity, sweat, and skin oils. The bond strength of adhesives decreases over time, and a second coat of adhesive applied 4 to 8 hours after the first coat may enhance retention. Adhesive retention may also be increased by applying NO-STING SKIN-PREP Protective Dressing (Smith & Nephew, Largo, FL, USA) to the skin before donning the prosthesis.[14–16] Double-sided tapes, adhesives, and engagement of undercuts do not provide adequate retention for patients with very active lifestyles or those who engage in contact sports and activities such as swimming. These patients should be considered for osseointegrated implants.

When osseointegrated implants are used, the implants are placed in the bone within or adjacent to the defect. After healing, the bone bonds with the implants. The implants remain within the bone and have extensions added to exit the skin. These extensions are termed abutments. Attachments are then added to the abutments and to the intaglio or inner side of the prosthesis. These attachments may be of a snap-on type with a female and male portion that join together in a method analogous to snap-on clothing, or magnets may be used alone or in conjunction with snap-type attachments.

Patients may have difficulties in placing the prosthesis in the proper position. This situation is especially true for those with manual dexterity or visual impairments and is further worsened by the visual field being blocked by the patient's hands during placement and removal of the prosthesis. The use of osseointegrated implants may reduce these problems by allowing for the fabrication of a prosthesis that self-aligns with magnets. For these reasons, a family member or a caregiver should be educated to assist in the donning and doffing of the prosthesis. In addition, there is a learning period in which the patient becomes familiar with the retentive properties of the prosthesis, anticipates the time for which an application of adhesive will last and the correct amount of adhesive to apply, and identifies activities that may dislodge the prosthesis. It is highly recommended that the patient learns to wear the prosthesis before venturing into public.

CARE AND MAINTENANCE OF FACIAL PROSTHESES

Facial prostheses should be removed daily for cleaning and skin care. The skin, and the osseointegrated implants, if present, should be cleaned with a mild soap and inspected for any changes such as redness, irritation, or ulceration. Adverse reactions need to be reported to the maxillofacial prosthodontist for evaluation and possible referral to a dermatologist. First, the prosthesis should be cleaned by rolling the adhesive toward the outer margins of the prosthesis for removal. Then it is cleaned with a mild soap and water, rinsed, and allowed to air dry. Patients should be instructed to store the prosthesis in an area away from children and pets. It is desirable to have the patient remove the prosthesis during sleep to avoid placing pressure on the defect and to allow the skin time to rest.

The lifespan of an adhesive-retained prosthesis is usually 1 to 3 years and that of a prosthesis retained by osseointegrated implants is 3 to 5 years. Over time, a prosthesis may be lost, damaged, or discolored by smoke and ultraviolet light or may

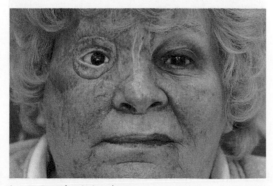

Fig. 4. Prosthesis in place.

become worn-out. The principle reason for replacement of a facial prosthesis is degradation in appearance because of changes in color and physical properties.[9,17] The costs of prosthesis fabrication and remakes are usually covered by medical insurance because a facial prosthesis is generally considered a durable medical equipment. A certificate of medical necessity may be required to establish the medical need for prosthesis fabrication.[9] It is always advisable to request a predetermination of benefits with the patient's insurance carrier before beginning prosthetic rehabilitation.

Even with the limitations of prosthetic rehabilitation, most patients wearing a prosthesis report that they use it on a regular basis and are overall satisfied with the results. Patients with osseointegrated implant–retained prostheses gave higher positive ratings when compared with patients with adhesive-retained prostheses, citing ease of placement and removal, frequency of wear at home, and quality of retention during various activities such as home chores and when perspiring, sneezing, or coughing.[18] Patients did express desires for prostheses that last longer and have improved color stability and enhanced retention.[19,20]

SURGICAL CONSIDERATIONS FOR AURICULAR, NASAL, AND ORBITAL DEFECTS

The primary goal of ablative surgery is disease control. After surgical resection, attention should be focused on preparing the defect site to enhance prosthetic rehabilitation. Small areas of tissue that are not supported by bone or cartilage should be removed because these are difficult to capture accurately in an impression and they interfere with adaptation of the margins of a prosthesis. Proper positioning and placement of a prosthesis is facilitated by negative space or a concave defect.[1] Facial prostheses may be used to replace lost auricular, nasal, and orbital structures. In addition, a facial prosthesis may be used to obdurate defects of the cheek and forehead. Principles of a successful prosthetic rehabilitation include avoiding margin placement over moveable tissues; engaging tissue undercuts, if possible; and performing skin grafting to form a stable base for the prosthesis.[4]

Auricular defects may be associated with congenital malformations, trauma, or ablative tumor surgery. The decision as to reconstruct surgically or prosthetically is based on the size and complexity of the defect. Large reconstructions may be difficult in this area. If prosthetic rehabilitation is the preferred treatment option,

preservation of the tragus may help to conceal and align the anterior margin of a prosthesis (**Fig. 5**).[1,4] Preservation of the inferior half of the pinnae is of limited to no use. When possible, maintaining the root of the helix may serve as a good landmark for prosthesis fabrication and alignment and assist with vertical support.[1] An auricular prosthesis may be retained with a medical grade adhesive or with osseointegrated implants, which have a high degree of success in the temporal bone.[4,21] Using 2 or 3 implants offers adequate retention. These implants may be placed in the 1-, 3-, and 5-o'clock positions for the left ear and the 7-, 9-, and 11-o'clock positions for the right ear.[4]

Nasal defects may be surgically reconstructed with regional skin flaps from the forehead or adjacent areas. These flaps may not match the color or texture of the surrounding skin. Therefore, in some cases, a prosthesis may yield a more aesthetic result.[4] Before a decision is made as to the best treatment option, retention of the prosthesis must be considered. Nasal prostheses are exposed to moist airflow, which decreases the effectiveness of adhesives, thus reducing retention and duration of wear. Consideration should

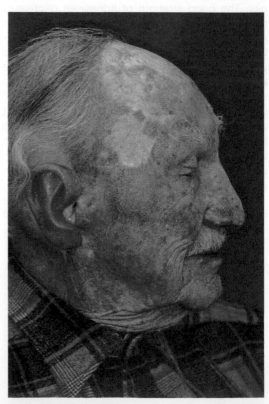

Fig. 5. Tragus retained to conceal and align the anterior margin of the prosthesis.

be given to holding the prosthesis in place with mechanical retention by engaging undercuts. In some instances, mechanical retention alone is adequate in retaining a nasal prosthesis.[21] Retention may also be possible with the placement of osseointegrated implants in the maxilla or glabella. During resection of the nasal bones, surgical techniques to avoid distortion of the contour and position of the cheek, lip, and nasolabial folds should be used.[4]

Orbital defects caused by ablative surgery may be divided into 2 groups. The first group is enucleation or evisceration in which the eyeball is removed and the remaining eye muscles and orbital contents are left intact. This type of defect is treated with an ocular prosthesis, commonly referred to as a glass eye, but is usually made from acrylic resin. The second group is orbital exenteration or removal of the entire eye and surrounding tissues. This type of defect is often reconstructed with a microvascular flap or by the fabrication of an orbital prosthesis that replaces the eye and the surrounding structures. Should the final treatment have a prosthetic component, adequate space for an aesthetic prosthesis should be present before performing prosthesis fabrication. Determination of this space is facilitated by preoperative evaluation with a standard-size ocular prosthesis that is held in place in front of the planned surgical site and the proposed margins are evaluated.[4] Small defects may not allow for adequate space for proper positioning or setting of the gaze of the ocular component of the orbital prosthesis; this inappropriateness may cause the eyes to appear crossed, looking in different directions, too close together, or not on the same horizontal plane (**Fig. 6**). In some instances, additional tissue may need to be removed to provide space. It is preferable to use split-thickness skin grafts for the lining of bony defects in this area. This type of graft affords more space and supplies a good tissue base for prosthesis support and retention.[1] Osseointegrated implants have been placed in the frontal bone for retention of orbital prosthesis, but long-term survival of implants in this area may be problematic.[22,23]

SUMMARY

Most patients requiring prosthetic facial rehabilitation have undergone ablative surgery for head and neck cancers.[1] These patients are best treated by a multidisciplinary approach involving the surgeons performing ablative and reconstructive surgery and the maxillofacial prosthodontist. Presurgical and postsurgical planning facilitates a more concerted effort between the various disciplines so that eradication of the disease and postsurgical outcome emerge favorably. In some instances, prosthetic rehabilitation is more desirable and has the potential to produce a better aesthetic result than surgical reconstruction. A prosthesis also allows for the surveillance of recurrent disease.[1–4] Aesthetics of a facial prosthesis may be enhanced through treatment planning with the surgeon as to which anatomic structures should be removed and which should be spared during ablative surgery. The patient's aesthetic and functional expectations need to be evaluated and in many instances, modified before treatment. If prosthetic rehabilitation is anticipated, patients and those around them must comprehend the limitations of the prosthesis, the daily maintenance involved, and the need for periodic remakes of the prosthesis. Because a facial prosthesis must be aesthetic and functional, it will never match the quality of the special effects created in Hollywood; instead a well-made prosthesis will pass "the grocery store or shopping mall test." Given these limitations, most patients report satisfaction with prosthetic rehabilitation. This situation is especially true when the prosthesis is retained by osseointegrated implants.[19,24]

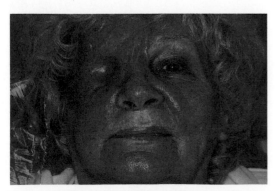

Fig. 6. A small surgical defect making it difficult to properly position the prosthetic eye.

REFERENCES

1. Lemon JC, Kiat-amnuay S, Gettleman L, et al. Facial prosthetic rehabilitation: preprosthetic surgical techniques and biomaterials. Curr Opin Otolaryngol Head Neck Surg 2005;13:255–62.
2. Parr GR, Goldman BM, Rahn AO. Maxillofacial prosthetic principles in the surgical planning for facial defects. J Prosthet Dent 1983;46:323–9.
3. Parr GR, Goldman BM, Rahn AO. Surgical considerations in the prosthetic treatment of ocular and orbital defects. J Prosthet Dent 1983;49:379–85.

4. Salinas TJ. Prosthetic rehabilitation of defects of the head and neck. Semin Plast Surg 2010;24(3): 299–308.

5. Roumanas ED, Freymiller EG, Chang TL, et al. Implant-retained prostheses for facial defects: an up to 14-year follow-up report on the survival of implants at UCLA. Int J Prosthodont 2002;15: 325–32.

6. Guttal SS, Patil NP, Shetye AD. Prosthetic rehabilitation of a midfacial defect resulting from lethal midline granuloma-a clinical report. J Oral Rehabil 2006;33: 863–7.

7. Thawley SE, Batsakis JG, Lindberg RD, et al. Comprehensive management of head and neck tumors. St Louis (MO): Elsevier; 1998. p. 526–7.

8. Harrison DF. Total rhinectomy-a worthwhile operation? J Laryngol 1982;96:1113–23.

9. Art as Applied to Medicine. The Facial Prosthetics Clinic of Johns Hopkins University Web site. Available at: http://hopkinsmedicine.org/medart/Prosthetics.htm. Accessed September 24, 2010.

10. Andres CJ, Haug SP, Munoz CA, et al. Effects of environmental factors on maxillofacial elastomers: part 1-literature review. J Prosthet Dent 1992;68: 519–22.

11. Wolfaardt J, Gehl G, Farmand M, et al. Indications and methods of care for aspects of extraoral osseointegration. Int J Oral Maxillofac Surg 2003;32: 124–31.

12. Beumer J, Ma T, Marunick, et al. Restoration of facial defects: etiology, disability, and rehabilitation. In: Beumer J, Curtis TA, Marunick MT, editors. Maxillofacial rehabilitation: prosthodontic and surgical considerations. St Louis (MO): Ishiyaku EuroAmerica; 1996. p. 377–453.

13. Heller HL, McKinstry RE. Facial materials. In: McKinstry RE, editor. Fundamentals of facial prosthetics. Arlington (TX): ABI Professional Publications; 1995. p. 79–97.

14. Kiat-amnuay S, Khan Z, Gettleman L. Protective skin dressing effects on adhesive retention of maxillofacial prostheses [abstract]. J Dent Res 1990;79:122.

15. Kiat-amnuay S, Gettleman L, Khan Z, et al. Effect of adhesive retention on maxillofacial prostheses. Part 1. Skin dressing and solvent removers. J Prosthet Dent 2000;84:335–40.

16. Kiat-amnuay S, Gettleman L, Khan Z, et al. Effect of adhesive retention on maxillofacial prostheses. Part 2. Time and reapplication effects. J Prosthet Dent 2000; 84:438–41.

17. Haug SP, Andres CJ, Moore BK. Color stability and colorant effect on maxillofacial elastomers. Part 1: colorant effect on physical properties. J Prosthet Dent 1999;81:418–22.

18. Chang T, Garrett N, Roumanas E, et al. Treatment satisfaction with facial prostheses. J Prosthet Dent 2005;94:275–80.

19. Markt JC, Lemon JC. Extraoral maxillofacial prosthetic rehabilitation at the M.D. Anderson Cancer Center: a survey of patient attitudes and opinions. J Prosthet Dent 2001;85:608–13.

20. Eriksson E, Branemark PI. Osseointegration from the prospective of the plastic surgeon. Plast Reconstr Surg 1994;93:626–37.

21. Secilmis A, Ozturk N. Nasal prosthesis rehabilitation after partial rhinectomy: a clinical report. Eur J Dent 2007;1:115–8.

22. Nishimura RD, Roumanas E, Sugai T, et al. Auricular prostheses and osseointegrated implants: UCLA experience. J Prosthet Dent 1995;73:553–8.

23. Toljanic JA, Eckert SE, Roumanas E, et al. Osseointegrated craniofacial implants in rehabilitation of orbital defects: an update of a retrospective experience in the United States. J Prosthet Dent 2005;94: 177–82.

24. Chang T, Neal G, Eleni R, et al. Treatment satisfaction with facial prostheses. J Prosthet Dent 2005; 94:275–80.

Setting up the Mohs Surgery Laboratory

Sharon L. Thornton, MD[a,b,*], Barbara Beck, HT/HTL(ASCP)[c]

KEYWORDS

- Mohs • Micrographic surgery • Laboratory
- Frozen sections • Histopathology

Mohs micrographic surgery has the highest cure rate for skin cancer, while preserving the surrounding normal tissue. The success rate of the procedure is dependent on microscopic examination of 100% of the surgical margin at the time of surgery. Accurate and precise preparation of horizontally cut quality frozen sections in the Mohs laboratory is essential.[1] A thoughtful approach is needed when designing a successful, efficient, and safe Mohs laboratory. The essential categories of development of the laboratory are planning and design, selection of proper equipment and supplies, training of laboratory personnel, adherence to regulatory standards of Clinical Laboratory Improvement Amendments (CLIA), and execution of an efficient and accurate daily routine.

DESIGN OF SPACE

The Mohs laboratory should be located close to the surgical suites to allow ease of transporting tissue from the patient's room to the laboratory. Grossing and inking of the Mohs specimen may take place in the surgical suite or the laboratory. Grossing and inking of the tissue in the patient's room is often beneficial for ensuring anatomic accuracy of mapping and inking of the specimen. A wheeled cart that can be readily moved from room to room may be used for the grossing and inking process in each room.

The laboratory should be organized to follow the flow of the specimen processing. Division of the laboratory into a workbench area and a microscope viewing area is helpful. Bench height laboratory stools and 91.5-cm (36-inch) countertops are used in the workbench area during the processing of tissue. Desk height stools and 76-cm (30-inch) countertops are placed in the microscope viewing area for the surgeon. Having a separate designated area within the laboratory for the surgeon's microscopic examination of the frozen sections is recommended. The surgeon's close proximity to the Mohs technician allows ease of communication regarding special considerations with specimen processing and need for recuts. A 2-headed microscope is helpful for teaching purposes. These microscopes are available with a side-by-side adapter and a face-to-face adapter. Counter space and laboratory design should be constructed according to the type of adapter that is used. With the advent of electronic medical records, it is helpful to have a computer easily accessible for the technician in the laboratory.

The specimens arrive in the laboratory and are placed on an open countertop near the cryostat. The cryostat must be located in an easily accessible area. A separate 20-A dedicated circuit is required. Two cryostats are often placed in the laboratory to have a backup cryostat should the main cryostat malfunction. Avoid placing the cryostat directly under an air vent, which could lead to problems with maintaining temperature and frost accumulation. A microscope near the cryostat and staining area is helpful for preview of the slides by the Mohs technician before staining. This process provides immediate feedback to the

Disclosures: The authors have nothing to disclose.
[a] Columbus Skin Surgery Center, Inc, 6670 Perimeter Drive, Suite 260, Dublin, OH 43016, USA
[b] Division of Dermatology, Department of Internal Medicine, The Ohio State University, Columbus, OH, USA
[c] Mohs Technical Consulting, Inc, 894 Buck Falls Road, Highlands, NC 28741, USA
* Corresponding author. Columbus Skin Surgery Center, Inc, 6670 Perimeter Drive, Suite 260, Dublin, OH 43016.
E-mail address: thorntonss@yahoo.com

Dermatol Clin 29 (2011) 331–340
doi:10.1016/j.det.2011.01.007

technician about the completeness of the epidermal edge in the sections. Additional sections can be taken at this point, as needed, rather than waiting for evaluation by the surgeon after staining.

Adequate chemical-resistant countertop space is needed for staining. Manual staining requires a linear arrangement of Coplin jars or staining dishes in an area with adequate ventilation and a fume hood, if hazardous chemicals are used. An automatic stainer can be fitted with an appropriate-sized fume hood. A fume hood with a back draft is available to fit under overhead cabinets, if required. The presence of a fan-powered exhaust vent that exhausts directly to the outdoors also helps to decrease any chemical odors generated in the laboratory.

A flammable liquid storage cabinet should be located in the laboratory for storage of flammable chemicals. The metal cabinet should be labeled clearly and placed away from exit doorways.

Other considerations for the laboratory are designated areas for biohazard disposal, an eyewash station, slide storage, supply storage, textbooks and other references, and a sink for hand washing near the exit.

EQUIPMENT

Basic equipment needs for the Mohs laboratory are the cryostat, staining equipment, and a microscope. The cryostat is the largest single purchase for the laboratory. The most commonly used brands of cryostats are made by Leica Microsystems (Bannockburn, IL, USA): TBS Minotome Plus (Triangle Biomedical Systems, Raleigh, NC, USA) and Microm.[2] The Microm cryostat has recently been replaced by the Avantik QS11 (Avantik Biogroup, Springfield, NJ, USA). Key components of a cryostat are the microtome, cryochamber, blade holder, handwheel, and freeze plate. Features for consideration are a motorized versus manual object head, Peltier cooling, ultraviolet disinfection, antiroll plate, and heat extractor. The cryostat should be kept between -20 and $-25^{\circ}C$. Two or 3 cryostats may be desirable based on the volume of cases and need for a backup cryostat. If you do not have a backup cryostat, CLIA require you to have documentation of your plan of action if your cryostat quits functioning.

An automatic stainer can reduce reagent waste, increase efficiency in the laboratory, and enable more consistent staining. A survey by Robinson[3] in 2001 reported that use of the automatic stainer, the Linistainer system, for routine slide preparation decreased staining variability by approximately 20% and reduced processing time by about 30%.

Other benefits of the automatic stainer were cited as increased technician availability for mapping tissue, increased caseload, ability to perform larger cases with more sections, and performing other laboratory techniques.[3] The most commonly used stainer is the Linistat (Thermo Scientific, Kalamazoo, MI, USA), which is 63.5 cm (25 inches) long. The average time for staining is less than 5 minutes. The stainer requires a supply line and drain tubing that may simply run into a sink. It may be connected directly under the sink, so that the sink can still be used for hand washing or for an attached eyewash. A fume hood is recommended over the automatic stainer. Supplies for manual staining are also recommended.

The microscope for the surgeon's examination of the prepared sections is the other major purchase for the Mohs laboratory. Recommended features of the microscope for reading of the slides include a 2 to $2.5\times$ low-power screening objective, $4\times$, $10\times$ and $40\times$ objectives, ceramic stage, 5-position turret, long-life bulb, flat field optics, and mechanical stage tension adjustment control. A tilting binocular tube can be helpful to prevent back and neck issues. As mentioned earlier, a dual-view side-by-side adapter or dual-view face-to-face adapter may be desired for teaching purposes.

Other equipment needs are a microscope for use by the Mohs technicians for reviewing slides for quality and completeness before presenting them to the surgeon, cryogen, any special embedding equipment, fire extinguisher, safety storage cabinet for flammable materials, and an eyewash station. A slide storage system is necessary to store biopsy and positive Mohs section slides indefinitely and negative Mohs section slides for 10 years.[4] All slides should be saved for at least 10 years.

SUPPLIES

An evolving list of supplies is useful to ensure adequate inventory and minimize excess. **Box 1** outlines the commonly needed supplies in the Mohs laboratory. The reagents vary based on the desired staining protocol. However, generally the following reagents are necessary: 95% alcohol, 100% alcohol, xylene or xylene substitute, hematoxylin, eosin, bluing reagent, optimal cutting temperature (OCT) compound or freezing matrix, cover slipping glue, positive charged slides, cover glass, and gauze. If you use disposable blades, it is suggested you keep an extra pack on hand. When ordering supplies, order several reagents at a time because there is a hazardous shipping charge on all chemicals shipped; this charge is the same whatever the amount of the shipment.

Box 1
Supplies needed for the Mohs laboratory

25-mm specimen chucks

30-mm specimen chucks

Scalpel

Forceps

Microtome lubricating oil

Microtome tools

Antiroll brushes

Diposable blades

Specimen storage tray

Charge slides

Coverslips

Petri dishes

Marking dyes

Cryospray or liquid nitrogen

Tissue freezing medium

OCT compound

Mounting medium

Reagents for staining

Slidefolders

Slide storage system

SPECIMEN PROCESSING

Several different methods of tissue processing in Mohs surgery have been developed through the years. The method of tissue processing must give optimal results for processing skin, including the epidermis, dermis, and adipose, in the least amount of time.[5] Some of the described techniques include heat extractor, glass microscope slide, Bard Parker scalpel handle, Miami Special (Delasco, Council Bluffs, IA, USA), Cryomold (Sakura Finetek, Torrance, CA, USA), forceps, American Optical tissue presser, and the cryoembedder (Cryoembedder, Salt Lake City, UT, USA).[5,6]

When processing tissue during a Mohs procedure the cryostat needs to be turned to −21

to −25°C. The micrometer setting is best set about 6 μm for skin sections. At this setting you can achieve a webbing effect in fatty specimens.

The tissue is brought to the laboratory in a secondary container along with a completed Mohs map. The map gives the location and a diagram of the Mohs layer. The map also contains the gross description of the specimen submitted to the laboratory. The Mohs map is marked with the time and technician's initials when the tissue arrives in the laboratory. The tissue may be processed as 1 section or divided, as needed. Several different methods have been described to aid in obtaining a complete margin and epidermal edge in frozen sections, such as beveled excision, ex vivo or in vivo relaxing incisions, mechanical tissue flattening, and division of the tissue.[5,7–10] The tissue may be carefully scored around the edges to place all the epidermis and deep margin completely down on the same plane. After the scoring is complete, the technician or surgeon dyes the tissue to ensure proper orientation when the surgeon is reviewing each section under the microscope. The dye and orientation are marked on the map for future review, and they must correspond correctly with the tissue so the surgeon can identify the location(s) of the remaining positive margin.

The surgeon marks the tissue with a notch at 12 o'clock to maintain orientation; the tissue is marked with red dye to the right of the notch at 12 o'clock, blue dye to the left of the 12 o'clock margin, and green dye at 6 o'clock; if needed, yellow dye and black dye can be added for layers containing several quadrants. All quadrants should have at least 3 focal points under the microscope, as seen in **Fig. 1**.

Each quadrant has its own differential markings. This method of inking is used so that if the tissue is flipped, it cannot be confused with another quadrant.

After the tissue has been marked with the dyes, the tissue is ready to be embedded. There are several techniques to embed the tissue or prepare the tissue to be sectioned in the cryostat. Three of the more commonly used techniques are discussed.

A 12 o'clock   **B** 12 o'clock  **C** 12 o'clock

Fig. 1. Representation of inking of the specimen. (*A*) Full specimen, 1 section. (*B*) Bisected specimen, 2 sections. (*C*) Divided specimen into quadrants based on size, 4 sections.

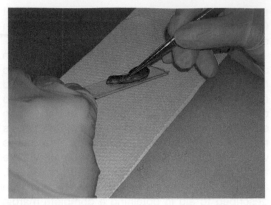

Fig. 2. Slide technique. Tissue is placed deep side down on the slide with all skin edges flattened against the slide.

The first technique is the slide technique. The tissue is placed deep side down on the slide, making sure all skin edges are flat against the slide (**Fig. 2**). A little OCT compound is placed around the tissue and this is snap frozen in liquid nitrogen (LN$_2$) for approximately 10 to 15 seconds. It may be placed in a small cup of LN$_2$ or frozen on the quick-freeze bar of the cryostat. There should be a little graying left on top of the OCT compound (**Fig. 3**). The specimen on the slide is then slightly thawed in the palm of the technician's hand and the button is slid off the slide (**Fig. 4**). A little OCT compound is placed on a chuck in the cryostat, and the button from the slide is inverted and placed on the chuck with OCT compound in the cryostat. The flat side is now in the up position, with the tissue ready for sectioning (**Fig. 5**). The heat sink that is in the cryostat is placed on top of the newly formed button and allowed to freeze. The chuck is ready to section in seconds (**Fig. 6**).

The next embedding technique is the heat extractor. After the epidermis is flat, and the tissue is dyed, the technician places the tissue deep margin down on the free-standing heat extractor of the cryostat and makes sure the epidermis is flat against the cold extractor (**Fig. 7**). A little

OCT compound is placed around the frozen specimen (**Fig. 8**). Then, a little OCT compound is placed on a chuck in the cryostat. As soon as the OCT compound starts to freeze and turn white, more OCT compound is added and the heat extractor is placed tissue down in the soft OCT compound. This compound is allowed to freeze for a minute (**Fig. 9**). The tissue and the extractor are pulled apart and the chuck is ready to section (**Fig. 10**).

The last embedding technique is the cryoembedder. The tissue is placed as flat as possible with the deep margin down. The side of the tissue that was the deepest part nearest the patient is placed down on the flat disc of the cryoembedder, which has been kept in the cryostat to remain as cold as possible. The epidermis is placed down against the disc so that the technician can obtain a full section of the epidermis on the first cut (**Fig. 11**). After the epidermis is teased out and the tissue is flat on the disc of the cryoembedder, a little OCT compound is placed around the tissue and allowed to freeze (**Fig. 12**). A chuck is placed in the holder in the cryostat and a little OCT compound is placed on the chuck (**Fig. 13**). Once the OCT compound on the chuck is partially frozen, a little more OCT compound is added to the chuck and the chuck is inserted into the other side of the cryoembedder (**Fig. 14**). Once the OCT compound on the chuck is partially frozen (holding onto the chuck), flip the cryoembedder and the chuck upside down and put it on top of the other side of the cryoembedder with the tissue. Once they have been placed on top of one another, flip both pieces of the cryoembedder and slightly spray them with the cryospray. Place the cryoembedder inside the cryostat and allow the button to freeze (**Fig. 15**). The chuck is now ready for sectioning (**Fig. 16**).

No matter which embedding technique is used, as soon as the chucks are prepared and cutting begins, it is essential to avoid cutting deep into the tissue. The technician should adjust the chuck in the cryostat knife to obtain a full section of the tissue. The technician needs to move the chuck

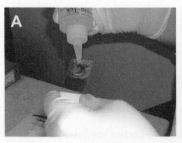
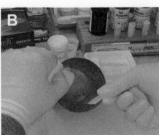

Fig. 3. Slide technique. (*A*) A small amount of OCT is placed around the specimen, (*B*) snap freezing of the tissue in liquid nitrogen.

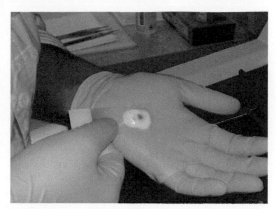

Fig. 4. Slide technique. Warming of the button to remove it from the slide.

holder and align the block evenly with the knife to avoid cutting too deep into the tissue. Every section is important to be able to determine the depth of the tumor. The technician should section just enough OCT compound and the first few sections off the block until a complete skin edge is obtained. Checking under the microscope for the epidermis at this point helps the technician get familiar with going deep into the blocks. If the technician checks microscopically for completeness of the skin edge before placing the slide on the stainer, time is saved for both the technician and the surgeon.

Special stains may be performed on frozen sections during Mohs micrographic surgery to enhance detection of residual tumors. In particular, poorly differentiated tumor cells, tumor cells among dense inflammatory infiltrate, tumors with perineural invasion, and tumor cells in fibrotic or connective tissue around blood vessels or within fascial planes may be difficult to detect.[11–14] Toluidine blue highlights basal cell carcinoma with a pink metachromatic appearance of the mucopolysaccharide stroma of basal cell carcinoma.[15] Mohs micrographic surgery for treatment of lentigo maligna and invasive melanoma is controversial, especially because of the difficulty in interpreting frozen sections in melanoma. Some

Mohs surgeons report usefulness of immunohistochemical stains, such as HMB-45, Mel-5, S-100, and Melan-A (MART-1), and microphthalmic transcription factor for the detection of melanoma.[11] Cytokeratin stains may be useful in identifying residual basal and squamous cell carcinoma, Ber-EP4 may aid in detection of residual basal cell carcinoma, and CD34 may help delineate residual dermatofibrosarcoma protuberans.[11] Techniques in immunostaining are continuing to evolve.

TROUBLESHOOTING TIPS FOR SPECIMEN PROCESSING

Refer to **Table 1**.

TRAINING OF LABORATORY PERSONNEL

In looking for a technician in the Mohs laboratory, it is helpful if the technician has some histology background, especially for troubleshooting regarding staining and cryostat sectioning. Histotechnicians are not always available. If you have a noncertified technician, the job description should be titled Mohs technician or laboratory technician. If you list your technician as "histotechnician" and your job description uses "histotechnician," CLIA may ask for their degree or certification. A histotechnician has a degree in histology and board certification; a laboratory technician or Mohs technician is not required to have a certificate.

Whether the technician is a certified histotechnician or someone trained in the office, it is crucial to have these persons trained by someone who specializes in this technical field. The surgeon undertakes a fellowship program specializing in the Mohs technique, and the technician should receive the same type of specialized training. Because the surgeon and technician work closely together, the technician needs to be a good communicator. The technician must pay close attention to detail and also multitask with ease. It is essential to have constant communication between the surgeon and the technician. The

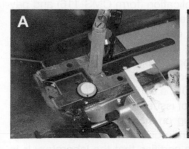
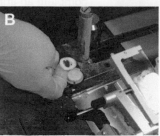

Fig. 5. Slide technique. (A) Preparing the chuck in the cryostat for placement of the button containing the specimen. (B) Placing inverted button onto the chuck.

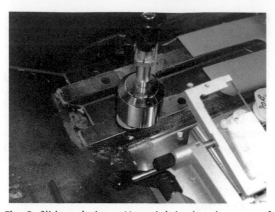

Fig. 6. Slide technique. Heat sink is placed on top of the newly formed button for flattening of the specimen as much as possible prior to sectioning.

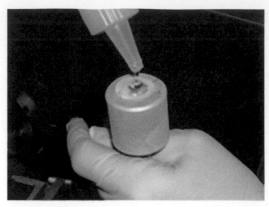

Fig. 8. Heat extractor technique. A small amount of OCT is placed to cover the tissue.

surgeon must explain each layer and orientation to the technician.

Mohs technicians may participate in training programs run by seasoned technicians, workshops at the annual American Society for Mohs Histotechnology, in-office training sessions conducted by the Mohs Histotechnology Quality Assurance training initiative program, the Fundamentals of Mohs Surgery training program at the annual meeting of the American Society of Mohs Surgery, and formal training sessions of private institutions or private consulting services.[16] In addition, technicians may find the knowledge of the surgeon and other Mohs technicians and resource textbooks to be helpful.

CERTIFICATION OF THE MOHS LABORATORY

In 1988, Congress passed CLIA, which established quality standards for all laboratory testing performed on specimens derived from the human body for purposes of providing information in the

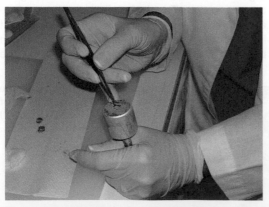

Fig. 7. Heat extractor technique. The tissue is placed deep side down directly on the heat extractor.

diagnosis, prevention, and treatment of disease, or impairment of or assessment of health. Subsequently, in 2003 the US Food and Drug Administration (FDA) released revised rules regarding many laboratory issues, including quality control, test method verification, patient test management, laboratory director educational requirements, record keeping, proficiency testing, and laboratory licensure.[17] CLIA require that all laboratories performing these tests be certified by the Secretary of the Department of Health and Human Services (DHHS). The Centers for Medicare and Medicaid Services (CMS), with the assistance of the FDA and the Centers for Disease Control and Prevention, administer the CLIA laboratory certification program for DHHS.[18] Although CLIA standards are national, they are enforced through state CLIA offices. The standards apply to all providers offering clinical laboratory services, and the regulations apply to laboratory testing in every setting, including the Mohs laboratory in physicians' offices.

CLIA regulations are organized based on the complexity of the laboratory procedures. The higher the complexity, the more stringent the regulations. Mohs micrographic surgery is categorized as a procedure of high complexity.

The first step in obtaining CLIA certification is to complete an application (form CMS-116) and pay the applicable fees. A high-complexity laboratory may apply for a certificate of compliance (COC) or a certificate of accreditation (COA). After receiving the application, CLIA issue a unique CLIA number and a certificate of registration. If applying for a COC, a survey is usually performed within 6 months of issue of the certificate of registration, depending on state guidelines. A COC is issued if CLIA standards are met during the survey. This COC, which certifies that the laboratory is in

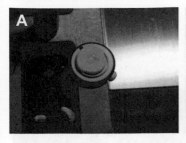
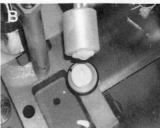

Fig. 9. Heat extractor technique. (*A*) Preparing the chuck in the cryostat with a small amount of OCT. (*B*) Placing the heat extractor with the tissue on top of the chuck in the cryostat.

compliance with all applicable CLIA requirements, is valid for 2 years. If applying for a COA, the laboratory must meet the standards of a nonprofit accreditation program approved by CMS. These standards have requirements that are equal to or exceed the standards of CLIA. The 6 CMS-approved accrediting organizations are the Joint Commission of Accreditation of Healthcare Organizations, College of American Pathologists, American Osteopathic Association, Commission on Office Laboratory Accreditation, American Association of Blood Banks, and American Society for Histocompatability and Immunogenetics. A COA also requires an on-site inspection to determine that all program requirements are met.

At the time of the survey, CLIA request access to the following materials: the laboratory written policy and procedures and records regarding equipment, quality control, quality assessment, test procedures, and proficiency testing. Personnel records and safety information are also reviewed. The surveyor interviews staff and observes the physical laboratory and its daily operations.

To satisfy CLIA regulations, every step of the testing process in the laboratory must meet standards and be documented, including personnel, facilities, reagents, equipment, laboratory procedures, reporting procedures, record keeping, and laboratory proficiency.[17] Personnel need to be adequately trained and knowledgeable of and proficient at their job duties in the laboratory. The responsible laboratory personnel are reported to CLIA on CMS form 209. Facilities must have sufficient space, lighting, ventilation, water, electrical outlets, and temperature and humidity regulation. Equipment housed in the facilities should be calibrated and monitored to ensure accurate performance. Maintenance logs should be kept to document this monitoring. Reagents arriving in the laboratory should be properly identified and labeled on receipt and then appropriately stored. The reagent logs should reflect this process, including documentation of receipt, appropriate identifiers, and expiration dates.

The laboratory procedure manual should document all laboratory procedures performed. The manual may be divided into a descriptive section of procedures and a logbook to track the daily routines. The descriptive portion should include policies and procedures for Mohs micrographic surgery and processing of Mohs frozen sections, quality control for Mohs slides and staining, equipment and reagent maintenance, process of quality assessment and proficiency testing, and training and personnel information. The logbook portion should include a case log, cryostat temperature and maintenance log, room temperature log, microscope maintenance log, autostainer

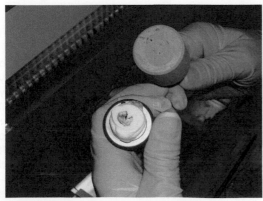

Fig. 10. Heat extractor technique. Removal of heat extractor.

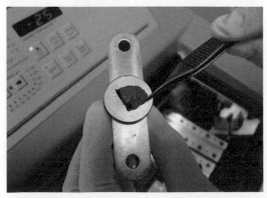

Fig. 11. Cryoembedder technique. Specimen is placed deep side down on the disk of the cryoembedder.

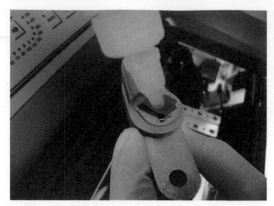

Fig. 12. Cryoembedder technique. A small amount of OCT is placed around the tissue.

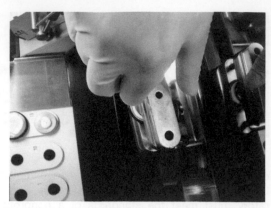

Fig. 14. Cryoembedder technique. The chuck is inserted into the bottom portion of the cryoembedder and then placed onto the disk with tissue.

maintenance log, reagent and stain rotation log, quality control form for slides, refrigerator temperature and maintenance (if needed), fume hood maintenance log, and proficiency testing results.

The purpose of quality control is to detect failures in the testing system and monitor the accuracy of testing over time.[17] One of the aspects of quality control is the monitoring of quality of the frozen sections in the Mohs laboratory. One method of detecting failures in the system is to process the first slide of the day as a quality control slide for review by the Mohs surgeon. The quality of the slide staining, completeness of the section, thickness of the section, and inking are evaluated. If any changes need to be made, they are recorded in the daily log of quality control slides. In addition, if any concerns arise in the processing of the slides, they are brought to the immediate attention of the laboratory director, the Mohs surgeon. The concern is clearly identified and appropriate remedial action is immediately taken. The issue is documented for quality assessment purposes and both the Mohs technician and

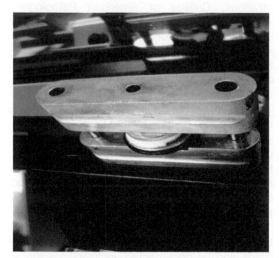

Fig. 15. Cryoembedder technique. Allowing the tissue to freeze, approximately 10–15 seconds.

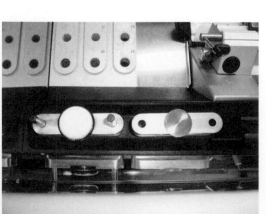

Fig. 13. Cryoembedder technique. Preparing the chuck in the cryostat with OCT.

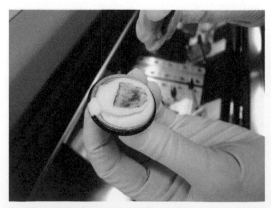

Fig. 16. Cryoembedder technique. Completed chuck is ready for sectioning.

Table 1
Troubleshooting tips for specimen processing

Problem	Cause	Remedy
Sections curl on anti-roll plate	Anti-roll plate protrudes too far beyond the cutting edge	Readjust anti-roll plate
Scraping noise during sectioning	Anti-roll plate protrudes too far beyond edge and is scraping against the specimen	Readjust anti-roll plate
Ridged sections	Knife/blade damaged Loose blade or specimen holder	Move blade to new area or change Check everything to tighten
Shatter in sections	Specimen insufficiently frozen onto disc Specimen disc not tight Loose blade or holder Blunt blade or knife Incorrect clearance angle	Refreeze specimen onto disc (be sure discs are at room temp Check disc Check tightness of blade and holder Change or move blade Reset angle/move disc angle slightly
Thick-thin sections	Incorrect temperature Hand wheel speed not uniform Specimen holder loose Check blade for build up on back Incorrect angle Specimen holder too far extended Dull blade	Most of the time it is too cold, warm disc slightly Turn hand wheel evenly, not too fast Tighten specimen holder and blade holder Slightly move disc to different angle Move holder back and readjust blade holder Move blade or replace
Specimen sticks or crumbles on the anti-roll plate	Anti-roll plate is too warm or incorrectly positioned Static electricity Tissue or OCT build up on corner or edge of anti-roll Dull blade	Cool down anti-roll plate or reposition plate Place dryer sheet in cryostat Slightly blow on specimen while sectioning Clean anti-roll plate with brush or wipe with gauze Change blade area or replace blade
Fatty sections	Specimen not cold enough	Freeze with cryo freeze or LN2 Rock and roll fly wheel, cut thicker section
Sections curl up when move anti-roll plate	Static electricity or air currents Anti-roll plate too warm	Place dryer sheet in cryostat Slightly blow on section prior to cutting Cool anti-roll plate with cryo freeze or LN2
Sections tear	Temperature too low for the tissue Dull area on blade, dirt, or build up on blade Leading edge of anti-roll plate damaged	Freeze with cryo freeze or LN2 Change or clean blade Replace the plate or turn

the Mohs surgeon sign the report. Other important areas of the quality control program are monitoring and maintenance of equipment, materials, and reagents. Documentation of such monitoring should be kept in the logbook portion of the procedure manual, as described earlier. A protocol should be in place for the malfunctioning of equipment.

Proficiency testing is an important part of the CLIA regulations. The standards require that the laboratory be tested for each examination or procedure conducted, except those for which a proficiency test cannot be reasonably developed. The testing should be performed quarterly, except if technical or scientific reasons allow a test to be performed less often, but not less than twice per year. For the Mohs laboratory, a Mohs surgeon can send random Mohs slides to another Mohs surgeon or dermatopathologist biannually or quarterly for blinded testing to fulfill the requirement. Similarly, anatomic and surgical pathology units throughout the United States use a quality assurance protocol, including peer review, which is recommended by the Association of Directors of Anatomic and Surgical Pathology.[19]

Failure to meet the requirements of CLIA may lead to sanctions, including suspension of the laboratory's certificate. The surveyor may also report deficiencies that need to be corrected.

LABORATORY SAFETY

Universal precautions should be followed in the Mohs laboratory as in the rest of the medical office. The workbench area of the laboratory should be considered contaminated. Biohazardous procedures include grossing of the specimen, cutting of the specimen in the cryostat, handling of the slides, and cleaning of the cryostat and laboratory. Personal protective equipment is required for these biohazardous procedures. Employees should receive training regarding exposure to blood-borne pathogens.

Hazardous chemicals are present in the laboratory. All chemicals must be clearly labeled, and material safety data sheets should be kept in the laboratory. Storage of all hazardous chemicals should be in lower cabinets, except flammable chemicals, which are stored in a metal cabinet for flammable materials. A spill kit should be kept in the laboratory beneath the sink in a lower cabinet. A fire extinguisher and eyewash station must be easily accessible.

The Occupational Safety and Health Administration oversees laboratory safety. The Mohs laboratory should have formal employee training and a written policy regarding exposure to blood-borne pathogens and safe use of chemicals used in the laboratory.

REFERENCES

1. Cottel WI, Bailin PL, Albom MJ, et al. Essentials of Mohs micrographic surgery. J Dermatol Surg Oncol 1988;14:11–3.
2. Fish FS III, editor. Manual of frozen section processing for Mohs micrographic surgery. Milwaukee (WI): American College of Mohs Surgery; 2008.
3. Robinson JK. Current histologic preparation methods for Mohs micrographic surgery. Dermatol Surg 2001; 27:555–60.
4. Hetzer MR. The Mohs laboratory. In: Snow SN, Mikhail GR, editors. Mohs micrographic surgery. 2nd edition. Madison (WI): University of Wisconsin Press; 2004. p. 329–37.
5. Miller LJ, Argenyi ZB, Whitaker DC. The preparation of frozen sections for micrographic surgery. J Dermatol Surg Oncol 1993;19:1023–9.
6. Hanke WC, Lee M. Cryostat use and tissue processing in Mohs micrographic surgery. J Dermatol Surg Oncol 1989;15:29–32.
7. Geisse JK. Mohs surgery: debulking specimens–to submit or discard–that is the question. Dermatol Surg 2000;26:399–400.
8. Wanitphakdeedecha R, Nguyen TH, Chen TM. In vivo intraoperative relaxing incisions for tissue flattening in Mohs micrographic surgery. Dermatol Surg 2008;34:1085–7.
9. Weber PJ, Moody BR, Dryden RM, et al. Mohs surgery and processing: novel optimization and enhancements. Dermatol Surg 2000;26:909–14.
10. Ladd S, Cherpelis BS. Scoring of Mohs tissue in one-piece processing to prevent tissue crumbling or detachment from the embedding medium while sectioning. Dermatol Surg 2009;35:1555–6.
11. Stranahan D, Cherpelis BS, Glass F, et al. Immunohistochemical stains in Mohs surgery: a review. Dermatol Surg 2009;35:1023–34.
12. Robinson JK, Gottschalk R. Immunofluorescent and immunoperoxidase staining of antibodies to fibrous keratin. Arch Dermatol 1984;120:199–203.
13. Mondragon RM, Barrett TL. Current concepts: the use of immunoperoxidase techniques in Mohs micrographic surgery. J Am Acad Dermatol 2000; 43:66–71.
14. Salmon RM. The use of monoclonal antibody stains in Mohs micrographic surgery. Australas J Dermatol 1997;38:44–5.
15. Humphreys TR, Nemeth A, McCrevey S, et al. A pilot study comparing toluidine blue and hematoxylin and eosin staining of basal cell and squamous cell carcinoma during Mohs surgery. Dermatol Surg 1996;22: 693–7.
16. Chen TM, Wanitphakdeedecha R, Whittemore DE, et al. Laboratory assistive personnel in Mohs micrographic surgery: a survey of training and laboratory practice. Dermatol Surg 2009;35:1746–56.
17. Sieck CK, editor. Clinical laboratory improvement amendments (CLIA) manual. Schaumburg (IL): American Academy of Dermatology Association; 2004.
18. Centers for Medicare and Medicade Services. Overview clinical laboratory improvement amendments. 2010. Available at: https://www.cms.gov/clia/. Accessed September 20, 2010.
19. Mariwalla K, Aasi SZ, Glusac EJ, et al. Mohs surgery histopathology concordance. J Am Acad Dermatol 2009;60:94–8.

Current Procedural Terminology Coding for Mohs Micrographic Surgery

Richelle M. Knudson, MD[a],*, Robert H. Cook-Norris, MD[a],
Jeremy S. Youse, MD[a], Randall K. Roenigk, MD[b]

KEYWORDS
- CPT codes • Mohs micrographic surgery • Reimbursement
- Dermatologic surgery • CPT code modifiers

CODING IN DERMATOLOGIC SURGERY

Knowledge about surgical current procedural terminology (CPT) coding is essential to every surgeon, because accurate coding allows for proper reimbursement, decreases the possibility of being audited, and decreases the likelihood of inadvertently misrepresenting a claim. It is also important to have proper documentation to substantiate submitted claims. Accurate coding and documentation promote the timely processing of claims and decrease the likelihood of having to appeal denied claims.

CPT CODES

The CPT codes are developed by the American Medical Association (AMA) and are used to describe the type of services provided to a patient. Each code consists of a combination of numbers that defines a specific medical, surgical, or diagnostic service. These codes are universal and allow for accurate communication of information about medical services and procedures among medical providers, coders, accreditation organizations, and payers. The reimbursement to providers for services received by patients is determined by the CPT code(s) used.

The CPT system is a registered trademark of the AMA, which is responsible for assigning codes for newly developed services, revising current codes, and eliminating outdated codes. Codes are updated annually. Because the AMA has a copyright on the CPT codes, free use and distribution of these codes is not permitted. The AMA charges a license fee to associate relative value units (RVUs) with CPT codes. Software and several books and manuals are also available to aid those who use CPT codes. The AMA receives approximately $70 million annually from these licensing fees and the sale of reference materials.

RESOURCE-BASED RELATIVE VALUE SCALE

The Resource-based Relative Value Scale is used to determine how much medical providers are reimbursed. This scale is used to assign an RVU to procedures performed by a physician. To determine the payment, the value is adjusted according to the geographic region where the procedure is performed, and then multiplied by a fixed conversion factor. This fixed conversion factor changes every year. The conversion factor, as of June 1, 2010, is $36.8729. Prices are based on 3 factors: physician work

The authors have no conflict of interest.
[a] Department of Dermatology, Mayo School of Graduate Medical Education, College of Medicine, Mayo Clinic, 200 First Street SW, Rochester, MN 55905, USA
[b] Department of Dermatology, College of Medicine, Mayo Clinic, 200 First Street SW, Rochester, MN 55905, USA
* Corresponding author.
E-mail address: knudson.richelle@mayo.edu

Dermatol Clin 29 (2011) 341–355
doi:10.1016/j.det.2011.01.008
0733-8635/11/$ – see front matter © 2011 Elsevier Inc. All rights reserved.

Table 1
Common dermatology modifiers

Modifier	Title	Description	Applicable Global Period (d)	When It Cannot Be Used
Modifier -22	Increased procedural service	When a service that is provided requires substantially greater work than is typically required by the specific procedure code	0, 10, or 90	—
Modifier -24	Unrelated E/M service by the same physician during a postoperative period	Used in the postoperative period when an unrelated E/M service is provided by the same physician	10 or 90	Service related to postoperative care Unrelated service on same day as the procedure
Modifier -25	Significant, separately identifiable E/M service by the same physician on the day of a procedure or other service	Indicates that, on the day of a minor surgical procedure, a significant and separately identifiable E/M service is also provided	0 or 10	—
Modifier -51	Multiple procedures	Indicates that the same provider performs multiple procedures on the same operative day	—	—
Modifier -52	Reduced service	Indicates that a service performed is significantly less than what is required when normally performing the service	—	When a procedure is terminated When the patient is not able to pay the full charge Cannot be used with an E/M code
Modifier -54	Surgical care only	Used when postoperative care is provided by a physician who is not a member of the same group as the surgeon	10 or 90	With a procedure that does not have a global period With a procedure with a global period other than 10 or 90 days Should not be appended to an E/M code
Modifier -55	Postoperative management only	Used when the surgeon is providing outpatient postoperative care	10 or 90	—

Modifier				
Modifier -57	Decision to perform surgery	Used when the decision to perform surgery is made on the day before or the day of a major surgery	90	When a minor surgery is being performed Should not be used with a surgery that is preplanned or prescheduled
Modifier -58	A staged or related procedure or service	Indicates that the same physician provides a staged or related procedure during the postoperative period	—	To report treatment of a complication from the original procedure that requires returning to the operating room When an unrelated procedure is performed in the postoperative period
Modifier -59	Distinct procedural service	Used to indicate that 2 separate procedures or services, independent of each other, are performed on the same day	—	—
Modifier -76	Repeat procedure by the same physician	Used when the same physician performs a repeat procedure within the global period	—	If a service is repeated because of technical problems For services repeated for quality control If a different procedure is performed
Modifier -78	Procedure during the postoperative period	Used when an operative procedure that is related to the primary procedure is performed during the postoperative time frame	10 or 90	If a procedure is performed at a site other than the operating room or an ambulatory surgery center
Modifier -79	Unrelated procedure in the postoperative period	Indicates that an unrelated procedure is performed by the same physician during the postoperative period	—	—
Modifier -99	Multiple modifiers	Used if 2 or more modifiers are necessary on 1 line of service	—	—

Abbreviation: E/M, evaluation and management.

(PW; 52%), practice expense (PE; 44%), and malpractice expense (MP; 4%). The total RVUs equal the PW RVUs plus PE RVUs plus MP RVUs.

The PW RVU includes the time, technical skills, effort, mental effort, judgment, and stress involved in providing a service. At least every 5 years, each CPT code is reviewed to determine the work RVU for a particular service. At that time, it is determined whether the components of the service have changed since the value was last set and whether the value should increase or decrease. The PE RVU includes the costs of direct expenses (staff time, supplies, and equipment time) and indirect expenses (administrative expense and other overheads) to the physician providing any given service. The PE RVU assigned to a specific CPT code is often different when the procedure is performed in a facility setting, such as a hospital, versus a freestanding center. Generally, the PE compensation for a freestanding center is greater than that for a hospital setting. The MP RVU is usually the smallest component and includes payment for the cost of professional liability premiums.

GEOGRAPHIC PRACTICE COST INDEX

The Geographic Practice Cost Index (GPCI) is used to adjust for the regional and/or geographic differences in the cost of providing patient services. Each component of the RVU (PW, PE, and MP premiums) is adjusted according to the GPCI.

The Centers for Medicare and Medicaid Services is required by law to update the GPCI every 3 years. These changes can affect 1, 2, or all 3 components of the GPCI.

GLOBAL SURGICAL PACKAGE

Payment for all services associated with a procedure is bundled into a single package, called the global surgical package. The RVUs for a global surgical package include preoperative care, local infiltration or topical anesthesia, immediate postoperative care (dictation, notes, speaking with family), writing orders, and typical postoperative care. It also includes 1 related evaluation and management (E/M) encounter on the date before, or the same date as, the procedure, after the decision for surgery has been made. The global time period includes the time allowed for all work related to a procedure to be completed. During this time period, services that are unrelated to the original procedure may be provided along with services that are related. Therefore,

modifiers are used to communicate to payers which services are related and which services are not related.

CPT MODIFIERS

CPT modifiers are used to provide information to insurance payers beyond the CPT 5-digit procedure codes to assure that the provider is reimbursed correctly when more than 1 service, or a modification of the described service, is provided. The last step in the coding process is adding the modifier. More than 1 modifier can be used with a procedure code. Up to 4 modifiers are allowed, but Medicare and Medicaid or other payers may recognize only the first and second modifiers. Because of this, it is important to put the modifiers that affect reimbursement first. Although some modifiers may not affect reimbursement directly, they can determine whether a service is covered or denied. The functional modifier should be placed first, with the informational modifier placed second. Placing the informational modifier first may slow claim processing. It is essential to use modifiers appropriately to be reimbursed properly. Correct use of modifiers prevents charges of fraud and abuse. There are different rules for the proper use of modifiers between private payers, as well as Medicare, and it is important to be familiar with these different rules to submit accurate claims. An overview of the pertinent modifiers used in surgical dermatology is given in **Table 1**.

Modifier -24: Unrelated E/M Service by the Same Physician During a Postoperative Period

Modifier -24 is used in the postoperative period, which begins the day after a procedure, when an unrelated E/M service is provided by the same physician. Physicians in the same specialty and in the same group practice are required to bill as though they are the same physician. This modifier can be used during the postoperative period of a procedure code with a 10-day or 90-day global period. This modifier cannot be used for a service related to postoperative care (treatment of a wound infection) and cannot be used with an unrelated service on the same day as the procedure.

An example of an appropriate use of this code is a patient who had a basal cell carcinoma treated with Mohs micrographic surgery (MMS), and the resulting defect was repaired with a skin flap. At a 1-month follow-up visit the patient was noted to have a new lesion suspicious for nonmelanoma skin cancer, and a biopsy was performed. Modifier -24 can appropriately be added because this

Table 2
CPT codes for destruction

Code	Procedure	Global Period
17000	Destruction (eg, laser surgery, electrosurgery, cryosurgery, chemosurgery, surgical curettement), premalignant lesions (eg, actinic keratoses); first lesion	010
+17003	Second to 14th lesions, each listed separately in addition to code for first lesion	—
17004	Destruction (eg, laser surgery, electrosurgery, cryosurgery, chemosurgery, surgical curettement), premalignant lesions (eg, actinic keratoses); 15 or more lesions	010
17106	Destruction of cutaneous vascular proliferative lesions (eg, laser technique) <10 cm^2	090
17107	10.0–50.0 cm^2	090
17108	>50.0 cm^2	090
17110	Destruction (eg, laser surgery, electrosurgery, cryosurgery, chemosurgery, surgical curettement), of benign lesions other than skin tags or cutaneous vascular proliferative lesions; ≤14 lesions	010
17111	≥15 lesions	010
17250	Chemical cauterization of granulation tissue	000
17260	Destruction, malignant lesion (eg, laser surgery, electrosurgery, cryosurgery, chemosurgery, surgical curettement), trunk, arms or legs; lesion diameter ≤0.5 cm	010
17261	Lesion diameter 0.6–1.0 cm	010
17262	Lesion diameter 1.1–2.0 cm	010
17263	Lesion diameter 2.1–3.0 cm	010
17264	Lesion diameter 3.1–4.0 cm	010
17266	Lesion diameter >4.0 cm	010
17270	Destruction, malignant lesion (eg, laser surgery, electrosurgery, cryosurgery, chemosurgery, surgical curettement), scalp, neck, hands, feet, genitalia; lesion diameter ≤0.5 cm	010
17271	Lesion diameter 0.6–1.0 cm	010
17272	Lesion diameter 1.1–2.0 cm	010
17273	Lesion diameter 2.1–3.0 cm	010
17274	Lesion diameter 3.1–4.0 cm	010
17276	Lesion diameter >4.0 cm	010
17280	Destruction, malignant lesion (eg, laser surgery, electrosurgery, cryosurgery, chemosurgery, surgical curettement), face, ears, eyelids, nose, lips, mucous membrane; lesion diameter ≤0.5 cm	010
17281	Lesion diameter 0.6–1.0 cm	010
17282	Lesion diameter 1.1–2.0 cm	010
17283	Lesion diameter 2.1–3.0 cm	010
17284	Lesion diameter 3.1–4.0 cm	010
17286	Lesion diameter >4.0 cm	010

Table 3
CPT codes for incision and drainage

Code	Procedure	Global Period
10040	Acne surgery (marsupialization, opening or removal of multiple milia, comedones, cysts, pustules)	010
10060	Incision and drainage of abscess; simple or single	010
10061	Complicated or multiple	010
10080	Incision and drainage of pilonidal cyst; simple	010
10081	Complicated	010
10120	Incision and removal of foreign body, subcutaneous tissues; simple	010
10121	Complicated	010
10140	Incision and drainage of hematoma, seroma, or fluid collection	010
10160	Puncture aspiration of abscess, hematoma, bulla, or cyst	010
10180	Incision and drainage, complex, postoperative wound infection	010

new lesion is unrelated to the patient's previous surgery, is within the postoperative period, and requires another procedure.

Modifier -25: Significant, Separately Identifiable E/M Service by the Same Physician on the Day of a Procedure or Other Service

Modifier -25 is used to indicate that, on a day when a minor surgical procedure is performed, a significant and separately identifiable E/M service is also provided. A minor surgical procedure is considered to have a 0-day or 10-day global period. When using this modifier, it is not necessary that the diagnosis code for the E/M service is different than the diagnosis code for which the procedure is being done. This modifier can be used whether or not the E/M service and the procedure are performed by the same physician or practitioner. One such example would be a patient being evaluated for a lesion suspicious for a nonmelanoma skin cancer. An E/M service can be assigned for evaluation of the lesion and modifier -25 can be added if this lesion is biopsied.

Modifier -51: Multiple Procedures

Modifier -51 is used to indicate that the same provider performed multiple procedures on the same operative day. The rationale behind this modifier is that less physician work and less expense are required to perform multiple procedures on the same day than if the patient presents on a separate day for a separate primary service. Therefore, the secondary service is usually reimbursed at a lower rate. Medicare's multiple-surgery reduction rule is that the first procedure is reimbursed 100%. Any subsequent procedure is billed at 50%. If 6 or more procedures are performed on the same operative day, a report has

to be submitted with the claim. Some private insurance carriers may reimburse at only 25% for the third and subsequent procedures.

CODING FOR DESTRUCTION, INCISION AND DRAINAGE, BIOPSIES, AND INJECTIONS

CPT codes 17000 to 17286 are used for destruction (**Table 2**). Destruction can be undertaken by several means, including laser surgery, electrosurgery, cryosurgery, or surgical curettement. For benign lesions (codes 17000–17004), the specific code used depends on the number of lesions destroyed and the location of the lesion. For malignant lesions (codes 17260–17286), the specific code used depends on the size of the lesion and its location. There are also specific codes for the destruction of cutaneous vascular proliferations, based on the area in square centimeters.

Incision and drainage procedure codes (10060–10180) are based on the lesion that is incised and drained (abscess, pilonidal cyst, foreign body,

Table 4
CPT codes for biopsy

Code	Procedure	Global Period
11100	Biopsy of skin, subcutaneous tissue and/or mucous membrane (including simple closure), unless otherwise listed; single lesion	000
+11101	Each separate/additional lesion (list separately in addition to code for primary procedure)	

Table 5
CPT codes for removal of skin tags

Code	Procedure	Global Period
11200	Removal of skin tags, multiple fibrocutaneous tags, any area; ≤15 lesions	000
+11201	Each additional 10 lesions, or part thereof (list separately in addition to code for primary procedure)	

subcutaneous tissue, hematoma, seroma, bullae, or cyst) as well as whether the procedure is simple or complicated and single or multiple (**Table 3**).

The biopsy procedure codes (11100–11101) are used to indicate that the procedure performed to obtain tissue for pathologic examination is performed independently or is unrelated to other procedures or services provided at that time (**Table 4**). These details should be reported

Table 6
CPT codes for shaving of epidermal or dermal lesions

Code	Procedure	Global Period
11300	Shaving of epidermal or dermal lesion, single lesion, trunk, arms, or legs; lesion diameter ≤0.5 cm	000
11301	Lesion diameter 0.6–1.0 cm	000
11302	Lesion diameter 1.1–2.0 cm	000
11303	Lesion diameter >2.0 cm	000
11305	Shaving of epidermal or dermal lesion, single lesion, scalp, neck, hands, feet, genitalia; lesion diameter ≤0.5 cm	000
11306	Lesion diameter 0.6–1.0 cm	000
11307	Lesion diameter 1.1–2.0 cm	000
11308	Lesion diameter >2.0 cm	000
11310	Shaving of epidermal or dermal lesion, single lesion, face, ears, eyelids, nose, lips, mucous membrane; lesion diameter ≤0.5 cm	000
11311	Lesion diameter 0.6–1.0 cm	000
11312	Lesion diameter 1.1–2.0 cm	000
11313	Lesion diameter >2.0 cm	000

Table 7
CPT codes for injection

Code	Procedure	Global Period
11900	Injection, intralesional; ≤7 lesions	000
11901	>7 lesions	—
11950	Subcutaneous injection of filling material (eg, collagen); 1 mL or less	000
11951	1.1–5.0 mL	—
11952	5.1–10.0 mL	—
11954	>10.0 mL	—

separately when they are not considered to be components of other procedures and when they are performed on different lesions or different sites. The code used depends on the number of lesions biopsied. The CPT codes used for the removal of skin tags (codes 11200–11201) can be applied when the skin tags are removed by scissoring or any other sharp method, ligature strangulation, electrosurgical destruction, or a combination of treatment modalities, including chemical destruction or electrocauterization, with or without local anesthesia (**Table 5**). The CPT code used depends on the number of lesions removed. Shaving of epidermal or dermal lesions is described as the sharp removal by transverse incision or horizontal slicing. This procedure is done without a full-thickness dermal excision. The CPT codes (11300–11313) include local anesthesia and chemical cauterization or electrocauterization of the wound. The code used depends on the location of the lesion and its size (**Table 6**).

Table 8
CPT codes for debridement

Code	Procedure	Global Period
11000	Debridement of extensive eczematous or infected skin; ≤10% of body surface area	000
+11001	Add on for each additional 10% of body surface, or part thereof	—
11040	Debridement; skin, partial thickness	000
11041	Skin, full thickness	000
11042	Skin and subcutaneous tissue	000

Intralesional injections (CPT codes 11900–11901) are coded according to the number of lesions injected, whereas subcutaneous injection of filling material, such as collagen, is coded according to the volume used (CPT codes 11950–11954) (**Table 7**).

Debridement of the skin can be partial thickness or full thickness and can also involve subcutaneous tissue (CPT codes 11040–11042). When eczematous or infected skin is debrided, the specific CPT code used (11000–11001) depends on the amount of body surface debrided (**Table 8**).

CODING FOR BENIGN AND MALIGNANT EXCISIONS

CPT codes 11400 to 11446 are used for the excision of benign lesions (**Table 9**). CPT codes 11600 to 11646 are used for the excision of malignant lesions (**Table 10**). The code used depends on the site and the excised diameter. The excised diameter includes the diameter of the clinically apparent lesion plus the margin necessary to completely excise the lesion (**Fig. 1**).

CODING FOR MMS

Because the surgeon acts as both the surgeon and the pathologist when performing MMS, the codes used when billing for MMS cannot be used if the pathology specimen is evaluated by another physician. If this is the case, the surgeon can bill for only the excision and the repair (**Table 11**).

Table 9
CPT codes for excision of benign lesions

Code	Procedure	Global Period
11400	Excision, benign lesion including margins, except skin tag (unless listed elsewhere), trunk, arms, or legs; excised diameter ≤0.5 cm	010
11401	Excised diameter 0.6–1.0 cm	010
11402	Excised diameter 1.1–2.0 cm	010
11403	Excised diameter 2.1–3.0 cm	010
11404	Excised diameter 3.1–4.0 cm	010
11406	Excised diameter >4.0 cm	010
11420	Excision, benign lesion including margins, except skin tag (unless listed elsewhere), scalp, neck, hands, feet, genitalia; excised diameter ≤0.5	010
11421	Excised diameter 0.6–1.0 cm	010
11422	Excised diameter 1.1–2.0 cm	010
11423	Excised diameter 2.1–3.0 cm	010
11424	Excised diameter 3.1–4.0 cm	010
11426	Excised diameter >4.0 cm	010
11440	Excision, other benign lesion including margins, except skin tag (unless listed elsewhere), face, ears, eyelids, nose, lips, mucous membrane; excised diameter ≤0.5 cm	010
11441	Excised diameter 0.6–1.0 cm	010
11442	Excised diameter 1.1–2.0 cm	010
11443	Excised diameter 2.1–3.0 cm	010
11444	Excised diameter 3.1–4.0 cm	010
11446	Excised diameter >4.0 cm	010

Table 10
CPT codes for excision of malignant lesions

Code	Procedure	Global Period
11600	Excision, malignant lesion including margins, trunk, arms, or legs; excised diameter ≤0.5 cm	010
11601	Excised diameter 0.6–1.0 cm	010
11602	Excised diameter 1.1–2.0 cm	010
11603	Excised diameter 2.1–3.0 cm	010
11604	Excised diameter 3.1–4.0 cm	010
11606	Excised diameter >4.0 cm	010
11620	Excision, malignant lesion including margins, scalp, neck, hands, feet, genitalia; excised diameter ≤0.5 cm	010
11621	Excised diameter 0.6–1.0 cm	010
11622	Excised diameter 1.1–2.0 cm	010
11623	Excised diameter 2.1–3.0 cm	010
11624	Excised diameter 3.1–4.0 cm	010
11626	Excised diameter >4.0 cm	010
11640	Excision, malignant lesion including margins, face, ears, eyelids, nose, lips; excised diameter ≤0.5 cm	010
11641	Excised diameter 0.6–1.0 cm	010
11642	Excised diameter 1.1–2.0 cm	010
11643	Excised diameter 2.1–3.0 cm	010
11644	Excised diameter 3.1–4.0 cm	010
11646	Excised diameter >4.0 cm	010

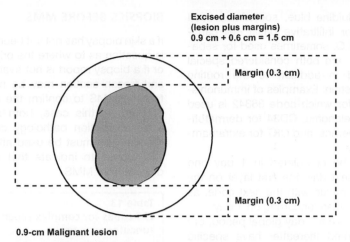

Fig. 1. Measuring the excised diameter of a malignant or benign lesion. Diameter of lesion plus the narrowest margin required equals the excised diameter.

CPT codes 17311 and 17313 are used for the first layer of MMS. Code 17311 is used for tumors on the head, neck, hands, feet, genitalia, and any location involving major nerves or vessels, tendon, bone, cartilage, or muscle, whereas code 17313 is used for tumors of the trunk, arms, and legs. These codes include the work involved before the procedure (explanation of the procedure, informed consent, and preparing the patient for surgery), during the procedure (tumor debulking, excision of the specimen, mapping, color coding the specimens, preparing the tissue for evaluation with routine staining, microscopic evaluation of the specimens, and mapping of positive margins), and after the procedure (discussion of postsurgical wound care). These codes include up to 5 tissue blocks, although the number of slides per block does not affect coding.

CPT codes 17312 and 17314 are used for each additional stage after the first stage. Code 17312 is used for tumors on the head, neck, hands, feet, genitalia, and any location involving major nerves or vessels, tendon, bone, cartilage, or muscle, whereas code 17314 is used for tumors of the trunk, arms, and legs. These codes include up to 5 tissue blocks. These codes are reimbursed at a lower rate than codes 17311 and 17313, because the additional work includes only reexcision of positive margins, processing of the specimens, and microscopic evaluation of the specimens.

CPT code 17315 is used if more than 5 tissue blocks are needed in any stage. This code is used for each additional tissue block. It is an add-on code and is used only in conjunction with codes 17311–17314.

Special CPT codes are used if any additional stains, other than routine stains, are used. Each additional stain must be coded separately. CPT code 88314 is used for a special stain on frozen section, code 88342 is used for an immunohistochemical stain, and code 88311 is used for

Table 11 CPT codes for MMS		
Code	Procedure	Global Period
17311	Mohs micrographic technique, of the head, neck, hands, feet, genitalia, or any location with surgery directly involving muscle, cartilage, bone, tendon, major nerves, or vessels; first stage, ≤5 tissue blocks	000
+17312	Each additional stage after the first stage, ≤5 tissue blocks (list separately in addition to code for primary procedure)	—
17313	Mohs micrographic technique, of the trunk, arms, or legs; first stage, ≤5 tissue blocks	000
+17314	Each additional stage after the first stage, ≤5 tissue blocks (list separately in addition to code for primary procedure)	—
+17315	Mohs micrographic technique, each additional block after the first 5 tissue blocks, any stage (list separately in addition to code for primary procedure)	—

decalcification. Toluidine blue, sometimes used for morpheaform or infiltrative basal cell carcinomas, and oil red O, sometimes used for sebaceous carcinomas, are both considered special stains when used in addition to the routine hematoxylin-eosin stain. Examples of immunohistochemical stains for which code 88342 is used are MART-1 for melanoma, CD34 for dermatofibrosarcoma protuberans, and CK7 for extramammary Paget disease.

If MMS cannot be completed in 1 day and continues on the next day, the first layer on the next day should continue with the next code, as if the whole surgery were occurring on 1 day.

All MMS codes have a 0-day global period, but the repairs performed thereafter have specific global periods.

BIOPSIES BEFORE MMS

If a skin biopsy has not yet been performed, if there is question as to where the original biopsy site is, or if a biopsy report is not available, a skin biopsy and frozen section may be needed before performing MMS to confirm the diagnosis, the site, or both. In this case, both a skin biopsy and a frozen-section pathology code can be used. Modifier -59 must be used after each of these 2 CPT codes to indicate that these services are distinct from MMS.

Table 12
CPT codes for intermediate repair of skin and subcutaneous tissue

Code	Procedure	Global Period
12031	Repair, intermediate, wounds of scalp, axillae, trunk and/or extremities (excluding hands and feet); ≤2.5 cm	010
12032	2.6–7.5 cm	010
12034	7.6–12.5 cm	010
12035	12.6–20.0 cm	010
12036	20.1–30.0 cm	010
12037	>30.0 cm	010
12041	Repair, intermediate, wounds of neck, hands, feet and/or external genitalia; ≤2.5 cm	010
12042	2.6–7.5 cm	010
12044	7.6–12.5 cm	010
12045	12.6–20.0 cm	010
12046	20.1–30.0 cm	010
12047	>30.0 cm	010
12051	Repair, intermediate, wounds of face, ears, eyelids, nose, lips and/or mucous membranes; ≤2.5 cm	010
12052	2.6–5.0 cm	010
12053	5.1–7.5 cm	010
12054	7.6–12.5 cm	010
12055	12.6–20.0 cm	010
12056	20.1–30.0 cm	010
12057	>30.0 cm	010

Table 13
CPT codes for complex repair of skin and subcutaneous tissue

Code	Procedure	Global Period
13100	Repair, complex, trunk; 1.1–2.5 cm	010
13101	2.6–7.5 cm	010
+13102	Each additional 5 cm or less (list separately in addition to code for primary procedure)	—
13120	Repair, complex, scalp, arms, and/or legs; 1.1–2.5 cm	010
13121	2.6–7.5 cm	010
+13122	Each additional 5 cm or less (list separately in addition to code for primary procedure)	—
13131	Repair, complex, forehead, cheeks, chin, mouth, neck, axillae, genitalia, hands and/or feet; 1.1–2.5 cm	010
13132	2.6–7.5 cm	010
+13133	Each additional 5 cm or less (list separately in addition to code for primary procedure)	—
13150	Repair, complex, eyelids, nose, ears and/or lips; ≤1.0 cm	010
13151	1.1–2.5 cm	010
13152	2.6–7.5 cm	010
+13153	Each additional 5 cm or less (list separately in addition to code for primary procedure)	—
13160	Secondary closure of surgical wound or dehiscence, extensive or complicated	090

CODING FOR RECONSTRUCTION

Several types of repairs are available when planning a closure, including second intent healing, layered closure (simple, intermediate, and complex), adjacent tissue transfer or rearrangement (flaps), grafts (split, full, and composite), combined repairs, and staged repairs. There are also a few special sites to consider, including the lip and the eyelid.

Layered Closures

The specific code used for a layered closure, whether simple, intermediate, or complex, depends on the site and length or sum of lengths.

Simple closures are used for superficial wounds, for which 1-layered closure is sufficient. Simple repair codes (12001–12021) are used. These codes include reimbursement for anesthesia and cauterization. If more than 1 simple closure is performed within 1 anatomic group, only 1 code is used, chosen according to the sum of the lengths of all closures. Reimbursement for a simple closure is included in the code for benign and malignant excisions, and a separate simple repair code is not required.

Intermediate closures are used for defects that require a layered closure because of involvement of deeper layers such as the subcutaneous tissue, necessity of closing dead space, and necessity of providing prolonged support to decrease tension on the suture line. Intermediate repair codes

Table 14
CPT codes for adjacent tissue transfer or rearrangement (skin flaps)

Code	Procedure	Global Period
14000	Adjacent tissue transfer or rearrangement, trunk; defect ≤10 cm^2 or less	090
14001	Defect 10.1–30.0 cm^2	090
14020	Adjacent tissue transfer or rearrangement, scalp, arms and/or legs; defect ≤10 cm^2	090
14021	Defect 10.1–30.0 cm^2	090
14040	Adjacent tissue transfer or rearrangement, forehead, cheeks, chin, mouth, neck, axillae, genitalia, hands and/or feet; defect ≤10 cm^2	090
14041	Defect 10.1–30.0 cm^2	090
14060	Adjacent tissue transfer or rearrangement, eyelids, nose, ears and/or lips; defect ≤10 cm^2	090
14061	Defect 10.1–30.0 cm^2	090
14301	Adjacent tissue transfer or rearrangement, any area; defect 30.1–60.0 cm^2	090
14302	Each additional 30.0 cm^2, or part thereof (list separately in addition to code for primary procedure)	090
14350	Filleted finger or toe flap, including preparation of recipient site	090

Table 15
CPT codes for special pedicle flaps

Code	Procedure	Global Period
15570	Formation of direct or tubed pedicle, with or without transfer; trunk	090
15572	Scalp, arms, or legs	090
15574	Forehead, cheeks, chin, mouth, neck, axillae, genitalia, hands, or feet	090
15576	Eyelids, nose, ears, lips, or intraoral	090
15600	Delay of flap or sectioning of flap (division and inset); at trunk	090
15610	At scalp, arms, or legs	090
15620	At forehead, cheeks, chin, neck, axillae, genitalia, hands, or feet	090
15630	At eyelids, nose, ears, or lips	090
15650	Transfer, intermediate, of any pedicle flap, any location	090
15731	Forehead flap with preservation of vascular pedicle (eg, axial pattern flap, paramedian forehead flap)	090
15732	Muscle, myocutaneous, or fasciocutaneous flap; head and neck	090
15734	Trunk	090
15736	Upper extremity	090
15738	Lower extremity	090
15740	Flap; island pedicle	090

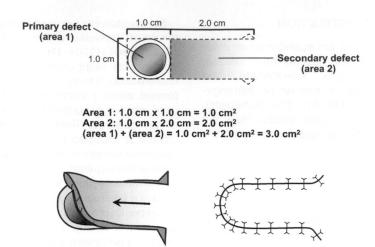

Area 1: 1.0 cm x 1.0 cm = 1.0 cm²
Area 2: 1.0 cm x 2.0 cm = 2.0 cm²
(area 1) + (area 2) = 1.0 cm² + 2.0 cm² = 3.0 cm²

Fig. 2. Measuring the area of an advancement flap.

(12031–12057) are used in this situation. A contaminated wound requiring extensive cleaning is considered an intermediate repair, even though a single-layer closure is used (**Table 12**).

Complex closures are used for defects requiring more than a layered closure. This technique includes such things as extensive undermining or retention sutures. Add-on codes based on site are used in addition to complex repair codes (13100–13160) for repairs beyond the first 7.5 cm in length. Each additional 1 to 5 cm can be reported (**Table 13**).

Adjacent Tissue Transfer or Rearrangement (Flaps)

When coding for adjacent tissue transfer or rearrangement, reimbursement for the excision is also included (**Tables 14** and **15**). Therefore, the

excision is not reported separately. The site and size of the flap (centimeters squared) are used for coding. The size of the primary defect of the excision is measured, along with the size of the secondary defect necessary to design the flap, which is achieved by multiplying the longest axis of repair by the widest perpendicular axis. These measurements are then added together to determine the size of the flap in centimeters squared. Skin rearrangement codes include CPT codes 14000 to 14350 (**Figs. 2** and **3**).

A few special circumstances exist. If the secondary defect is closed with a skin graft, a graft code is billed along with the skin rearrangement code. If a donor site is repaired with a graft or a flap, the graft or flap is considered an additional procedure. A few flaps have codes assigned according to the site and not the size, including a pedicle flap (code 15740), direct or tubed pedicle

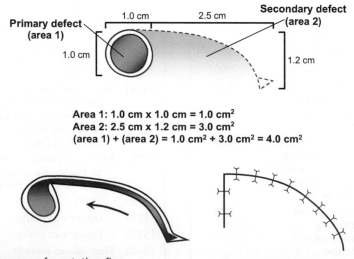

Area 1: 1.0 cm x 1.0 cm = 1.0 cm²
Area 2: 2.5 cm x 1.2 cm = 3.0 cm²
(area 1) + (area 2) = 1.0 cm² + 3.0 cm² = 4.0 cm²

Fig. 3. Measuring the area of a rotation flap.

(codes 15570–15576), delay of flap and sectioning of flap (codes 15600–15630), and myocutaneous flap (codes 15732–15738).

Skin Grafts

The size and location of the defect and the type of graft (full thickness, split thickness, allograft, xenograft, or skin substitute) are used to code skin grafts appropriately. When a full-thickness skin graft is performed, the code used includes closure of the donor site. However, if a graft or flap is necessary for closing the donor site, then this is coded as a separate additional procedure. When a skin graft is performed, the excision of the initial lesion is coded separately (**Table 16**).

If a defect is closed with a combination of different closure types (partial primary closure, flap, and/or graft), modifier -59 should be added to discern that these are separate procedures. Xenografts, allografts, skin substitute, full-thickness grafts, and split-thickness grafts all have add-on codes that are not subject to the multiple-surgery reduction rule. According to this rule, the most valuable procedure, which is reported first, is generally reimbursed at 100%. Each additional procedure, which is valued lower, is subject to the multiple-surgery reduction rule, modifier -51.

Table 16
CPT codes for grafts

Code	Procedure	Global Period
15200	Full-thickness graft, free, including direct closure of donor site, trunk; $\leq$20 cm^2	090
+15201	Each additional 20 cm^2, or part thereof (list separately in addition to code for primary procedure)	—
15220	Full-thickness graft, free, including direct closure of donor site, scalp, arms, and/or legs; $\leq$20 cm^2	090
+15221	Each additional 20 cm^2, or part thereof (list separately in addition to code for primary procedure)	—
15240	Full-thickness graft, free, including direct closure of donor site, forehead, cheeks, chin, mouth, neck, axillae, genitalia, hands, and/or feet; $\leq$20 cm^2	090
+15241	Each additional 20 cm^2, or part thereof (list separately in addition to code for primary procedure)	—
15260	Full-thickness graft, free, including direct closure of donor site, nose, ears, eyelids, and/or lips; $\leq$20 cm^2	090
+15261	Each additional 20 cm^2, or part thereof (list separately in addition to code for primary procedure)	—
15400	Xenograft, skin (dermal), for temporary wound closure, trunk, arms, legs; first 100 cm^2 or less, or 1% of body area of infants and children	090
+15401	Each additional 100 cm^2, or each additional 1% of body area of infants and children, or part thereof (list separately in addition to code for primary procedure)	—
15420	Xenograft, skin (dermal), for temporary wound closure, face, scalp, eyelids, mouth, neck, ears, orbits, genitalia, hands, feet, and/or multiple digits; first 100 cm^2 or less, or 1% of body area of infants and children	090
+15421	Each additional 100 cm^2, or each additional 1% of body area of infants and children, or part thereof (list separately in addition to code for primary procedure)	—
15430	Acellular xenograft implant; first 100 cm^2 or less, or 1% of body area of infants and children	090
+15431	Each additional 100 cm^2, or each additional 1% of body area of infants and children, or part thereof (list separately in addition to code for primary procedure)	—

Staged Repairs and Scar Revision

Modifier -58 is used when a staged or related procedure is performed during the global period. It is used when a staged procedure is planned, when the staged procedure is more extensive than the original procedure, or for therapy after a diagnostic surgical procedure.

If a patient has an unsatisfactory scar after treatment of a skin cancer, scar revision may be undertaken. If this occurs outside the global period, it cannot be reported with the original tumor diagnosis. However, reimbursement is unlikely to result by coding the procedure as scar revision along with a history of skin cancer. An appeal may be necessary for reimbursement to occur.

Lip and Eyelid Reconstruction

Several special codes are used when lip or eyelid reconstruction takes place (Tables 17 and 18). It is important to be aware of the different codes for these special sites.

If a lesion is excised from the upper lip, more than half the vertical height of the lip is involved, and full-thickness repair is necessary for closure, and this could be billed either as a complex closure or a cheiloplasty of more than one-half the vertical height. Usually reimbursement for cheiloplasty codes is higher than that for complex closure.

Table 17
CPT codes for lip reconstruction

Code	Procedure
40500	Vermilionectomy (lip shave), with mucosal advancement
40510	Excision of lip; transverse wedge excision with primary closure
40520	V-excision with primary direct linear closure
40650	Repair lip (cheiloplasty), full thickness; vermilion only
40652	Up to half the vertical height
40654	More than half the vertical height, or complex
40525	Excision, full thickness, reconstruction with local flap
40527	Excision, full thickness, reconstruction with cross-lip flap
40812–40816	Excision of lesion of mucosa and submucosa, vestibule of mouth, with simple or complex repair

Table 18
CPT codes for some cutaneous eyelid excision and repair

Code	Procedure
67930	Suture of recent wound, eyelid, involving lid margin, tarsus and/or palpebral conjunctiva direct closure; partial thickness
67935	Full thickness
67961	Excision and repair of eyelid, involving lid margin, tarsus, conjunctiva, canthus or full thickness, may include preparation for graft or flap; up to one-fourth of lid margin
67966	More than one-fourth of lid margin

When the eyelid is reconstructed, different codes are used depending on how much of the eyelid is involved. A different code is used when up to one-fourth of the lid margin (code 67961) and when more than one-fourth of the lid margin (code 67966) are involved.

RECONSTRUCTIVE VERSUS COSMETIC REPAIR

Reconstructive surgery has been defined by the AMA as surgery performed on a structural abnormality caused by disease, infection, congenital deformity, trauma, or tumors. Reconstructive surgery is medically necessary and is performed to improve function. Cosmetic surgery has been defined as the reshaping of a normal part of the body to improve the patient's appearance and self-esteem.

Repairs are considered to be reconstructive when a defect is caused by removal of cancer, when the repair improves function, and when repair is necessary to allow for a normal appearance. Generally, reconstructive procedures that are performed because of underlying tumors, infection, or disease are reimbursed.

Table 19
CPT codes for hair transplant grafts

Code	Procedure	Global Period
15775	Punch graft for hair transplant; 1–15 punch grafts	000
15776	>15 punch grafts	000

Table 20
CPT codes for dermabrasion and chemical peels

Code	Procedure	Global Period
15780	Dermabrasion; total face (eg, for acne scarring, fine wrinkling, rhytides, general ketosis)	090
15781	Segmental, face	090
15782	Regional, other than face	090
15783	Superficial, any site (eg, tattoo removal)	090
15786	Abrasion; single lesion (eg, keratosis, scar)	010
+15787	Each additional 4 lesions or less (list separately in addition to code for primary procedure)	—
15788	Chemical peel, facial; epidermal	090
15789	Dermal	090
15792	Chemical peel, nonfacial; epidermal	090
15793	Dermal	090

Table 21
CPT codes for onabotulinumtoxinA (Botox) for the treatment of hyperhidrosis

Code	Procedure	Global Period
64650	OnabotulinumtoxinA for treatment of hyperhidrosis, axillary	010
64653	OnabotulinumtoxinA for treatment of hyperhidrosis, other	010

CODING FOR HAIR TRANSPLANTATION, DERMABRASION, CHEMICAL PEELS, AND HYPERHIDROSIS

The CPT code used for hair transplant grafts (codes 15775–15776) depends on the total number of punch grafts performed. Hair transplantation has a 0-day global period (**Table 19**). Both dermabrasion and chemical peels have a 90-day global period. The CPT code used for dermabrasion (codes 15780–15787) as well as chemical peels (codes 15788–15793) depends on the location and the depth (**Table 20**). The treatment of hyperhidrosis with onabotulinumtoxinA (Botox) has a 10-day global period, and the specific CPT code used depends on whether the location is axillary or elsewhere (**Table 21**).

SUMMARY

Knowledge of the different CPT codes and modifiers is important. It is imperative that the procedures performed are coded accurately and that the codes appropriately reflect the procedures that were performed. Accurate and appropriate coding allows for proper reimbursement and decreases the likelihood of inadvertently misrepresenting a claim. Adequate documentation is also essential, because this substantiates submitted claims and promotes their timely processing.

FURTHER READINGS

American Medical Association. CPT (professional edition). Chicago: AMA; 2010.

Current Procedural Terminology. Available at: http://www.ama-assn.org/ama/pub/physician-resources/solutions-managing-your-practice/coding-billing-insurance/cpt.shtml. Accessed October 10, 2010.

Derm Coding Consult. Available at: http://www.aad.org/members/publications/consult.html. Accessed October 10, 2010.

Index

Note: Page numbers of article titles are in **boldface** type.

Dermatol Clin 29 (2011) 357–363
doi:10.1016/S0733-8635(11)00034-9
0733-8635/11/$ – see front matter © 2011 Elsevier Inc. All rights reserved.

derm.theclinics.com

Moving?

Make sure your subscription moves with you!

To notify us of your new address, find your **Clinics Account Number** (located on your mailing label above your name), and contact customer service at:

Email: journalscustomerservice-usa@elsevier.com

800-654-2452 (subscribers in the U.S. & Canada)
314-447-8871 (subscribers outside of the U.S. & Canada)

Fax number: 314-447-8029

**Elsevier Health Sciences Division
Subscription Customer Service
3251 Riverport Lane
Maryland Heights, MO 63043**

*To ensure uninterrupted delivery of your subscription, please notify us at least 4 weeks in advance of move.

ELSEVIER

Printed and bound by CPI Group (UK) Ltd, Croydon, CR0 4YY

03/10/2024

01040359-0003